# Atlas of Endoscopic Airway Surgery

# Atlas of Endoscopic Airway Surgery


## Douglas R. Sidell, MD, FAAP, FACS

**Professor**
Department of Otolaryngology–Head and Neck Surgery
Division of Pediatric Otolaryngology
and by courtesy, Pediatrics and Cardiology
Stanford University
**Director**
Pediatric Aerodigestive and Airway Reconstruction Center
Lucile Packard Children's Hospital Stanford
Palo Alto, California

## Karthik Balakrishnan, MD, MPH, FAAP, FACS

**Professor**
Department of Otolaryngology–Head and Neck Surgery
Division of Pediatric Otolaryngology
and by courtesy, Pediatrics and Pediatric Cardiology
Stanford University
**Susan B. Ford Surgeon-in-Chief**
Stanford Medicine Children's Health
Lucile Packard Children's Hospital
Palo Alto, California

## Kara D. Meister, MD, FACS, FAAP

**Assistant Professor**
Department of Otolaryngology–Head and Neck Surgery
Stanford University
Palo Alto, California



ELSEVIER

Elsevier
1600 John F. Kennedy Blvd.
Ste 1800
Philadelphia, PA 19103-2899

ATLAS OF ENDOSCOPIC AIRWAY SURGERY ISBN: 978-0-443-10568-5



For accessibility purposes, images in electronic versions of this book are accompanied by alt text descriptions provided by Elsevier. For more information, see https://www.elsevier.com/about/accessibility.

Books and Journals published by Elsevier comply with applicable product safety requirements. For any product safety concerns or queries, please contact our authorised representative, Elsevier B.V., at productsafety@elsevier.com.

Publisher's note: Elsevier takes a neutral position with respect to territorial disputes or jurisdictional claims in its published content, including in maps and institutional affiliations.



**Notice**

Practitioners and researchers must always rely on their own experience and knowledge in evaluating and using any information, methods, compounds or experiments described herein. Because of rapid advances in the medical sciences, in particular, independent verification of diagnoses and drug dosages should be made. To the fullest extent of the law, no responsibility is assumed by Elsevier, authors, editors or contributors for any injury and/or damage to persons or property as a matter of products liability, negligence or otherwise, or from any use or operation of any methods, products, instructions, or ideas contained in the material herein.

*Content Strategist:* Jessica McCool
*Senior Content Development Specialist:* Kate Mannix
*Content Development Manager*: Meghan Andress
*Publishing Services Manager:* Deepthi Unni
*Senior Project Manager:* Kamatchi Madhavan
*Senior Book Designer:* Amy Buxton
*Illustrator:* Chris Gralapp



Printed in India

Last digit is the print number: 9 8 7 6 5 4 3 2 1

# Contributors


**Juan L. Anton-Pacheco, MD, PhD**
Department of Pediatric Surgery
Hospital Universitario 12 de Octubre
**Associate Professor**
Department of Pediatrics
Universidad Complutense de Madrid
Madrid, Spain

**Karthik Balakrishnan, MD, MPH, FAAP, FACS**
**Professor**
Department of Otolaryngology–Head and Neck Surgery
Division of Pediatric Otolaryngology and by courtesy, Pediatrics and Pediatric Cardiology
Stanford University
**Susan B. Ford Surgeon-in-Chief**
Stanford Medicine Children's Health
Lucile Packard Children's Hospital
Palo Alto, California

**Nancy M. Bauman, MD**
**Professor**
Department of Otolaryngology
George Washington University
**Attending Physician**
Department of Otolaryngology
Children's National Hospital
Washington, District of Columbia

**Sergio Bottero, MD**
Laryngotracheal Team Director
Airway Surgery Unit
Bambino Gesù Children's Hospital IRCCS
Rome, Italy

**Dinesh Khatri Chhetri, MD**
**Professor**
Department of Head and Neck Surgery
University of California, Los Angeles
Los Angeles, California

**John Dahl, MD, PhD, MBA**
**Associate Professor**
Department of Otolaryngology–Head and Neck Surgery
University of Washington
Seattle, Washington

**Alessandro De Alarcon, MD, MPH**
**Professor**
Department of Pediatric Otolaryngology
Cincinnati Children's Hospital Medical Center
**Professor**
Department of Otolaryngology
University of Cincinnati
Cincinnati, Ohio

**Alexandra G. Espinel, MD**
**Associate Professor of Surgery and Pediatrics**
Department of Pediatric Otolaryngology
Children's National Hospital
Washington, District of Columbia

**Catherine K. Hart, MD, MS**
**Professor**
Department of Pediatric Otolaryngology–Head and Neck Surgery
Cincinnati Children's Hospital Medical Center
University of Cincinnati College of Medicine
Cincinnati, Ohio

**Kate Heathcote, MBBS, FRCS**
**Consultant Laryngologist**
Department of Otolaryngology
University Hospitals Dorset
Bournemouth, United Kingdom

**Andy Inglis, MD**
**Retired**
Department of Otolaryngology
University of Washington
Seattle, Washington

**Romaine F. Johnson, MD, MPH**
**Professor**
Department of Otolaryngology–Head and Neck Surgery
UT Southwestern Medical Center
Dallas, Texas

**Kara D. Meister, MD, FACS, FAAP**
**Assistant Professor**
Department of Otolaryngology–Head and Neck Surgery
Stanford University
Palo Alto, California

**Julina Ongkasuwan, MD**
**Professor, Chief of Laryngology**
Department of Otolaryngology–Head and Neck Surgery
Baylor College of Medicine/Texas Children's Hospital
Houston, Texas

**Shazia Peer, MBBCh, FC(ORL)SA, MMED(Otol)UCT**
**Professor**
Department of Surgery
Division of Otorhinolaryngology
University of Cape Town
**Head of Clinical Services**
Department of Surgery
Division of Pediatric Otorhinolaryngology
Red Cross War Memorial Children's Hospital
Cape Town, South Africa

**Diego Preciado, MD, PhD, FACS, FAAP**
**Chief, Pediatric Otolaryngology**
Children's National Hospital
Professor (with tenure) of Surgery and Pediatrics
George Washington University School of Medicine
Washington, DC

**Scott Rickert, MD**
**Division Chief**
Department of Pediatric Otolaryngology
New York University Langone
New York, New York

**Michael J. Rutter, BHB, MBChB, FRACS**
**Professor of Pediatric Otolaryngology**
Division of Otolaryngology
Cincinnati Children's Hospital Medical Center
**Professor of Pediatric Otolaryngology**
Department of Otolaryngology
University of Cincinnati
Cincinnati, Ohio

**Douglas R. Sidell, MD, FAAP, FACS**
**Professor**
Department of Otolaryngology–Head and Neck Surgery
Division of Pediatric Otolaryngology and by courtesy, Pediatrics and Cardiology
Stanford University
**Director**
Pediatric Aerodigestive and Airway Reconstruction Center
Lucile Packard Children's Hospital Stanford
Palo Alto, California

**Nicholas James Smith, MD**
**Clinical Associate Professor**
Department of Pediatric Otolaryngology
Children's of Alabama
Birmingham, Alabama

**Rakesh Srivastava, MBBS, MS**
**Consultant Laryngologist**
Department of Otorhinolaryngology
Sushrut Institute of Plastic Surgery and Trauma Center
Lucknow, India

**Briac Thierry, MD, PhD**
**Airway Surgeon**
Department of Pediatric Otolaryngology
Hopital Necker–Enfants Malades – Assistance Publique Hôpitaux de Paris
Paris, France

**Dana Mara Thompson, MD, FACS**
**Chair**
Department of Pediatric Otolaryngology
Ann & Robert H. Lurie Children's Hospital of Chicago
**Professor**
Department of Otolaryngology
Northwestern University Feinberg School of Medicine
Chicago, Illinois

**Marilena Trozzi, MD, PhD**
**Head of Airway Surgery Unit**
Department of Specialty Pediatric Surgery
Bambino Gesù Children's Hospital
Rome, Italy

**Taher Valika, MD**
**Attending Physician**
Division of Otolaryngology–Head and Neck Surgery
Ann & Robert H. Lurie Children's Hospital of Chicago
Feinberg School of Medicine
Department of Otolaryngology–Head and Neck Surgery
Northwestern University
Chicago, Illinois

**Michelle Wyatt, MA (Cantab), FRCS (ORL-HNS)**
**Pediatric Otolaryngologist**
Department of Pediatric Otolaryngology
Great Ormond Street Hospital for Children
London, United Kingdom

**Carlton J. Zdanski, MD, FAAP, FACS**
**Chief**
Division of Pediatric Otolaryngology
**Associate Professor**
Department of Otolaryngology–Head and Neck Surgery
**Surgical Director**
The North Carolina Children's Airway Center
University of North Carolina School of Medicine
Chapel Hill, North Carolina

# Foreword

Airway reconstruction has evolved significantly over the past five decades. Surgeons now have a large inventory of endoscopic tools to use. Glass rod telescopes and video recording have been available since 1970, but there is an increasing availability of endoscopic tools such as airway balloons, surgical robots, and electrosurgical instruments. These tools demand that surgeons possess the expertise and setup to match the needs of individual patients. Certainly, the surgeon must be comfortable with the full range of open-operative techniques, including graft expansion, resection, and slide operations. However, more and more complex airway procedures now have an endoscopic analog, demanding a continued learning curve of surgical expertise.

This textbook serves as an important resource for residents and fellows, junior surgeons, and experienced airway surgeons for whom endoscopic airway procedures are a component of their practice. Each chapter covers a key concept of an endoscopic airway procedure and serves as a useful reference and review tool for both a novice and a senior surgeon. The authors and editors clearly delineate key points of patient selection, informed consent, equipment and setup, operative techniques, and perioperative management. Review of the relevant chapters in this text before performing a given operation will give the surgeon added confidence to attain the best outcome for the patient. It also serves as a foundation for development of further endoscopic techniques.

Many important developments in open and endoscopic airway surgery have come out of the Cincinnati Children's Hospital Medical Center Airway and Aerodigestive and Esophageal Center Programs that I founded, and subsequently from programs led by Cincinnati graduates and their fellows, who have become experienced and valued colleagues in pediatric airway care. I am particularly proud that this textbook's surgical editors and many of its chapter authors are part of this long and vibrant legacy.

A pedagogical maxim is that great teachers should be outshone by their students. This book is the perfect example of this guiding principle in teaching.

**Robin T. Cotton, MD (happily retired)**

# Preface

The practice of airway surgery, and particularly pediatric airway surgery, is demanding. Surgeons must understand the physiology of multiple organ systems, particularly respiratory and cardiac; be able to take on the lifelong commitment needed to care for airway patients; and understand the balance of risk and benefit in terms of all critical airway functions, namely breathing, swallowing, and voice. Intraoperatively, surgeons must of course understand anatomy, normal and abnormal physiology, and operative technique to achieve intraoperative success for their patients. However, perhaps to a unique degree, they must be able to apply all of this expertise in fragile patients, balancing planning with adaptation and improvisation, and, in the case of congenital airway anomalies, creating structures that the patient did not previously develop. The endoscopic airway surgeon has an even more demanding task in that all of these skills must often be applied while the patient is breathing spontaneously with an unprotected airway, while working within the limitations of pulmonary reserve in unhealthy pediatric and adult patients.

In this context, we saw utility in a textbook that captures fundamental and cutting-edge endoscopic airway procedures in a straightforward, practical, and visual way. This book offers several strengths. First, it is focused on the components of airway surgery practice that both beginning and experienced learners often find most challenging: patient selection, choosing between different methods of accomplishing the same operation, and intraoperative technique. Second, each chapter has been written by one or more master surgeons, allowing the reader to benefit by learning directly from experts without involvement of more junior authors. Third, the surgeon editors, all of whom are highly experienced airway surgeons, have added "pearls of wisdom" to each chapter, adding nuance that allows the reader to benefit from multiple experts' knowledge. Fourth, readers will learn from the work of one of the finest medical illustrators in the field. Fifth, each chapter is pragmatic and includes not only detailed steps of technique but also information about informed consent discussion, equipment, and operative room setup.

We feel strongly that in order to provide patients with the best possible care, airway surgeons must master both open and endoscopic methods. This textbook represents the collected endoscopic surgical expertise of the editors and that of our colleagues, teachers, and friends, brought together with care and dedication. We sincerely hope that readers at all levels of learning and expertise will find content of value, whether they are preparing to do an operation for the first time, brushing up on their knowledge before doing a familiar procedure, preparing to teach others, or building an endoscopic airway program.

We are grateful to Kate Mannix for her guidance and grace through the long process of developing this book; to Chris Gralapp for her extraordinary vision and skill in creating the illustrations; to our teachers and mentors; to our patients; to our families; and to the Kuo-Patch family for supporting our work on this textbook. For the readers who have taken the time to read this preface, we are honored to have you as colleagues in this challenging and ever-evolving field. Please do not hesitate to contact us if we can collaborate or be of assistance as you continue to advance endoscopic airway surgery.

**Douglas R. Sidell**
**Karthik Balakrishnan**
**Kara D. Meister**

# Contents

# Video Contents

## Chapter 2 Pediatric Airway Endoscopy

2.1 Professor Nancy Bauman provides an overview of common equipment used in endoscopic airway diagnostic evaluation and surgery, including suspension laryngoscopes, rigid bronchoscopes, and essential associated equipment. Prof. Bauman also discusses key points in the setup and use of these instruments, as well as clinical pearls for the surgeon to consider when using them.

## Chapter 12 Endoscopic Management of Subglottic Cysts

12.1 Subglottic cyst visualized using a 4 mm Hopkins rod telescope. The patient also has low-grade subglottic stenosis and tracheostomy in place.

12.2 Bugbee cautery of subglottic cyst using a 3.5 mm rigid bronchoscope.

## Chapter 13 Endoscopic Radial Incision, Dilation, and Injection for Stenosis

13.1 Balloon dilation before performed as initial intervention.

13.2 Steroid injection using an orotracheal injector needle.

13.3 Endoscopic division of scar bands using Blitzer blade.

13.4 Balloon dilation follows intervention.

## Chapter 14 Endoluminal Airway Stents

14.1 Silicone stent placed in the trachea of a patient with malacia.

14.2 Metallic stent inserted in the trachea of a patient with malacia.

14.3 Biodegradable stent placement in the trachea: Endoscopic technique.

14.4 Biodegradable stent insertion in the right main bronchus: Endoscopic technique.

14.5 Balloon dilation of a severe tracheal stenosis followed by the insertion of a biodegradable stent.

14.6 Biodegradable stent placement in a patient with tracheomalacia.

## Chapter 16 Endoscopic Management of Collapse at the Tracheostomy Site

16.1 Dynamic collapse with inspiration at tracheostomy site.

16.2 Suprastomal granuloma causing airway obstruction.

16.3 Endoscopic visualization - excision of anterior suprastomal collapse.

## Chapter 17 Endoscopic Management of Anterior Glottic Webs

17.1 Laryngeal commissure open split.

## Chapter 21 Endoscopic Tumor Resection

21.1 Coblator resection of tumor.

21.2 Laser resection of synovial sarcoma.

21.3 Bronchoscopic laser excision of tracheal tumor.

21.4 Cryoablation of tumor.

## Chapter 22 Recurrent Respiratory Papillomatosis

22.1 FFL of patient with recurrent glottic papillomata.

22.2 Topicalization of local anesthetic onto glottis/subglottis.

22.3 Pledget application followed by second look.

22.4 Debulking cold steel with Kleinsasser forceps.

22.5 Microdebrider. Console with settings including skimmer blade inset showing aperture.

22.6 Debriding of papillomata obstructing posteriorly.

22.7 Coblation technique.

22.8 Coblating papillomata from ventricle.

22.9 Papilloma extraction through stoma.

22.10 Second look to assess distal airway using telescope. Dynamic obstruction.

22.11 Second look to assess distal airway using telescope. Ball-valving of papillomata.

# SECTION I

# Introduction to Airway Endoscopy

# 1 Introduction

KARA D. MEISTER, KARTHIK BALAKRISHNAN, AND DOUGLAS R. SIDELL

The pediatric aerodigestive tract is a complex region, containing a high density of interdependent neurovascular and musculoskeletal structures. It can house several distinct and overlapping pathologies, and access is challenging with inherent risks. Importantly, the pediatric airway surgeon must balance the critical functions of breathing, swallowing, and voice. Wherein one function may be improved, the same intervention may be to the detriment of another one of these functions. The surgeon's task is to balance the function of all three to obviate the pathology and meet the goals of the patient.

Many children, especially those under 2 years of age with a history of prematurity or other comorbidities, may have significant pulmonary, cardiopulmonary, or neurologic considerations that influence the preoperative, intraoperative, and postoperative decision making and management. Consideration of preoperative microbiology cultures, especially in those with multiple exposures to hospital settings or indwelling devices such as tracheostomy tubes, can drive perioperative antimicrobials. Children also may not easily cooperate with awake airway surveillance, such as flexible laryngoscopy, and the expectations for repeated procedures in the operating room must be established with the family prior to embarking on a surgical plan. Preoperative preparation is critical. This often involves consultation with colleagues in pulmonary medicine, gastroenterology, and speech/swallow therapy. If available, a comprehensive aerodigestive consultation may improve surgical outcomes. In addition, a complete evaluation of the patient's readiness for surgery, including nutrition status, and the consideration of social factors should be conducted. The surgeon should be aware of his or her institutional or systems-based considerations and constraints in the intraoperative and postoperative management of pediatric airway patients. The team surrounding the pediatric airway patient is critically important.

Contraindications to endoscopic airway surgery in children are related to patient comorbidities, such as body habitus or cervical spine problems preventing adequate exposure, and disease characteristics. Patients with significant cardiopulmonary disease are at increased risk for hypercarbia, metabolic acidosis, and postoperative respiratory complications requiring unanticipated airway intervention. Pediatric airway surgeons and care teams should have an open dialogue with pediatric intensivists and respiratory therapists to facilitate optimal patient care.

Disease-specific factors such as large masses, some cases of malignancy, or a need for open surgical placement of an anterior graft may limit the working space and reconstructive options for endoscopic surgery. As such, patients with these characteristics may best be served with an open surgery. Regardless of specific factors, when an endoscopic approach has been selected, the patient and family should be counseled that there is always the possibility of converting to an open approach if the planned procedure cannot be safely and effectively performed. There are several nuances of the pediatric larynx and aerodigestive system that must be considered. First, the anatomy of the pediatric larynx is more compact and there is less space for performing surgery. There is also less space to accommodate tissue edema. As such, gentle tissue handling is critical, despite the second-order haptics of endoscopic surgery. This is achieved through attention to tissue edema, operative duration, local tissue dehydration, and local tissue injury. Improving spatial orientation over time can facilitate these procedures. With experience, mastering relationships in the axial, coronal, and sagittal planes can translate into a robust three-dimensional understanding of the anatomy of the pediatric airway.

This atlas is designed primarily to assist the pediatric airway surgeon in developing an appropriate mental model to approach the technical considerations involved with pediatric airway endoscopic procedures. However, surgical skill is gained primarily through experience in the operating room and taking critical account of one's own experiences and outcomes. Pediatric airway surgery, whether open or endoscopic, is an iterative process. The surgeon should keep an eye on one's own outcomes and quality. Several axioms and principles of surgery are apropos to endoscopic airway surgery:

- Take great care to **maintain hemostasis**, both to keep a clean field with adequate endoscopic visualization and to prevent aspiration of blood
- **Adequate exposure/visualization** of the surgical field is key, and considering different exposures via altering the laryngoscope size and shape or the angle of an endoscope can be greatly beneficial and well worth the time investment
- **Gentle tissue handling** is key, as edema can exponentially narrow the airway and propagate obstructive complications into the postoperative period. Similarly, cautery and other tissue coagulation devices such as laser or coblation will all create some degree of devitalized tissue that may not be readily apparent during the procedure but can create pathology or complications in the days, weeks, or months following the thermal insult
- **Keep calm** and conduct yourself as a leader. Establish every endoscopic airway procedure as a shared-airway case with anesthesia; the surgeon should have a plan and several backup plans for airway management.

## Development of This Atlas

This case-based endoscopic pediatric airway surgery atlas is unique in that it is grounded in the experiences of senior surgeons from around the world and includes their perspectives and voices on operative techniques, pearls, and illustrative intraoperative pictures. As such, the authors, editors, and illustrator reviewed photographs, in-person observations, and surgical videos to create artwork that distills the key elements of each representation. We are so honored to have a leading group of world experts in open and endoscopic surgery contribute to this book. Most significantly, we are grateful for a generous donation in honor of a beloved patient that made this atlas a reality and perpetuates his legacy.

# 2

# Pediatric Airway Endoscopy

ALEXANDRA G. ESPINEL AND NANCY M. BAUMAN

## Introduction

Direct laryngoscopy and bronchoscopy (DLB) is a quintessential procedure for pediatric airway surgeons and has an extensive list of indications (Box 2.1). The procedure is sometimes also known as microdirect laryngoscopy and bronchoscopy, abbreviated MLB or MDLB. Whether the DLB is an elective, urgent, or emergent procedure, the surgeon's tone influences that of the entire operating room (OR); maintaining a calm demeanor and an organized thought process is critical for the welfare of the patient. This state is achieved with fastidious preparation and knowledge of equipment. This understanding also ensures that all diagnostic information is collected during the procedure.

Herein we present equipment and technique considerations for performing DLB as a freestanding diagnostic procedure or as a component of an endoscopic therapeutic procedure. Advantages and limitations of flexible versus rigid procedures are also reviewed.

## Preoperative Planning

When planning airway endoscopy, the surgeon must be circumspect and anticipate all evaluations and interventions that the patient may require in order to obtain informed consent, prepare equipment, and prime the OR personnel. When obtaining informed consent, risk of ventilation concerns, injury to adjacent structures (including the teeth), and the possibility of requiring postoperative airway support should be considered. Neck stability must also be assured.

A well-prepared airway surgeon prepares not only for the diagnostic endoscopy but also for potential airway interventions that can be conducted in the same setting. Preparing for possible dilation, steroid injection, sclerotherapy, biopsy, laser, coblation, cautery, and/or microdebridement, might spare the patient a subsequent trip to the OR without significantly prolonging the duration of the diagnostic procedure. Given the additional time, manpower, and equipment needed for use of the laser, these surgical tools are not typically prepared for prior to routine diagnostic endoscopy (Pearl 2.1).

**• BOX 2.1 Indications for Direct Laryngoscopy and Bronchoscopy**

Determine etiology of respiratory or laryngeal symptoms, including stridor
- Assess status of known airway anomalies
- Provide access for endoscopic airway procedures
- Assess upper airway collapse (drug-induced sleep endoscopy (DISE))
- Secure potentially compromised airway
- Survey established tracheotomy tube
- Gauge the severity of intubation trauma
- Plan an open-airway reconstructive procedure

**PEARL 2.1**

The airway surgeon is wise to develop an airway management ladder or sequence of escalating intervention options, tailored to the individual patient's airway pathology and overall physiology.

Patients with tracheotomy may have a suprastomal granuloma that can be removed at the time of tracheotomy surveillance. Removing this tissue can allow a better assessment of the suprastomal airway if considering decannulation and permit patients to better tolerate capping or use of the Passy Muir valve. While the microdebrider can be used to remove an immature, soft suprastomal granuloma, the reverse Kerrison rongeur (Fig. 2.1) is preferred in cases of mature granulomas (Pearl 2.2).

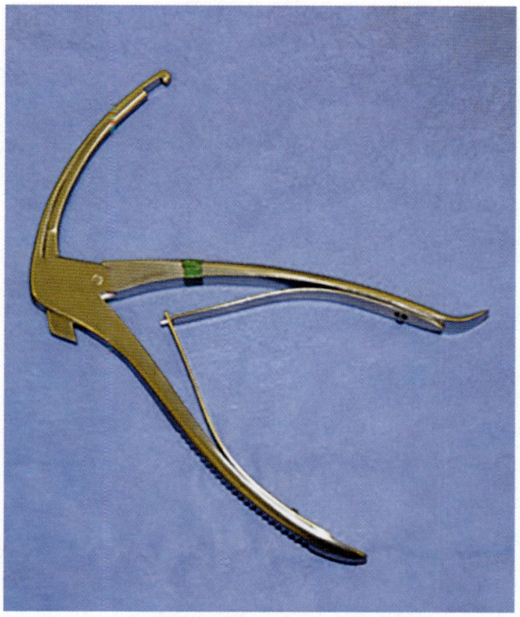

**• Fig. 2.1** *Curved* Kerrison Rongeur is ideal for removing suprastomal granuloma via tracheotomy stoma and should be readily available during all tracheotomy surveillance DLB's. *DLB*, Direct laryngoscopy and bronchoscopy.

**PEARL 2.2**

It is important to differentiate between anterior suprastomal collapse and the presence of a suprastomal granuloma or fibroma. While suprastomal granulomas/fibromas may be obstructive and result in improvement when excised, suprastomal collapse of the native airway may require different management entirely. As such, indiscriminate excision of suprastomal granulation that also results in excision of anterior suprastomal trachal collapse, may result in the loss of peristomal tracheal framework stability, thus worsening peristomal collapse at the time of decannulation.

The endoscopist should also consider the role of esophagoscopy, particularly for patients with dysphagia or external compression of the posterior trachea, and in workup of airway inflammatory conditions such as recurrent croup. Noting the nature and site of concomitant esophageal compression can differentiate an aberrant pulmonary sling that compresses the anterior esophagus from a retroesophageal subclavian artery that compresses the posterior esophagus.

The surgeon is responsible for ensuring that necessary equipment is available, correctly assembled, and in working order prior to the patient entering the surgical suite. One should ensure there are telescopes, laryngoscopes, and bronchoscopes of the appropriate size (Table 2.1), and that the telescopes are free of cracks (Fig. 2.2). Additionally, preservative-free lidocaine, ventilating supplies, tooth/alveolar guard, white-balanced camera, recording equipment, and, if indicated, suspension apparatus and microscope should be readied.

These preparations can help ensure that the endoscopy is comprehensive and diagnostic without unnecessary intraoperative delays due to equipment concerns or lack of planning for potential interventions.

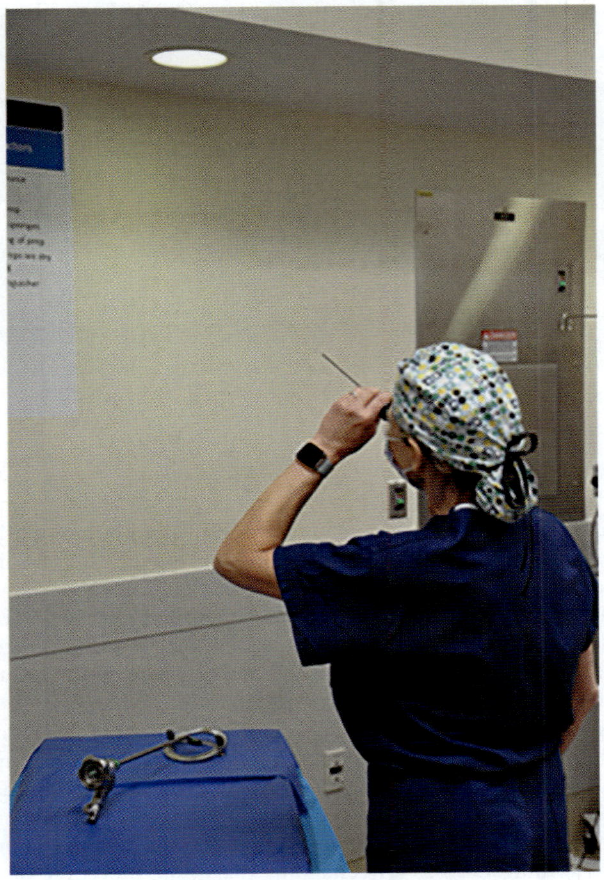

• **Fig. 2.2** All necessary equipment for DLB should be procured and checked before the patient enters the operating room suite to avoid intraoperative delays. Hopkins rod telescopes should be checked for cracks and flaws by gazing through the telescope directed at an overhead light. *DLB*, Direct laryngoscopy and bronchoscopy.

**TABLE 2.1 Age-Appropriate Endotracheal Tube and Bronchoscope Sizes[b]**

| Age | Cricoid Airway Diameter (mm) | UNCUFFED ENDOTRACHEAL TUBE SIZE: Inner Diameter (ID) (mm) | UNCUFFED ENDOTRACHEAL TUBE SIZE: Outer Diameter (OD) (mm) | BRONCHOSCOPE SIZE[a]: Size | BRONCHOSCOPE SIZE[a]: ID (mm) | BRONCHOSCOPE SIZE[a]: OD (mm) |
|---|---|---|---|---|---|---|
| Premature <30 weeks | 4.0 | 2.5 | 3.6 | 2.5 | 3.2 | 4.0 |
| Premature >30 weeks | 4.0–4.5 | 3.0 | 4.3 | 3.0 | 4.2 | 5.0 |
| Term Newborn | 4.5 | 3.5 | 4.9 | 3.0 | 4.2 | 5.0 |
| 6 months | 5.0 | 3.5 | 4.9 | 3.0 | 4.2 | 5.0 |
| 1 year | 5.5 | 4.0 | 5.6 | 3.5 | 4.9 | 5.7 |
| 2 years | 6.0 | 4.5 | 6.2 | 3.5 | 4.9 | 5.7 |
| 3 years | 7.0 | 5.0 | 6.9 | 4.0 | 5.9 | 6.7 |
| 5 years | 8.0 | 5.5 | 7.5 | 5.0 | 7.0 | 7.8 |
| 10 years | 9.0 | 6.5 | 8.9 | 5.0[a] | 7.0 | 7.8 |
| 14 years | 11.0 | 7.5 | 10.2 | 5.0[a] | 7.0 | 7.8 |

[a]A larger bronchoscope may be necessary if intermittent positive pressure ventilation (IPPV) is being used and air leak is present.

[b]Modified from Londino AV, Jagannathan N. Anesthesia in diagnostic and therapeutic pediatric bronchoscopy. *Otolaryngol Clin North Am.* 2019;52(6):1037–1048.

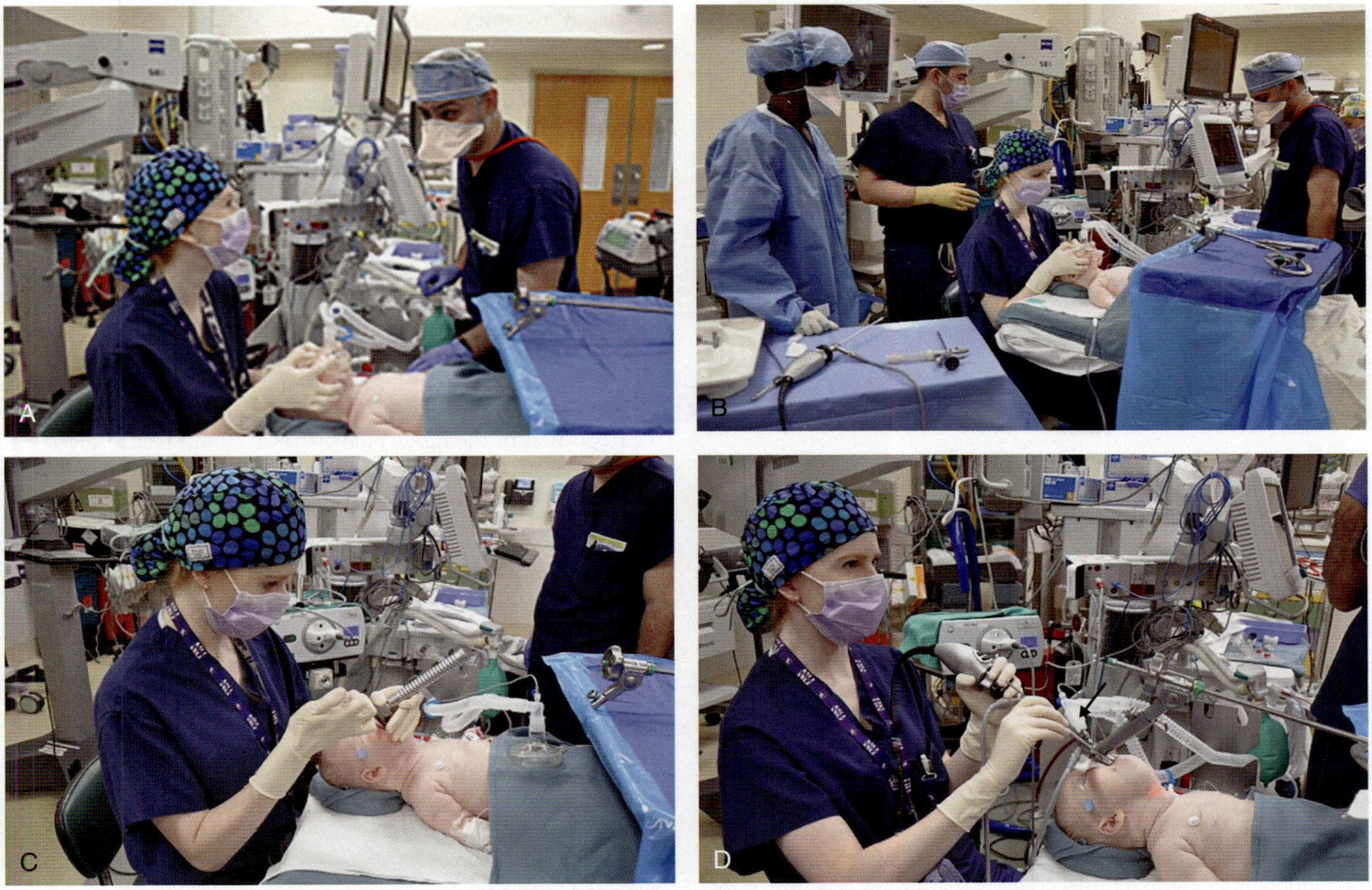

• **Fig. 2.3** (A) Communication of anesthetic and surgical plan between endoscopist, anesthetist, and entire operating room team is critical to ensure a safe and smooth DLB. *DLB*, Direct laryngoscopy and bronchoscopy. (B) The patient's chest should be visible to allow for assessment of chest wall excursion and access to auscultation. (C) Preservative-free topical lidocaine is applied to the supraglottic structures, particularly the laryngeal surface of the epiglottis, to blunt vagally-mediated reflexive laryngospasm and bronchospasm. The patient is mask-ventilated for 3–4 minutes to allow the topical medication to take effect before proceeding. (D) Suspension laryngoscopy facilitates simultaneous imaging of the airway along with measuring of the interarytenoid height and palpation of the arytenoid cartilages. The ventilating cap from a 3.0 oral endotracheal tube (*arrow*) fits snugly into the side ventilating pipe of the laryngoscope to allow for insufflation of oxygen, heliox, or volatile anesthetic agents.

## Equipment

A variety of laryngoscopes are available to accommodate the diverse anatomic variations and pathology of the pediatric airway. The most commonly used pediatric laryngoscopes are manufactured by Storz (Karl Storz Endoscopy, Tutlehiem, Germany) and Pilling (Teleflex Medical, Wayne, Pennsylvania). The authors are most familiar with Storz laryngoscopes and herein describe key considerations (see Video 2.1 for additional details).

Storz pediatric laryngoscopes are illuminated with either a side fiber-optic light pipe or a superior prismatic light deflector uniquely designed for each style of laryngoscope. The universal Benjamin-Havas light clip illuminates any laryngoscope and is useful if a laryngoscope and its corresponding illumination device are inadvertently separated, as can often occur during the sterilization process. The fiber-optic light cable that connects the laryngoscope light tube to the light source is a series of fragile microglass tubules bound with a flexible protective coating and must be handled with care. Light-emitting diode (LED) light sources are cooler, more energy efficient, and more durable than traditional xenon and halogen light sources.

The ventilating cap of a 3.0 pediatric endotracheal tube can be attached to the ventilating pipe of most laryngoscopes (Fig. 2.3) and provides a universal connection to facilitate oxygen, heliox, and/or volatile anesthetic delivery (Pearl 2.3).

**PEARL 2.3**

For greater length and flexibility, a cut portion of a 6.0 or 6.5 endotracheal tube along with its adapter may also be used.

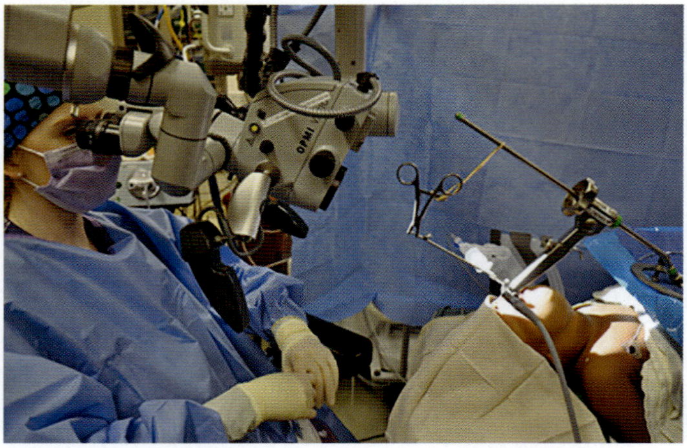

• **Fig. 2.4** The Lindholm laryngeal retractors placed in inverted fashion and secured to suspension bar to improve exposure of glottis, subglottis, and trachea.

For diagnostic laryngoscopy, the Lindholm, Storz Standard slotted, or Parsons slotted laryngoscopes are available in multiple sizes to accommodate preterm to adolescent patients and can be handheld or suspended. The slotted laryngoscopes allow for introduction of a bronchoscope when handheld. The laryngoscope is removed once the tip of the bronchoscope enters the subglottis. For operative laryngoscopy, the wide mouth of the Lindholm laryngoscope provides a favorable binocular view and ample space to manipulate microlaryngeal instruments. The tip of the Lindholm laryngoscope is placed in the vallecula and manipulated until the epiglottis is erect and adherent to the laryngoscope's internal edge. Distraction of the posterior false vocal folds by the Lindholm laryngeal spreaders (Fig. 2.4) improves exposure of the glottis and the posterior glottis, facilitates measuring the interarytenoid height,[1] provides surgical access to the subglottis virtually eliminating the need for subglottiscopes, and may even provide access to the proximal and mid trachea.

A shoulder roll can facilitate exposure for bronchoscopy but is generally not helpful for exposure in direct laryngoscopy.

## Anesthetic Considerations

While communication with the anesthesia team is essential in all surgical procedures (Fig. 2.3), it is particularly critical in airway endoscopy, as both teams share management of the airway. The anesthetic plan as well as the planned operative procedure, including interventions and anticipated surgical time, should be discussed. Whether the endoscopy is performed while the patient breathes spontaneously under total intravenous anesthesia (TIVA) or while the patient is apneic, intravenous access must first be secured. Preservative-free lidocaine is then applied topically to the supraglottis and glottis to blunt the vagally mediated afferent limbs of laryngospasm. Even patients with a tracheotomy tube may benefit from the use of topical laryngeal lidocaine to reduce the risk of bronchospasm that reflexively accompanies laryngospasm. When anesthetizing the larynx, it is important to allow time for the topical agent to take effect, as the onset of action of topical lidocaine to the larynx has been reported to be between 3 and 5 minutes. The patient can be mask ventilated and preoxygenated during this time.

Total intravenous anesthesia (TIVA) with spontaneous ventilation is generally preferred over apnea for diagnostic DLB, as it permits a dynamic view of the airway. It is important to achieve an appropriate plane of anesthesia in which the patient is relaxed and not reacting to the procedure but is still breathing spontaneously, so airway dynamics can be assessed. If the anesthetic plane is too light, the patient can contract the laryngeal muscles making exposure and evaluation difficult and potentially inducing laryngospasm. Propofol, delivered via an infusion pump, is ideal for TIVA and is augmented with intravenous fentanyl or morphine. A propofol starting point of 400 mcg/kg is generally indicated with titration to achieve the desired plane of anesthesia. The experienced airway surgeon recognizes the signals that the airway is ready for inspection, including the presence of nonlabored respirations and subtle abduction and adduction of the vocal folds synchronized with inspiration and expiration, respectively.

If performing endoscopy under apnea, the surgeon must be efficient in the endoscopic evaluation, as time is limited by the patient's ability to remain without breath. In these situations, it is important to be cognizant of the lag in reporting with pulse oximetry.

Regardless of the mode of anesthesia, equipment to mask ventilate, or intubate should be readily available should the patient need additional airway support.

## Systematic Review of the Airway During Direct Laryngoscopy and Bronchoscopy

When assessing the airway, it is best to proceed in a systematic approach so that critical findings are not overlooked and assessment can be easily interpreted by other providers managing the airway. A comprehensive operative report (Box 2.2) records these findings in detail.

### • BOX 2.2 Documentation Checklist for Direct Laryngoscopy and Bronchoscopy[a]

Anesthesia Information

- Description of breathing (spontaneous, supplemental oxygen, positive pressure, intubated)

**Airway Exposure**

- Grade of view (Cormack-Lehane classification)
- Laryngoscope type and size used
- Maneuvers to improve view (i.e., cricoid pressure)

**Anatomic Structures**

- Supraglottis
  - Aryepiglottic folds
  - False vocal cords
  - Interarytenoid area (include if palpated or not)
- Glottis
- Subglottis (if SGS, grade)
- Trachea (normal/abnormal)
  - Tracheomalacia (present/absent); (include severity and location)
  - External compression (include location and severity)
  - Complete tracheal rings (presence or absence)
  - Tracheoesophageal fistula (presence or absence)
  - Other (secretions, cobblestoning)

**Other**

- Desaturations (severity, management)
- Complications (injury, obstruction, teeth)
- Extubated or intubated at end of procedure

*SGS*, Subglottic stenosis

[a]Modified from Neocleous P, Dzioba A, Strychowsky J, et al. Documentation in pediatric microlaryngoscopy/bronchoscopy: international modified delphi consensus. *Laryngoscope*. 2023;133(5):1234–1238.

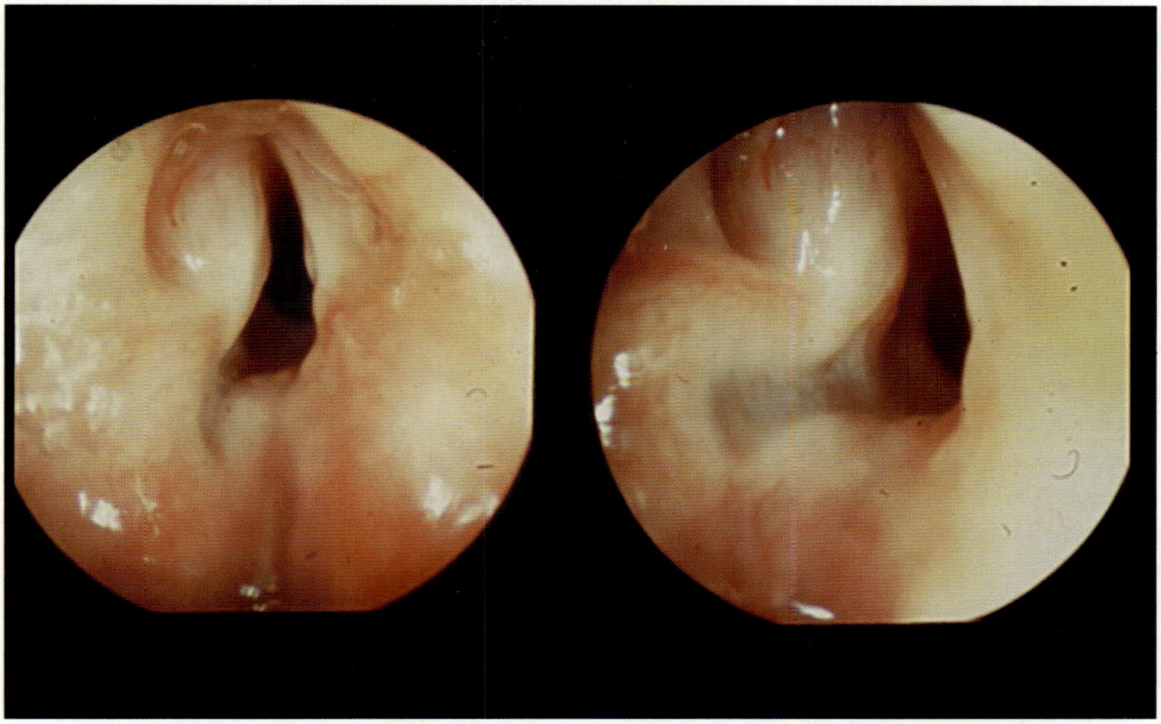

• **Fig. 2.5** View of a healed cricoarytenoid joint furrow secondary to intubation trauma with zero degree (*left*) and 30 degree (*right*) Hopkins rod telescope. Note improved visualization of depth of furrow, which extends to cricoid cartilage, with a 30-degree telescope.

The airway assessment begins proximally with the supraglottis then extends distally to terminate in the bronchi. Secretions should be gently suctioned, as they can obscure pathology. We highlight significant aspects of this exam that can be overlooked. Beginning in the supraglottis, the interarytenoid region should be evaluated, palpated, and measured relative to the height of the ventricle and the true and false vocal folds, to assess for laryngeal cleft. This maneuver typically requires suspension. Palpating the cricoarytenoid joints to determine stiffness or fixation is also beneficial, particularly when evaluating intubation trauma. The posterior glottic area requires close assessment, as congenital or acquired interarytenoid pathology can be easily overlooked. In addition to grading the percent of subglottic or tracheal stenosis, the length of the stenosis and distance of the stenosis the vocal folds, carina, and, if present, the tracheostoma should be measured. This is valuable information when planning an airway reconstruction.

Vocal fold activity can be affected by general anesthesia, even in a spontaneously ventilating patient, and is best assessed prior to induction of general anesthesia. Options for assessment include transnasal fiber-optic flexible laryngoscopy, translaryngeal ultrasound, or, in a cooperative patient, transoral exam with a rigid 70-degree telescope.

## Direct Laryngoscopy

Professor Bruce Benjamin, the "father" of laryngeal photography, advocated three-stage rigid laryngoscopy beginning with naked-eye examination of the larynx with an intubating laryngoscope to obtain an airway overview, determine ease of laryngeal exposure and apply topical preservative-free lidocaine (Stage 1).

The larynx is examined with a magnifying rigid telescope in Stage 2, and photo/video documentation is obtained. Regarding diagnostic (nonoperative) laryngoscopy, each pediatric otolaryngologist has the routine practice of suspending or not suspending. While some surgeons suspend routinely in diagnostic cases citing the benefits of having both hands free and a stable "straight shot" view of the airway once suspended, others only suspend when performing an endoscopic intervention. Angled telescopes (30, 45, or 90 degree) can provide a three-dimensional view of airway pathology, particularly the cricoarytenoid joints and posterior glottic scars (Fig. 2.5; Pearl 2.4).

When indicated, surgical intervention of the larynx, Stage 3, is performed with an operating microscope or handheld magnifying telescope as described in detail in subsequent chapters.

**PEARL 2.4**

Seventy- and 90-degree telescopes also allow the surgeon to look along the free edge of the vocal folds and to make a more thorough assessment of the anterior commissure; this is particularly helpful in patients with dysphonia.

While flexible laryngoscopy allows dynamic assessment of the supraglottis and vocal folds without general anesthesia, it is generally inferior to rigid laryngoscopy in evaluating the posterior glottis and subglottis (Table 2.2).

**TABLE 2.2 Flexible Versus Rigid Endoscopy**

| | Flexible Endoscopy | Rigid Endoscopy |
|---|---|---|
| **General Considerations** | | |
| Anesthesia | None, topical, general | General[a] |
| Ventilation | Spontaneous | Spontaneous, apneic, jet, intubation[b] |
| May administer oxygen/volatile agent through sideport | No | Yes |
| Location Performed[c] | OR, clinic, bedside, intensive care unit | OR, intensive care unit |
| Perform DISE exam | Yes | No |
| **Laryngeal Examination** | | |
| Assess supraglottic dynamics | Yes | May be affected by laryngoscope or anesthesia |
| Assess vocal cord dynamics | Yes | May be altered by anesthesia |
| Palpate cricoarytenoid joints | No | Yes |
| Assess posterior glottis | Limited | Yes |
| Assess interarytenoid region | No | Yes |
| Size subglottis | No | Yes |
| Enables endoscopic procedure | Yes, limited | Yes |
| Allows foreign body removal | Yes, limited | Yes |
| Exposes upper esophageal sphincter | No | Yes, via Benjamin lift |
| Allows tracheoscopy | Yes[d] | Yes |
| Facilitates Intubation | Yes, if ETT placed over scope | Yes |
| **Tracheobronchial Exam** | | |
| Assess tracheobronchial dynamics | Yes | May be affected by anesthesia |
| Assess anatomy | Yes | Yes |
| Allows cannulation of TEF | Yes | Yes |
| Enables endoscopic procedure | Yes (limited) | Yes |
| Allows foreign body removal | No | Yes |
| Allows stent placement | Yes | Yes |
| View of secondary and tertiary bronchioles | Yes | Limited, depending on patient size |

[a]Newborn infants may tolerate endoscopy without anesthesia; this can be the safest approach for a precarious airway.
[b]Intubation often prohibits view of pediatric larynx.
[c]Institution dependent.
[d]If properly anesthetized.
*DISE*, Drug-induced sleep endoscopy; *ETT*, endotracheal tube; *OR*, Operating room; *TEF*, tracheoesophageal fistula.

## Bronchoscopy

Diagnostic bronchoscopy can be performed with a rigid or fiberoptic telescope. Advantages and limitations of rigid versus flexible fiber-optic bronchoscopy are outlined (see Table 2.2). Historically speaking, diagnostic rigid bronchoscopy was completed by introducing a ventilating bronchoscope past the topically anesthetized larynx exposed with a handheld (nonsuspended) laryngoscope (Fig. 2.6). This method of rigid bronchoscopy remains advantageous for patients unable to tolerate short lapses in ventilation during bronchoscopy or who need procedures that are most easily performed through a rigid bronchoscope, including saline lavage of the distal airway. However, with advances in fiber-optics and anesthesia delivery, particularly the advent of TIVA, the tracheobronchial tree is now usually examined by passing a 0-degree Hopkins rod telescope through a handheld or suspended laryngoscope while the patient ventilates spontaneously or endures brief periods of apnea (Pearl 2.5). The mode of ventilation depends on the surgeon's preference, the patient's underlying respiratory status and the experience and comfort of the anesthesiologist.

> **PEARL 2.5**
>
> Some surgeons will place an endotracheal tube through the nose or mouth into the pharynx to provide supplemental oxygen and anesthetic gas. High-flow nasal cannula may also be useful, though it may obscure dynamic upper airway collapse.

A static view of the tracheobronchial tree can be performed under apnea or under any mode of ventilation. However, a dynamic view of the tracheobronchial tree is necessary to assess for tracheomalacia or bronchomalacia and requires

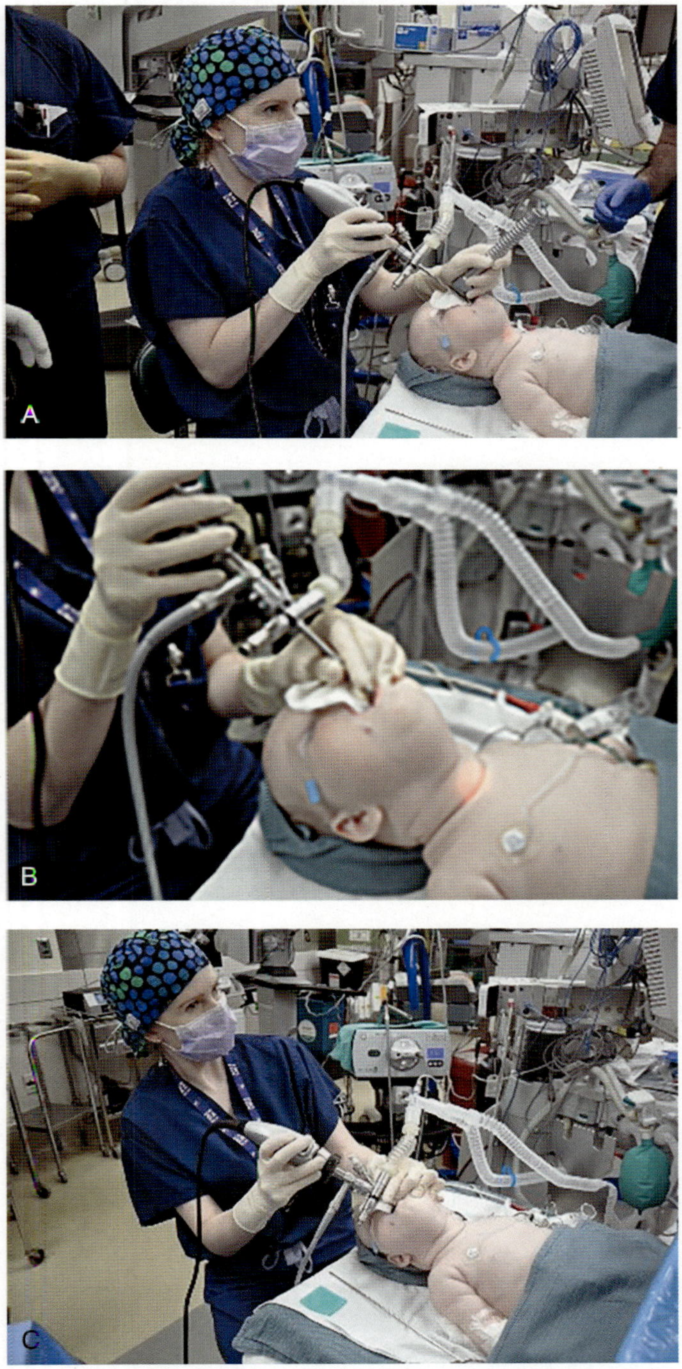

• **Fig. 2.6** (A) The bronchoscope is inserted through the handheld laryngoscope (*left*) and the laryngoscope is removed once the bronchoscope enters the trachea. (B) The middle finger rests between the bronchoscope and the patient's alveolar ridge (*right*) to avoid injury to the alveolar ridge. (C) The patient's head is gently rotated to the *right* to improve visibility of the distal *left* airway and vice versa.

spontaneous ventilation (Pearl 2.6). During bronchoscopy, the internal configuration of the trachea can be assessed, the cartilaginous:membranous ratio measured (normal 4.5:1), the character of secretions noted, and the presence of congenital or acquired stenoses or other airway anomalies ascertained, including tracheoesophageal fistula and tracheal compression.

**PEARL 2.6**

When performing a dynamic evaluation of the airway, flexible bronchoscopy is often a preferred method due to the reduced anesthetic requirement during this procedure.

"Three-phase bronchoscopy" where the airway is first examined statically, then under spontaneous ventilation, and finally under a light plane of anesthesia such that the endoscope can induce a cough provides the most physiologic assessment of the tracheobronchial tree. This three-phase approach is particularly helpful in assessing the severity of tracheomalacia and in identifying candidates for anterior aortopexy or posterior tracheopexy.

Depending on the indication for bronchoscopy and the intraoperative findings, the patient may benefit from culture of airway secretions, lavage of secondary bronchioles, mucosal biopsy of cilia, removal of suprastomal granuloma, dilation, catheterization or endoscopic closure of tracheoesophageal fistula, or biopsy of pathology. Pathology of the tracheobronchial tree should be categorized as intraluminal versus extraluminal, vascular versus nonvascular, congenital versus acquired, percent of airway obstruction, and location of pathology with distance measured relative to undersurface of vocal folds and carina, as the latter will aid in surgical planning. Likewise, for tracheal stenosis, the number of tracheal rings involved, length of stenosis, and distances from vocal cords and carina need to be determined.

## Archiving Airway Images

"A picture is worth a thousand words," and a detailed DLB operative report is similarly enhanced with airway photos. Airway videos provide a dynamic view of the airway and even more detail than a still image. Before taking a photo or video, the endoscopist should ensure that the image is color-accurate, focused, and ideally positioned in the composite. Images collected during the case can be printed and shared with caretakers and medical providers to aid in understanding pathology. Images uploaded to an institution's Health Insurance Portability and Accountability Act (HIPAA)-compliant electronic medical record (EMR), server, tower, or cloud storage allow easy access for subsequent comparison between procedures and for academic presentations. Establishing a HIPAA-compliant, facile method of archiving and retrieving high-quality images and videos is an expensive endeavor but one that serves patients and providers well. In the absence of such a system, a snapshot of the images taken with an institution's EMR capture mobile application provides an easy method to archive static images that can be shared with other providers and used for comparison at subsequent procedures; however, images may appear distorted, and resolution is usually too low to be used for academic presentations. Alternatively, images and videos are often saved by the endoscopist to a removable disk drive and can be downloaded to a password-protected computer or secure cloud-based storage. This latter method of archiving is relatively inexpensive and easy; however, it requires a commitment to download, label, and fastidiously catalog each image to facilitate subsequent access. Least advantageous is the senior author's experience of stacking printed images in a drawer and/or on a series of removable disk drives that never get downloaded to organized folders.

## Conclusion

Direct laryngoscopy and bronchoscopy is an essential procedure for both airway examination and interventions. A well-planned systematic approach not only facilitates a complete, efficient exam but also prioritizes patient safety. Obtaining and archiving high-quality, well-composed images and videos facilitates patient care and sharing of knowledge in academic settings.

## References

1. Coppes S, Padia R, Horn D, et al. Standardizing laryngeal cleft evaluations: reliability of the interarytenoid assessment protocol. *Otolaryngol Head Neck Surg.* 2019;160(3):533–539. doi:10.1177/0194599818806283.

# 3

# Image Recording and Archiving

RAKESH SRIVASTAVA

## Introduction

Often words cannot describe what the human eye will see. Visual documentation has been the cornerstone of medical education and experience for centuries. The digital imaging era commenced in 1979 with the invention of the charge-coupled device (CCD). Later, complementary metal-oxide semiconductors (CMOS) were introduced. CMOS image sensors offer high-quality images at faster frame rates and lower fabrication costs. Digital imaging and archiving of endoscopy have been in use since the early 21st century. More recently, chip-on-tip flexible endoscopes and rigid glass rod telescopes with high-definition (HD) cameras have been important in the assessment of airway and upper aerodigestive tract anatomy and pathology. These images and videos can be stored and analyzed.

Endoscopic airway assessment in the pediatric age group is challenging due to shorter apnea time and may be made more challenging due to airway pathology. Airway examination must be done efficiently and should be recorded. This recording facilitates a more detailed assessment of the patient through the surgeon's subsequent review, assessment of patient changes over time, discussion with patients and families, discussion with clinical and research teams, medical education, and academic and documentation for medicolegal purposes.

Digestive tract examination is an essential constituent of airway assessment, including evaluation of swallow function in many patients. The reflexive and voluntary actions of over 30 nerves and muscles produce the coordinated movements of swallowing within a few seconds. Functional endoscopic evaluation of swallowing (FEES) or video fluoroscopic swallow study (VFSS), also known as modified barium swallow study or MBSS, are dynamic comprehensive examinations of swallowing. These tests are also performed very quickly; subsequent review of video recording and still images is an integral part of the interpretation. Replay of these recorded videos during various phases of swallowing helps us in the interpretation of dysphagia scores and recommendations regarding management. These videos help in that they involve collaboration with a speech-language pathologist and/or occupational therapist during the swallow assessment. Slow-motion and freeze-frame review of video by a full team of experts is very helpful.

Airway surgeries are complex and need planning and explanation prior to surgical intervention. At a tertiary care center, this author counsels the caregiver and family members. Counseling addresses disease pathology, progress, complexities (voice, airway, and swallowing), treatment options (risks and benefits as well as alternative treatment options), staging for malignancy, when applicable, and expected results. Depending on the context, financial implications of airway surgeries are also explained. This detailed counseling for airway surgery relies heavily on images and videos of the airway.

## Technique and Technology of Archiving

When assessing laryngeal and particularly glottic lesions, I favor 4k contrast-enhanced laryngoscopy (narrow-band imaging) for better image quality and demarcation of capillaries in case of airway papillomas. Juvenile or adult airway papilloma scoring may be done most accurately through a review of archived images.

Images may be captured during endoscopy with the help of a built-in capture button (snapshot) on the endoscopy camera head, by using the snapshot option in the software application, or by using a foot pedal during the procedure. Various HD capture cards are available. The author prefers to use a Blackmagic Video Assist HD recorder in the operating room and VisualScopy software with an external HD capture card in the office setting. Conversion between video formats (like .mov to mp4 or WMV) can be done with various online conversion software packages (like Format Factory or HandBrake), which are often free of charge for the user. HandBrake is a free and open-source tool for video conversion to/from any format. Snapshots are taken by foot control during endoscopy or by playing video in VLC or Windows Media Player and using the snipping tool. The snipping tool is the Microsoft Windows screenshot utility tool. Blackmagic Video Assist records videos to flash memory (SDXC) in a .mov format; these are later transferred to a computer. I prefer to use DaVinci Resolve for video editing. Various other methods of video archiving are available, such as the Smith and Nephew system (660 HD system), Dax Medical Video Archive, HD, and 4k capture systems (Blackmagic, Microware, Corsair, AverMedia, etc.). Given the rapid pace of technologial advancements, new and updated software and hardware are frequently introduced. Consequently, there is considerable variability among institutions and clinicians. While the software mentioned in this chapter reflects the author's preferences, each clinician should select tools that best suit their practice and patients, ensuring compliance with institutional, local, and federal privacy regulations.

The ideal endoscopy archiving system (laptop/desktop) has a compact design, touchscreen monitor, speaker, 1TB internal storage (SSD or HDD), core i7 processor, standard internal storage of at least 12 TB (6 TB recording and 6 TB auto backup), multiple ports for HDMI, USB-3 data transfer, VGA output, video grabber, and wired or reliable Wi-Fi network connection. Recently, I started archiving endoscopy using a Fujitsu UH-X (11th Gen Core i7 with Iris Xe Graphics). The software should capture details of the patient's records, serial endoscopy pictures, file convertor (pdf/jpg), and include editing and sharing options (email/social media like WhatsApp). The sharing of patients' pictures or images via email and social media or messaging platform is not permitted in many countries, protected by laws such as the Health Insurance Portability and Accountability Act (HIPPA) in the US and the General Data Protection Regulation (GDPR) in Europe. The clinician should be aware of policies and laws at their institution and within their country.

## Storage

Clinical imaging makes up 70% of all data stored by healthcare organizations. The average image size ranges from 64 kB to 300 MB. Hospital patient archiving and communication system (PACS) stores patient images and related data, with cloud storage for images over time. I store my data in network access storage (NAS). Fast disks (SSD/SAS) are used for the application, database, and image short-term cache. Health Level Seven International (HL7) and Fast Interoperability Resources (FHIR) are standards for the exchange, integration, sharing, and retrieval of electronic health information. Health Level Seven International focuses on the standardization of data formats and protocols for health data exchange.

The database and image application portion are usually connected via a fiber channel. I use NAS in the office for archiving. The advantages are larger storage, multiple users of big files, easy remote access, automated backup, and data protection. When data are stored on a laptop or desktop alone, there is a risk of a sudden loss of data or violation of patient confidentiality due to unauthorized access. Network access storage has a simple server setup and private cloud, and hence fewer chances of corruption. The author indexes images in Excel sheets and stores data from various periods in cloud space categorized by the year of capture. The preferred snapshot image format is JPEG. The PNG format has a higher quality but uses more storage space.

Video files are archived in the cloud. These files can be used at a later date for comparing surgical outcomes. MOV files are safe, efficient, and of high quality. For non-Apple devices, MP4 has greater flexibility in data storage and transmission, and provides enhanced high-resolution content through the use of the latest codec H264. Both MOV and MP4 formats are interconvertible using various converter tools as noted earlier.

Picture archiving and communication systems (PACS) provide storage and access to medical images in hospitals. PACS comprises four major components: (1) image acquisition devices (imaging modalities); (2) communication networks; (3) PACS archive and server; and (4) integrated display workstations. PACS can be further connected to radiology information systems and hospital information systems. The disadvantages of PACS are their cost, the need for specialized personnel for installation and maintenance, training of users, the possibility of breakdown, and system-wide data security challenges.

The hospital maintaining the PACS must have a reliable intranet that is capable of transmitting text, images, full-motion video, and sound. The network communication standard is called transfer control protocol/internet protocol (TCP/IP), and all devices on the network must use this standard for communication. This streamilined data sharing improves coordination among airway surgeons, anesthetists, neonatologists, intensivists, pulmonologists, and various other specialties involved in each patient's care.

## Why Do We Need Archiving?

Archived images and videos are useful records for discussion and to guide patient care decisions during interdisciplinary airway clinics (IAC). Interdisciplinary airway clinics frequently use clinical vignettes (and their associated archived images and videos) to discuss surgical planning, perform risk–benefit analysis, and discuss past or potential future complications. The data archive is also important in meeting regulatory requirements, and can support research aimed at improving patient care.

Images or videos archived can be presented to the patient and their family to assist in surgical or postoperative counseling, discussing potential risk factors and management options. In addition, patients and their families can be shown similar cases and their management for comparative purposes.

Archiving helps the surgeon revisit past exams in cases of revision surgery, and supports a detailed understanding of the patient in cases of treatment failure. The review of serial endoscopic airway evaluations may also provide information to the treating clinician about wound healing and the status of recovery following airway surgery.

In situations where difficult or complex pathology exists, an image or video of a pathological lesion or process can be discussed with other airway experts through social media platforms with written consent from the patient or caregiver.

Archived data can also be used for academic purposes, including publication, teaching, giving oral presentations, and developing algorithms for deep learning. The author currently uses these stored images obtained in both white light and narrow-band imaging for deep learning. An extended application, tele-endoscopy, is promising. It is a digital video transport system (DVTS) that utilizes stored data for deep learning algorithms. VIDIZMO is one such software, which searches the content in a video by "Audio to text," "Video analysis," and "Metadata." Audio-to-text converts all spoken words into text, after which search engines can read through them easily. In video analysis, artificial intelligence (AI) can point out what is happening in a video by detecting a person's face or objects. Metadata allows tagging of a video, such that later, search engines will detect the content within the video.

## Summary

Airway counseling and communication are integral parts of airway management, especially for the parents of the pediatric patient. Diseases and their progression may be well explained through serial endoscopy pictures and videos. Complex pathology involving all three major functions of the larynx (voice, airway, and swallowing) can better be described through a review of archived images and video.

Also specific to the pediatric patient, the child may allow for endoscopic examination only once. Video storage allows for multiple replays of the same video at various speeds, and can help us understand the nature of the pathology or detect any synchronous airway lesion without performing prolonged or repeated awake endoscopy.

The concept of sharing pictures and videos among the team of consultants is important and may guide the discussion of treatment planning, consent, anesthesia aspects, and postoperative management.

Lastly, deep learning and artificial intelligence applications prove promising at current state, and are expected to improve dramatically in the coming years.

# SECTION II

# Surgery for Dysphagia and Aspiration

# 4

# Endoscopic Laryngeal Cleft Repair

DOUGLAS R. SIDELL AND KARTHIK BALAKRISHNAN

## Background

Laryngeal clefts represent any deficiency in the posterior tracheoesophageal septum, with or without cricoid or tracheal involvement. The majority of patients present with signs and symptoms associated with aspiration, although redundant mucosa in some clefts may predispose to obstructive airway symptoms such as stridor. Laryngeal clefts are diagnosed by means of endoscopy and palpation of the cleft site in the operating room, although a small percentage of cases may be visualized in the awake patient via nasal endoscopy. Laryngeal clefts are most frequently classified by means of the Benjamin-Inglis classification, or a derivative thereof. Short clefts (e.g., Type 1 and 2) may involve the interarytenoid space alone or a portion of the cricoid plate. Longer clefts (e.g., Types 3 and 4) may extend into the cervical or thoracic trachea or into mainstem bronchus (Fig. 4.1).

Under all circumstances, a deficiency exists that is associated with the interarytenoid musculature, with further extension dependent on the degree of posterior tracheoesophageal tissue deficiency (Fig. 4.2).

This chapter focuses on the endoscopic repair of the laryngeal cleft, performed most commonly for Types 1, 2, and select Type 3 clefts.

## Operative Endoscopic Assessment

### Patient Selection

Patients with clinical suspicion of laryngeal cleft based on clinical history and instrumental swallow evaluation will benefit from formal endoscopic assessment.

### Key Aspects of the Consent Process

Standard risks of operative airway endoscopy should be discussed, including:

- Risks of general anesthesia
- Risks of injury to oral, pharyngeal, and airway structures.

### Equipment

- Appropriately sized laryngoscope
- Hopkins rod telescope (0 degree)
- Equipment to spray medications on larynx
- Right-angled probe or small endoscopic alligator forceps

The reference standard for diagnosis of laryngeal cleft or laryngotracheoesophageal cleft is rigid airway endoscopy performed under general anesthesia; flexible bronchoscopy is notably less sensitive even in the most skilled hands. Steps to this assessment are as follows.

1. Patient positioning: The patient is positioned supine with head at the top of the table. The table is turned 90 degrees with the patient's left side toward the anesthesiology provider. No shoulder roll is used. If the patient's head tends to roll to one side or the other, a rolled towel or gel donut can be placed around the head. With young infants and patients with trisomy 21, take particular care not to overextend the neck. When properly exposed, the glottis and posterior supraglottis should be readily visible and accessible surgically. Appropriate laryngeal exposure can be seen in Fig. 4.3 (normal larynx) and Fig. 4.4 (laryngeal cleft).
2. Under telescopic or microscopic visualization and after application of topical laryngeal anesthetic, use a rigid right-angle probe or small alligator forceps to gently push the arytenoid cartilages apart and palpate the interarytenoid area (Fig. 4.5 showing the schematic view and Fig. 4.6 showing an alligator forcep probing a type 2 cleft).
3. Evaluate the inferior/caudal depth of the interarytenoid space relative to the glottis.
4. Palpate the cricoid in the posterior midline to determine whether there is any submucous absence of cartilage, indicating a submucous extension of the cleft. It may be helpful to pass a right-angle probe into the esophagus to palpate the posterior cricoid, ensuring there is no submucosal cartilaginous defect.

Suspension laryngoscopy may be beneficial because it allows the surgeon to elevate the larynx and visualize the esophageal inlet and posterior aspect of the cricoid; however, this is not mandatory. In addition, a laryngeal spreader can be placed if desired.

## Operative Approach

### Patient Selection

Endoscopic repair of laryngeal cleft is well suited for type 0 through type 2 clefts, with some type 3 clefts amenable depending on the patient's ease of laryngeal exposure and cardiopulmonary reserve. Otherwise, selection criteria are similar to those for endoscopic injection.

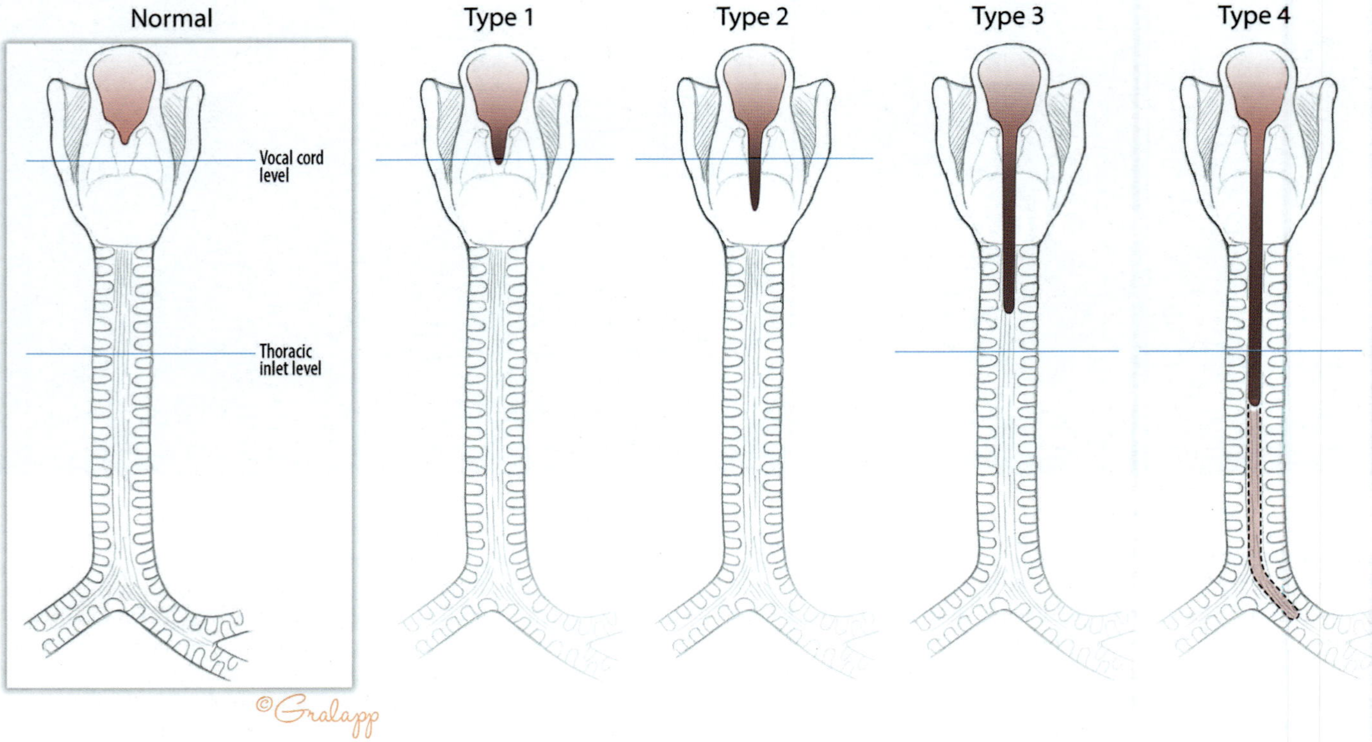


• **Fig. 4.1** Artist rendering depicting the Benjamin-Inglis classification for laryngeal and laryngotracheal clefts. (© 2024 Chris Gralapp.)

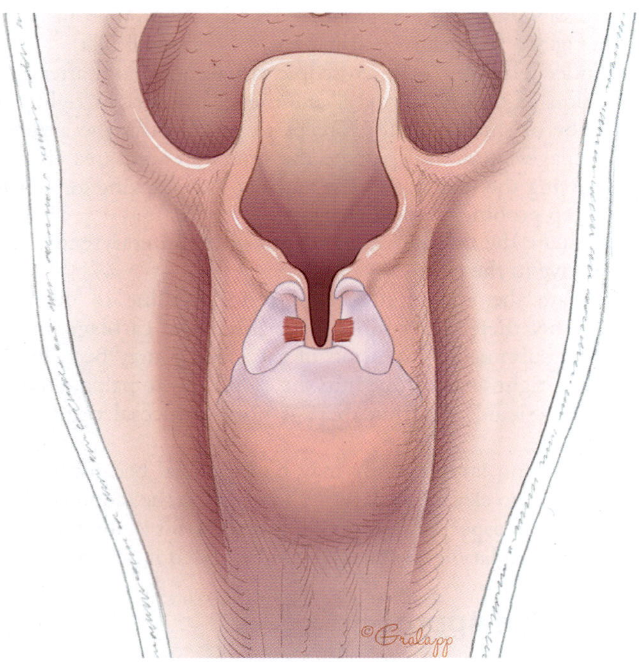


• **Fig. 4.2** Artist rendering depicting the deficiency of the interarytenoid musculature in a patient with a laryngeal cleft. (© 2024 Chris Gralapp.)

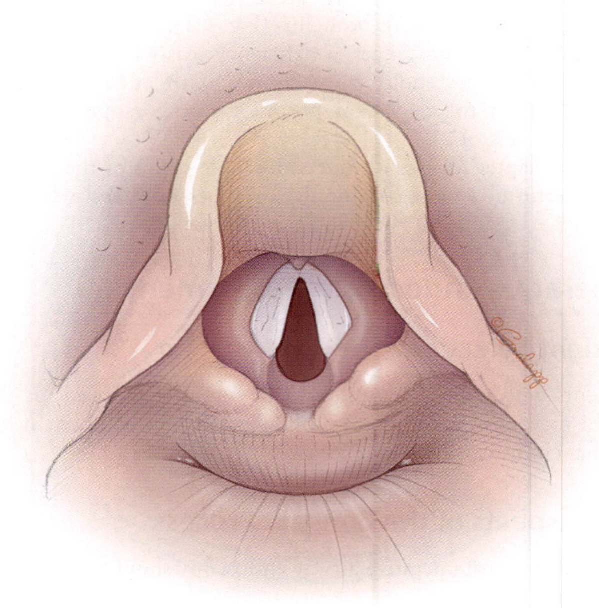


• **Fig. 4.3** Artist rendering depicting a normal larynx. (© 2024 Chris Gralapp.)

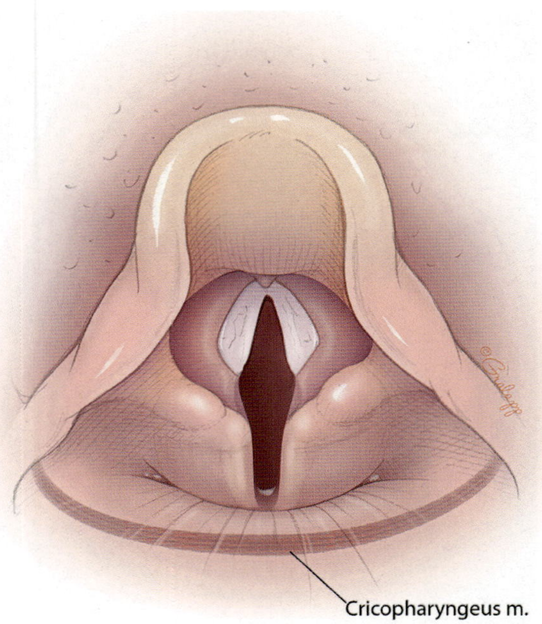


• **Fig. 4.4** Artist rendering depicting a laryngeal cleft. The cricopharyngeus musculature visible at the esophageal inlet. (© 2024 Chris Gralapp.)

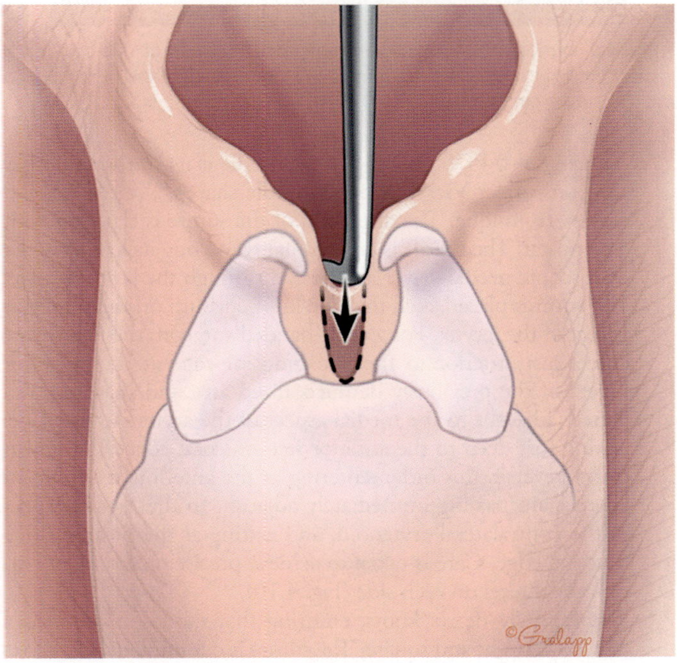

• **Fig. 4.5** Schematic view of the right-angle probe used to palpate the interarytenoid space when evaluating a patient for a laryngeal cleft. (© 2024 Chris Gralapp.)

## Key Aspects of the Consent Process

Same as endoscopic injection, with additional risks, including

- Airway fire if the laser is used
- Complete or partial dehiscence of the repair proximally (resulting in recurrent cleft) or distally (resulting in tracheoesophageal fistula)
- Posoperative stridor usually resolving in 12 to 24 hours; may last longer in patients with hypotonia or other neurologic problems

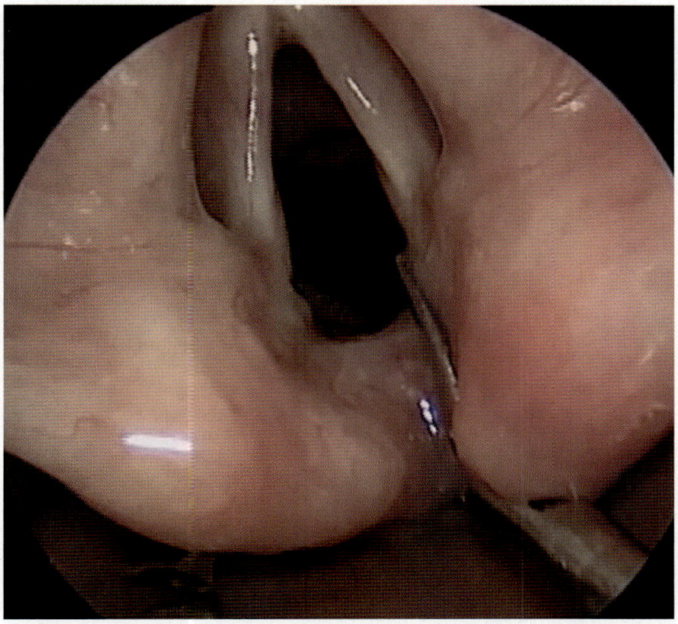

• **Fig. 4.6** Intraoperative image demonstrating the use of an alligator forceps to palpate a type 2 laryngeal cleft. A notch in the superior aspect of the cricoid cartilage is palpable. This cannot be identified by visualization alone, and differentiates a type 1 cleft from a type 2 cleft (as identified in this patient).

- Supraglottic stenosis (theoretical; despite extensive experience with endoscopic cleft repair, we have never seen this occur)
- Temporary worsening of swallow for 1 to 2 weeks

## Equipment

As with endoscopic injection above. Additional equipment includes:

- Operating microscope (required)
- Laryngeal spreaders (required)
- Equipment to demucosalize edges of the cleft, either with $CO_2$ laser or cold microlaryngeal instruments
- If laser is used, correct laser safety equipment, generator, and micromanipulator compatible with the operating microscope are needed
- Endoscopic needle driver and knot pusher
- Appropriate suture. Our preference is 4-0 PDS on an RB-1 taper needle. For a type 1 cleft, three to four sutures will likely be required
- Microlaryngeal instruments, including right and left grasping forceps and right and left curved scissors
- Laryngeal injection equipment (optional)

## Steps

1. Patient positioning: As discussed earlier, Fig. 4.7 demonstrates an example of the suspension laryngoscopy setup.
2. Laryngeal exposure: As discussed earlier, the surgeon must obtain an adequate view of the entire larynx, including epiglottis, aryepiglottic folds arytenoids, interarytenoid space, and postcricoid. The latter can be achieved by placing a blunt-tipped rigid suction behind the cricoid and gently pushing the larynx anteriorly. See Figs. 4.3 and 4.4 demonstrating adequate exposure.
3. Laryngeal spreaders: Placed as described earlier.
4. Visualization: The operating microscope provides hands-free visualization and depth perception. Focal length set to 400 mm.

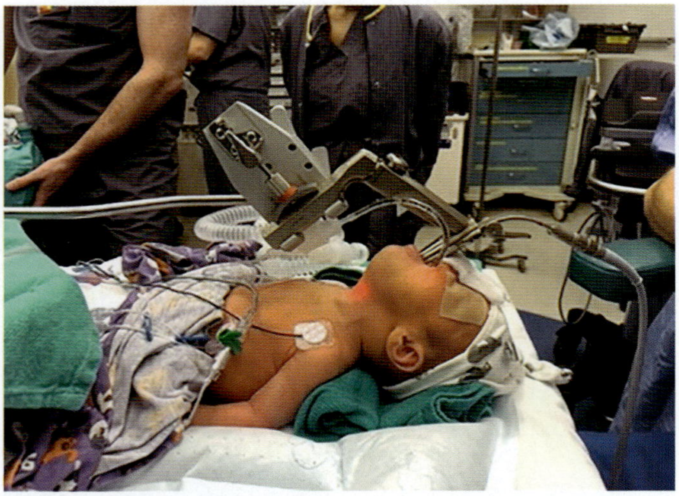

• **Fig. 4.7** Intraoperative image demonstrating a typical suspension laryngoscopy setup for an infant undergoing endoscopic laryngeal cleft repair.

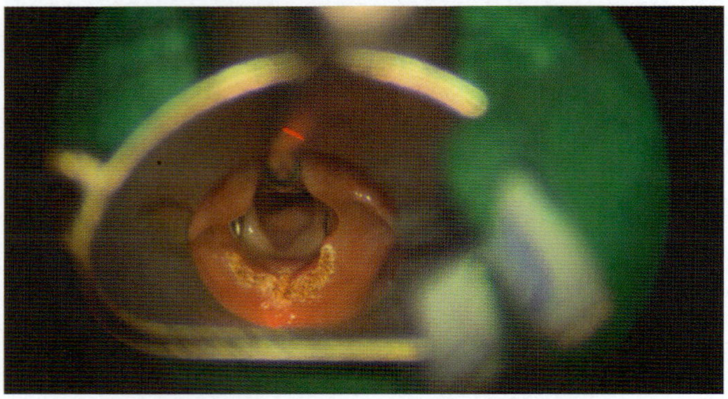

• **Fig. 4.8** Intraoperative image demonstrating the use of a $CO_2$ laser to remove the interarytenoid and cleft mucosa prior to suture closure.

5. Laser: If laser is to be used, the appropriate generator and micromanipulator should be attached to the microscope and correct function confirmed. Laser safety precautions should include protecting the patient with wet eye pads and wet towels to minimize the risk of laser scatter and burns. Any exposed tissue can be damaged by the laser, including the teeth. Inspired oxygen fraction should be confirmed 30% or less. The laser should be tested to confirm correct function and good alignment with the visible aiming beam and good function of any protective shutter. All personnel in the operating room should wear appropriate eye protection. If the surgeon plans to use a telescope and camera instead of a microscope, an appropriate laser filter should be placed between the camera head and telescope.
6. Demucosalization: Some surgeons prefer to inject the submucosal plane with lidocaine/epinephrine along the edges of the cleft to achieve some hydrodissection and hemostasis. Laser (Fig. 4.8) or laryngeal forceps and microscissors (Fig. 4.9) both effectively remove mucosa from the edges of the cleft, including the medial aspects of both arytenoids all the way to the distal apex of the cleft. Inspired oxygen fraction must be kept below 30% while the laser is used, to minimize risk of airway fire. After lasering, any charred mucosa is wiped away using an oxymetazoline pledget, which can also achieve hemostasis if cold instruments are used.

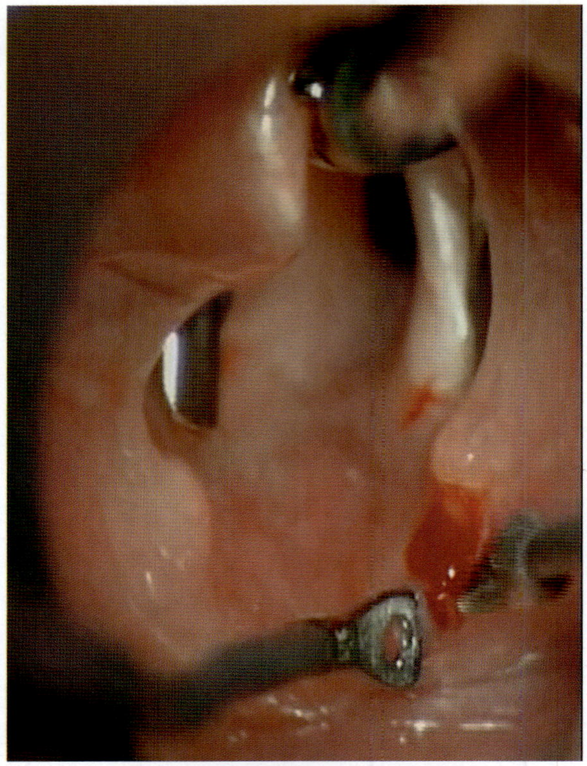

• **Fig. 4.9** Intraoperative image demonstrating the use of microlaryngeal instruments (microscissors) to remove the interarytenoid and cleft mucosa prior to suture closure.

7. Suturing: 4-0 PDS on RB-1 taper needle is used, though other surgeons prefer Vicryl or other needle shapes. We use a mass-closure technique. The distal end of the suture is clamped with a hemostat. The needle is grasped halfway along its length in the endoscopic needle driver and passed through the laryngoscope. The sutures placed such that the knot ends up on the posterior aspect of the larynx. For a right-handed surgeon, the first throw enters just anterior to the free mucosal edge at the posterior aspect of the previously demucosalized area and passes immediately adjacent to the medial aspect of the arytenoid cartilage, exiting just deep to the anterior free mucosal edge. The return throw reverses this order, entering at the anterior free mucosal edge, again passing immediately adjacent to the medial aspect of the contralateral arytenoid, and exiting at the posterior free mucosal edge. Care is taken to achieve precise matching of craniocaudal level on each side (Fig. 4.10).

We typically tie six knots, ensuring that the knots are placed down tight and square. The suture is cut immediately above the knot; longer suture tails may lead irritate the posterior pharyngeal wall and cause granulation.

The first suture is placed immediately at the inferior apex of the cleft, and subsequent sutures are separated by about 1 mm each. The topmost suture should be passed through the cuneiform/corniculate complex because the mucosa at the arytenoid peak is quite thin and tears easily, leading to dehiscence of this stitch. During closure, it is prudent to intermittently palpate the postcricoid space to ensure that the posterior pharyngeal mucosa is not incorporated. This is more important for deeper (e.g., Type 2 and 3) laryngeal clefts (Fig. 4.11). Fig. 4.12 demonstrates a freshly repaired type 1 cleft and the endolaryngeal view of the repair.

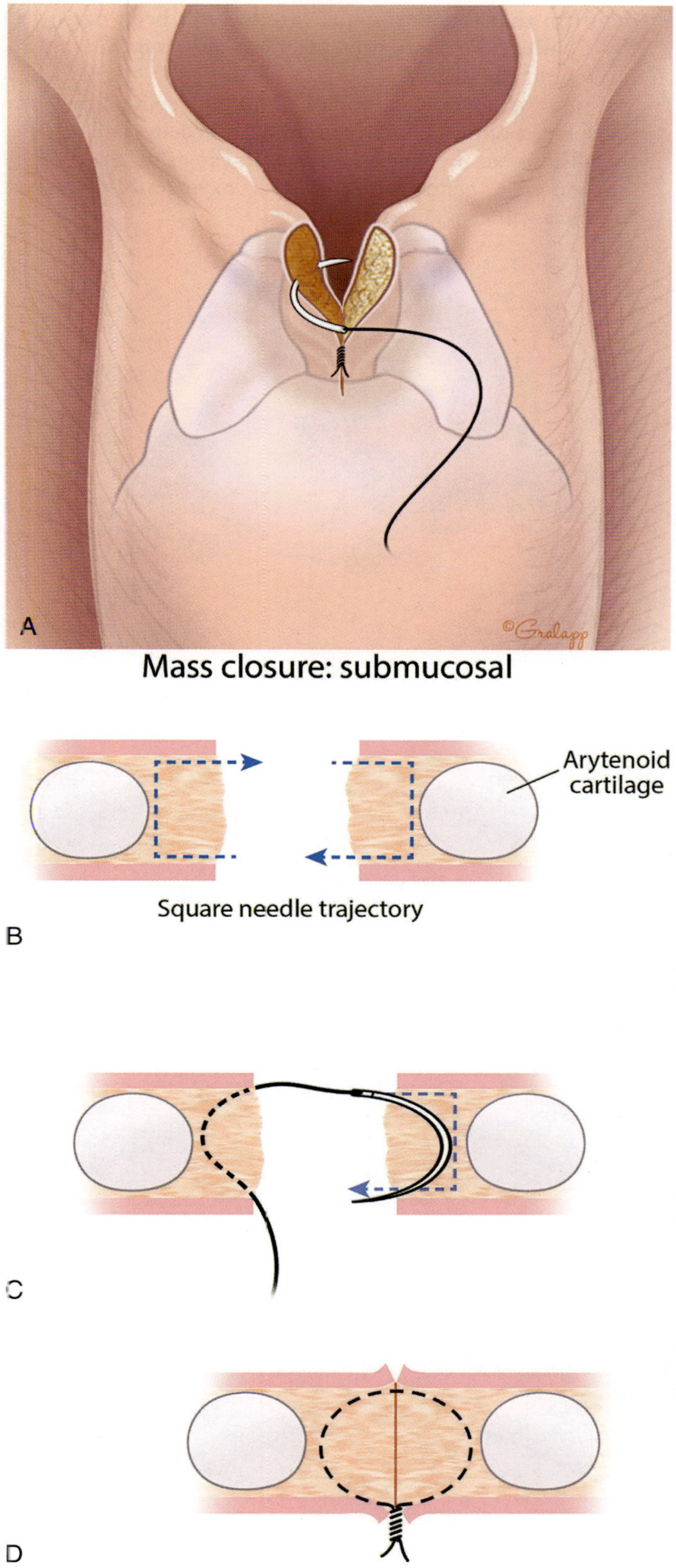


• **Fig. 4.10** Artist rendering demonstrating the suture closure pattern when completing a "mass closure" endoscopic cleft repair. The needle orientation and trajectory are shown. (© 2024 Chris Gralapp.)

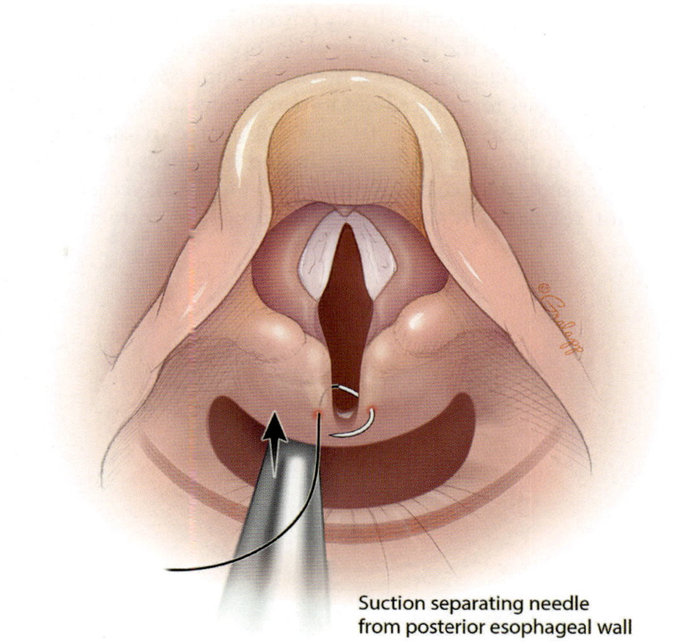


• **Fig. 4.11** Artist rendering demonstrating the use of a rigid suction to palpate the postcricoid space during closure of deeper clefts, ensuring that the posterior pharyngeal muscosa is not incorporated into the closure. (© 2024 Chris Gralapp.)

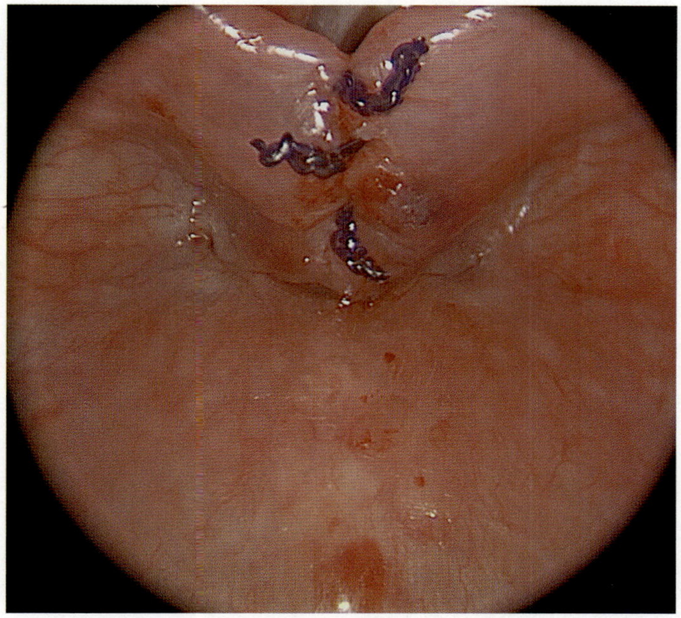

• **Fig. 4.12** Intraoperative image demonstrating the immediate postoperative result following closure of a laryngeal cleft.

8. Supraglottoplasty: Once the cleft has been sutured, we invariably find that the arytenoids are tipped slightly forward and the aryepiglottic folds appear short, creating an iatrogenic laryngomalacia. We create a small releasing incision in each

aryepiglottic fold immediately posterior to the epiglottis. This can be done at the beginning of the operation (after injection but prior to cleft closure) if needed to improve exposure. This often allows for reduced tension on the upcoming closure.

9. Photodocumentation: 0- and 70-degree telescopes are used to document the repair and examine the trachea to ensure that suctioning of any blood or secretions is not required. It is worth examining the endolarynx to confirm that the glottic aperture has not been narrowed by a suture inadvertently catching and medializing an arytenoid cartilage.
10. Hemostasis: If needed, topical 1:50,000 epinephrine can be sprayed onto the larynx to minimize edema and achieve hemostasis at the operative site. If extensive bleeding is encountered, gentle pressure with oxymetazoline-soaked pledgets will generally stop it.

# 5

# Transoral Robotic Surgery for Pediatric Upper Airway Pathology

CARLTON J. ZDANSKI

## Introduction

The FDA granted clearance for treatment of benign and malignant tumors of the head and neck in adults using the surgical robot in 2009.[1] Prior to and since then, there have been multiple descriptions of off-label use for Transoral Robotic Surgery (TORS) in pediatric patients,[1–10] including the first use in pediatric laryngeal surgery.[11] The robot's bimanual, wristed instrumentation and three-dimensional endoscopic visualization allow access to critical out-of-line-of-sight structures compared to traditional endoscopic approaches to multiple upper airway pathologies. In 2016, one of the largest case series demonstrated the safety and efficacy of utilizing TORS in pediatric patients in the treatment of a wide variety of pathology, including type 1, 2, and 3 laryngeal clefts, aerodigestive tract strictures, lymphatic malformations, saccular cysts, and base of tongue hamartomas.[12] Other pathologies addressed include thyroglossal duct cysts,[13] lingual tonsillectomies,[5] soft palate sarcoma, and cordotomy, arytenoidectomy, and endoscopic posterior graft.[3]

## Patient Selection

Technically, any upper aero-digestive tract pathology could be considered for pediatric TORS. Patients should be considered on an individualized basis, and thorough, advanced planning for airway management and alternate surgical planning in the event that TORS cannot be successfully completed are requisite. In general, size alone is not a contraindication to pediatric TORS, with the smallest patient in one series who underwent saccular cyst excision weighing 2.5 kg.[12] This particular pathology is quite proximal in the airway and size may be a relative contraindication to more distal pathology (i.e., high-grade laryngeal clefts), and each patient should again be approached on an individualized basis. Size may affect the surgical technique available to the surgeon, as small patients may not be able to accommodate laser-safe endotracheal tubes if the laser is being utilized. Finally, the use of TORS in infants and children is not FDA approved and thus is an off-label use. This must be explicitly explained to patients and caregivers in the informed consent/assent process.

## Anesthetic Considerations

Airway management is critical in pediatric TORS as in all upper airway surgery. Consultation with the attending anesthesiologist and anesthesia team preoperatively to review the airway management plan is advised. Some patients may have existing tracheotomies, simplifying management. For patients with tracheotomies in place, laryngoscopy and bronchoscopy are performed at the beginning of the procedure to evaluate the airway and to place a laser-safe metal Jackson tracheotomy tube (or a laser-safe endotracheal tube) through the stoma to minimize the risk of airway fire. For patients without tracheotomies, consideration may be given to placing a temporary tracheostomy to safely complete TORS and/or for postoperative management. More commonly, the patient without a tracheotomy is intubated nasally or orally after laryngoscopy and bronchoscopy with a laser-safe endotracheal tube, if size permits and the use of the laser is planned. Generally, TORS will employ the use of a laser or monopolar cautery in some form, so all airway fire precautions should be employed. TORS requires the docking of a relatively large robot in a very small confined space, and spontaneous ventilation with a native airway is strongly discouraged.

## Technique

It is strongly advised that all pediatric TORS procedures employ a two-surgeon approach with a "robotic surgeon" at the surgical console and a "bedside surgeon" positioned at the head of the operating table responsible for protecting the airway as well as surgically assisting the robotic surgeon.

After the airway is controlled, the robot is docked. This may vary depending on surgeon preference and model of robot employed. For the da Vinci Si and Xi models (Intuitive Surgical, Sunnyvale, CA), the bed is essentially reversed such that the patient's head is at the foot of the bed. This allows for the base of the Xi and Si to roll underneath the bed for docking. The bed (including the base) may be turned 90 degrees from anesthesia, or alternatively, the base may be turned 45 degrees from anesthesia and the top with the patient unlocked and turned an additional 45 degrees (90 degrees total). For the da Vinci SP model, the bed may be left in a normal

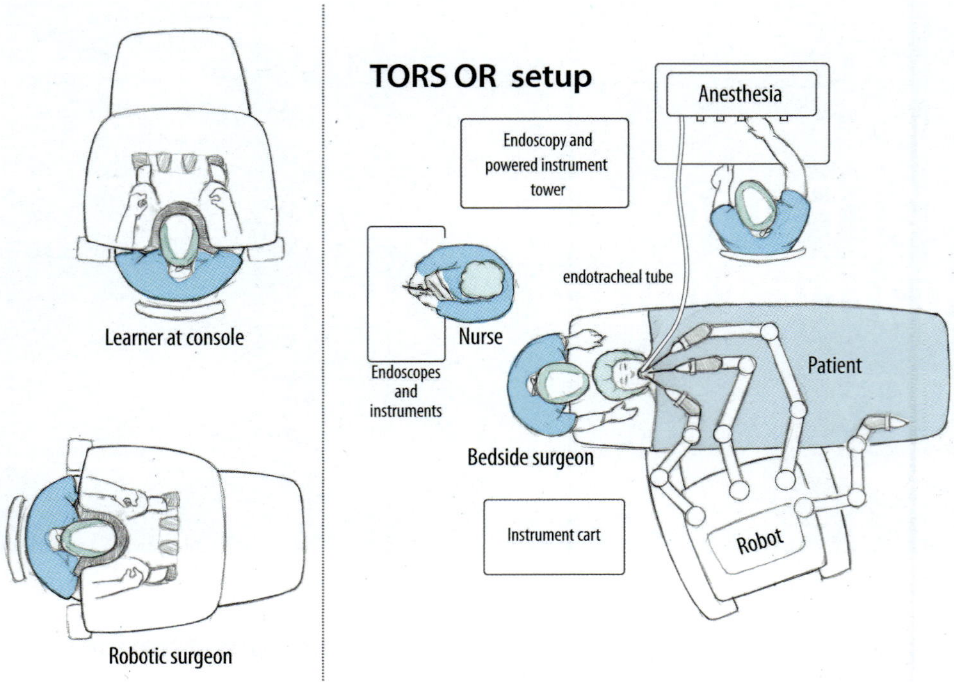


• **Fig. 5.1** Depicted is a representation of the surgical setup for the da Vinci Xi and Si surgical platform for TORS. If the da Vinci SP is utilized, the robot is positioned directly to the right of the patient's head rather than from the foot of the bed. *TORS*, Transoral Robotic Surgery. (© 2024 Chris Gralapp).

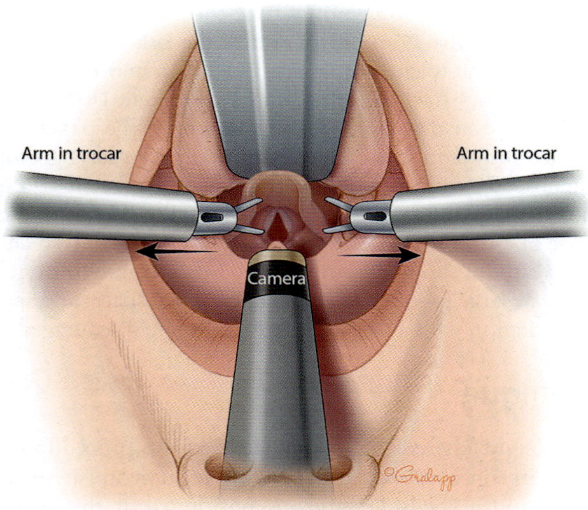


• **Fig. 5.2** The cannulae of the da Vinci Si and Xi can be used to carefully retract the cheeks of the oral cavity to improve exposure. (© 2024 Chris Gralapp).

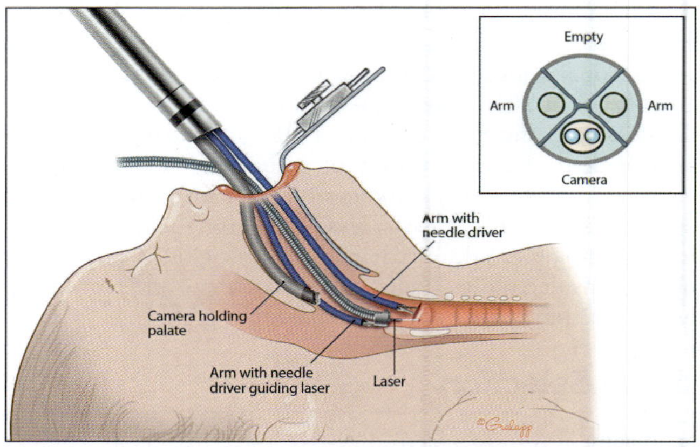


• **Fig. 5.3** The da Vinci SP camera is typically placed in the inferior port and can be used to carefully retract the soft palate to improve exposure. (© 2024 Chris Gralapp).

configuration turned 90 degrees from anesthesia or may also be reversed to allow easier access for the bedside surgeon.

A tooth or gum guard, custom or otherwise, may be advisable depending on the type of mouth gag employed (if at all). The use of a tongue stitch may be useful as well. In general, patients with base of tongue pathology did not require a mouth gag, only a tongue stitch; patients undergoing laryngeal cleft repair were suspended with a tonsil gag. This process is also quite individualized. Following optimal exposure, the robot is docked, and the operative canulae are brought into the field (Fig. 5.1). For the da Vinci Si and Xi models, the canulae can be used to carefully retract the cheeks of the oral cavity (Fig. 5.2). For the da Vinci SP model, the endoscope can be used to carefully retract the soft palate (Fig. 5.3).

## Select Procedures

### Laryngeal Cleft Repair

In general, the patient is suspended with a tonsil gag, including the endotracheal tube. If the laser is used, then a laser-safe tube is used to intubate the patient. If a standard endotracheal tube

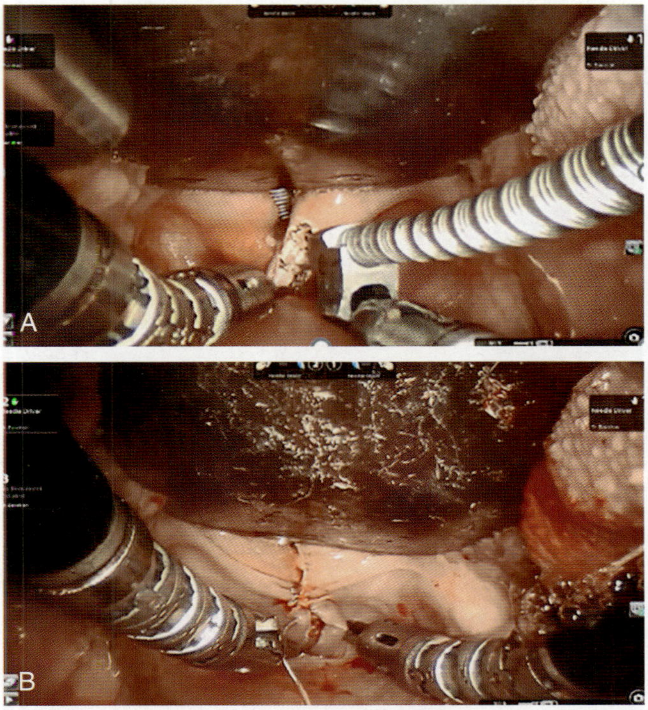


• **Fig. 5.4** (A) The cleft edges are resected using the laser or electrocautery and (B) the cleft is closed in layers. (From Worden CP, Prince AC, Kirse SN, et al. Pediatric robotic laryngeal cleft repair. *Otolaryngol Head Neck Surg*. 2024;171(1):254–260. doi:10.1002/ohn.723.)

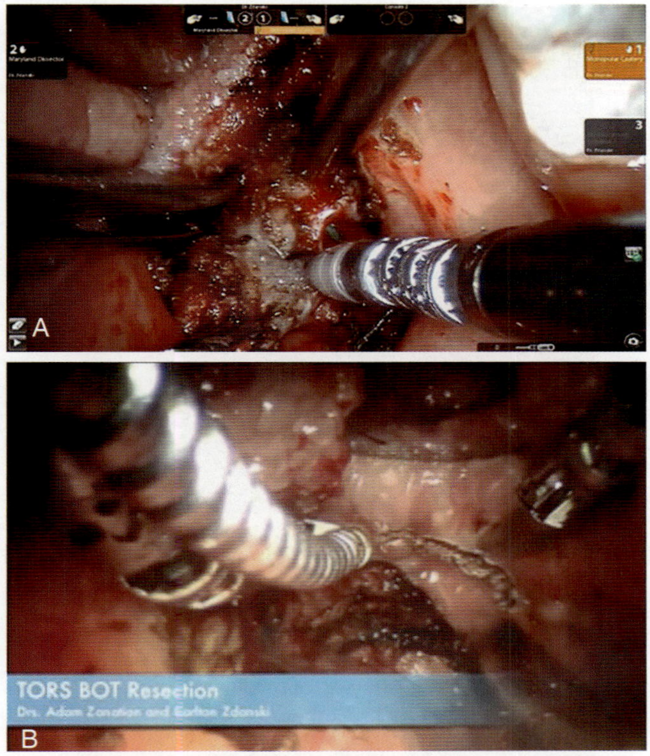


• **Fig. 5.5** (A) Base-of-tongue resection using monopolar cautery. (B) Base-of-tongue excision using $CO_2$ laser.

is used, then the monopolar cautery (paddle for the Si and Xi or monopolar scissors for the SP) may be used. If the patient has a tracheotomy, then placing a laser-safe tracheostomy or endotracheal tube is recommended. The cleft edges are then excised, and the cleft is closed in layers as opposed to mass closure (Fig. 5.4).

## Base-of-Tongue Resection

In general, the patient is not suspended with a gag, but a tongue stitch using a Mustard table to retract is helpful. The patient may be orally or naso-tracheally intubated depending on pathology and exposure. If the laser is used, then a laser-safe tube is used to intubate the patient, but we have found the monopolar cautery paddle to be the most effective instrument. The base-of-tongue pathology is addressed and any closure deemed necessary (if at all) is performed (Fig. 5.5).

## Endoscopic Posterior Laryngotracheoplasty

These patients have existing tracheostomies. It is recommended that patients undergoing TORS undergo endotracheal intubation or use a surgical airway as opposed to spontaneous ventilation with a native airway. The patient is suspended, typically with a tonsil gag, although individuals may require other means of suspension. The posterior cricoidotomy is performed using the laser, and then the graft is either sewn in place or "snap fit" into place and a stent placed (Fig. 5.6).

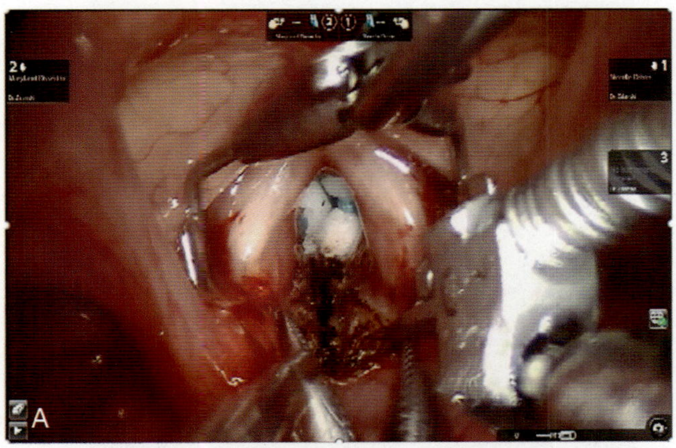


• **Fig. 5.6** (A) Posterior cricoidotomy using a laser. (B) Graft placement and suturing. (From Bann DV, Zdanski CJ. Endoscopic posterior laryngotracheoplasty. *Oper Tech Otolaryngol*. 2022;33(3):216–223.)

*Continued*

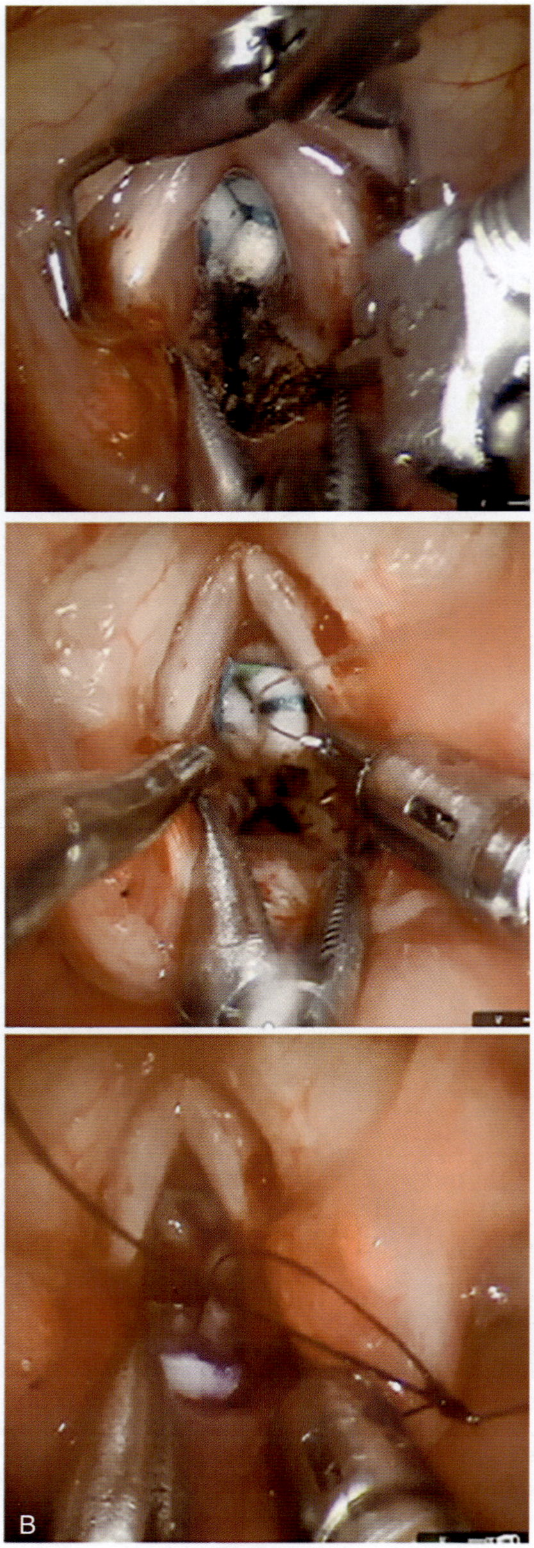


• **Fig.5.6—cont'd**

## Saccular Cyst Excision

The patient is intubated, but frequently these neonates are too small to safely accommodate a laser-safe endotracheal tube. A tongue stitch without a gag is employed and the cyst is completely excised (Fig. 5.7).

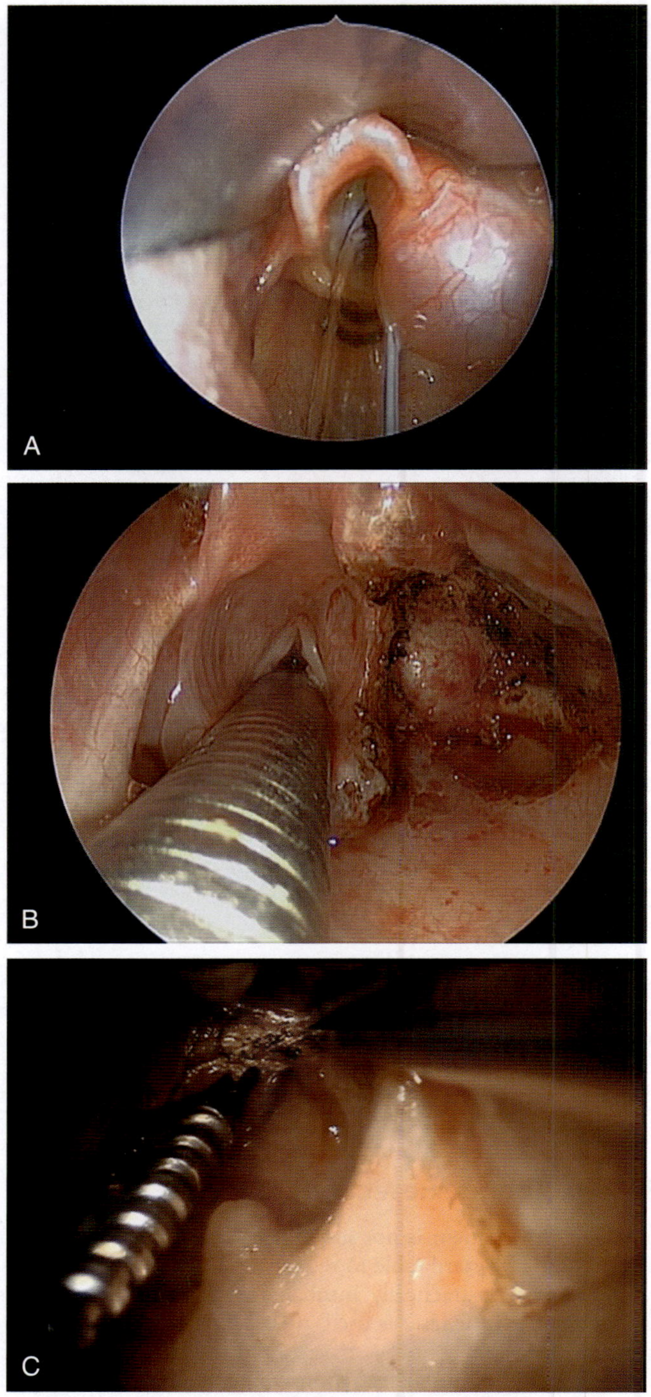


• **Fig. 5.7** (A) Saccular cyst preexcision. (B) Saccular cyst postexcision. (C) Saccular cyst undergoing excision. (From Zdanski CJ, Austin GK, Walsh JM, et al. Transoral robotic surgery for upper airway pathology in the pediatric population. *Laryngoscope*. 2017;127(1):247–251.)

## Conclusions

TORS in the pediatric population can be safely employed for a variety of airway pathology. Surgical planning, including airway management and alternate surgical plans in the event that the surgery cannot be completed with the robot, is paramount. Treatment planning is individualized based on specific patient and pathology characteristics. A two-surgeon approach, employing a bedside surgeon as well as a robotic surgeon, is strongly recommended.

## References


1. Chan JY, Richmon JD. Transoral robotic surgery (TORS) for benign pharyngeal lesions. *Otolaryngol Clin North Am.* 2014;47(3):407–413. doi:10.1016/j.otc.2014.02.003 PMID: 24882798.
2. Byrd JK, Leonardis RL, Bonawitz SC, Losee JE, Duvvuri U. Transoral robotic surgery for pharyngeal stenosis. *Int J Med Robot.* 2014;10:418–422.
3. Ferrell J, Roy S, Karni R, Yuksel S. Applications for transoral robotic surgery in the pediatric airway. *Laryngoscope.* 2014;124:2630–2635.
4. Kokot N, Mazhar K, O'Dell K, Huang N, Lin A, Sinha UK. Transoral robotic resection of oropharyngeal synovial sarcoma in a pediatric patient. *Int J Pediatr Otorhinolaryngol.* 2013;77:1042–1044.
5. Leonardis R, Duvvuri U, Mehta D. Transoral robotic-assisted lingual tonsillectomy in the pediatric population. *JAMA Otolaryngol Head Neck Surg.* 2013;139:1032–1036.
6. Leonardis R, Duvvuri U, Mehta D. Transoral robotic-assisted laryngeal cleft repair in the pediatric patient. *Laryngoscope.* 2014;124:2167–2169.
7. Thottam PJ, Govil N, Duvvuri U, Mehta D. Transoral robotic surgery for sleep apnea in children: is it effective? *Int J Pediatric Otorhinolaryngol.* 2015;79:2234–2237.
8. Wine T, Duvvuri U, Maurer S, Mehta D. Pediatric transoral robotic surgery for oropharyngeal malignancy: a case report. *Int J Pediatr Otorhinolaryngol.* 2013;77:1222–1226.
9. Worden CP, Prince AC, Kirse SN, et al. Transoral robotic surgery for pediatric upper airway pathology: an institutional update. *Int J of Pediatr Otorhinolaryngol.* 2024;184:112073. doi:10.1016/j.ijporl.2024.112073.
10. Worden CP, Prince AC, Kirse SN, et al. Pediatric robotic laryngeal cleft repair. *Otolaryngol Head Neck Surg.* 2024;171(1):254–260. doi:10.1002/ohn.723.
11. Rahbar R, Ferrari L, Borer J, Peters C. Robotic surgery in the pediatric airway: application and safety. *Arch Otolaryngol Head Neck Surg.* 2007;133:46–50.
12. Zdanski CJ, Austin GK, Walsh JM, et al. Transoral robotic surgery for upper airway pathology in the pediatric population. *Laryngoscope.* 2017;127(1):247–251. doi:10.1002/lary.26101.
13. Kayhan F, Kaya K, Koc A, Altintas A, Erdur O. Transoral surgery for an infant thyroglossal duct cyst. *Int J Pediatr Otorhinolaryngol.* 2013;77:1620–1623.

# 6

# Endoscopic Tracheoesophageal Fistula Repair

MICHAEL J. RUTTER AND KARTHIK BALAKRISHNAN

## Background

Tracheoesophageal fistula (TEF) most commonly occurs as a congenital anomaly, when the posterior tracheoesophageal septum forms with a focal defect, creating an abnormal collection between the airway and esophagus (Fig. 6.1). These fistulae can occur at any point along the trachea or proximal mainstem bronchi (broncho-esophageal fistula) but most commonly occur in the posterior membranous wall, at or just above the carina. A tracheoesophageal fistula may also be acquired after local trauma including button battery or caustic substance ingestion–related injury, iatrogenic injury related to instrumentation or surgery, neoplasm, ischemia, or infection.

Patients with TEF will often experience symptoms of dysphagia as well as recurrent respiratory infections (Fig. 6.2). It is rare for TEFs to be asymptomatic, so congenital occurrence is often detected early in life. The most common congenital type is a Type C TEF, meaning a TEF connecting to the distal esophagus, with a segment of esophageal atresia more proximally. Congenital "H" Type TEFs may also occur, either isolated or in addition to a Type C TEF. Repair of the fistula is indicated to decrease aspiration and promote pulmonary health.

Congenital TEFs are commonly, but not always, associated with esophageal atresia. Patients with TEF are also more likely to have a laryngeal cleft; these conditions may exacerbate dysphagia and feeding difficulties in patients with TEF.

Tracheoesophageal fistula repair is most often done through open or thoracoscopic approaches. However, carefully selected patients may be candidates for endoscopic repair as described in this chapter. The ideal candidate for endoscopic repair is a TEF with a long narrow tract running from proximally in the trachea to distally in the esophagus.

## Operative Endoscopic Assessment

### Patient Selection

Patients with clinical suspicion of TEF based on clinical history, instrumental swallow evaluation, and/or esophagram will benefit from a formal endoscopic assessment.

### Key Aspects of the Consent Process

Standard risks of operative airway endoscopy should be discussed, including:

- Risks of general anesthesia
- Risks of injury to oral, pharyngeal, airway, and esophageal structures
- The requirement for additional procedures should be discussed. While this procedure is frequently successful with one intervention, occasionally two or even three attempts at endoscopic closure may be required to achieve complete resolution of the fistula tract. Despite the return visits to the operating room, repeat endoscopic intervention is fast, low risk, and often carries a shorter total operating time (when performed two to three times) than a thoracoscopic closure

### Equipment

- Appropriately sized laryngoscope
- Hopkins rod telescope (0 degree; optional 30 degrees)
- Equipment to spray medications on larynx
- Right-angled probe or small endoscopic alligator forceps
- Small flexible suction catheter (optional)
- Appropriately sized flexible or rigid esophagoscope

As described in Chapters 2 and 4, a thorough diagnostic endoscopy of the airway, including assessment for laryngeal cleft, should be completed. Given that TEF involves both the trachea and esophagus and may be associated with other esophageal anomalies such as esophageal atresia or stricture, it is important to also perform esophagoscopy. The surgeon may want to perform this themselves or enlist a colleague from gastroenterology. Additional steps and considerations are as follows:

1. Close attention should be paid to the posterior tracheal wall, both in the midline and in the lateral grooves adjacent to the junction of the poster wall with the cartilage rings of the trachea. Any area that appears depressed or to be pulling secretions should be inspected carefully after clearing secretions with suction. These visual findings may indicate TEF. The surgeon should note that TEF may be quite small and not visually obvious until carefully probed, as shown in Fig. 6.1.
2. If TEF is suspected, carefully passing a thin, flexible suction catheter through the suspected opening may allow the surgeon

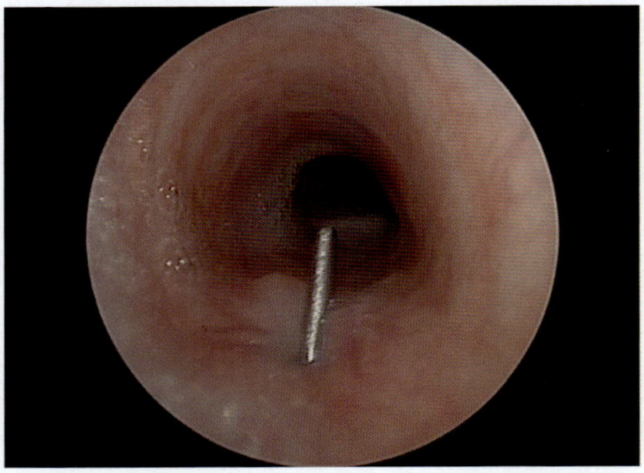

• **Fig. 6.1** Endoscopic view of tracheal lumen showing right-angle probe in the esophagus passing through a small H-type tracheoesophageal fistula into the airway.

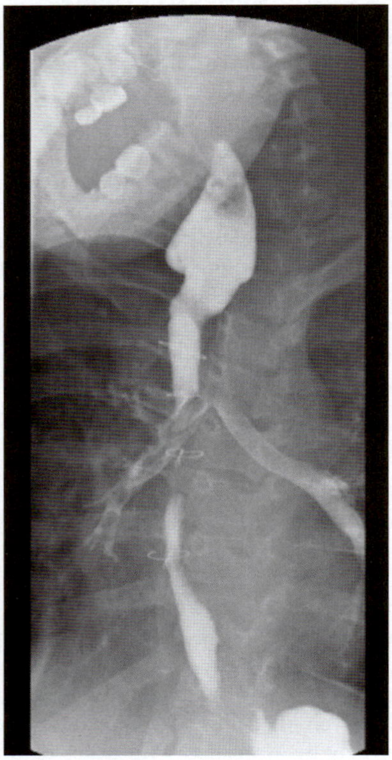

• **Fig. 6.2** Contrast esophagram showing secondary contrast bronchogram due to entry of contrast material into the airway via TEF. *TEF*, Tracheoesophageal fistula.

to assess whether a true fistula is present. If the catheter appears to pass without resistance for several centimeters beyond the apparent opening in the tracheal wall, the surgeon can consider leaving it in place to help identify the esophageal opening of the fistula on subsequent esophagoscopy. Some surgeons prefer to use a flexible guidewire or small Fogarty embolectomy catheter for this purpose.

3. Once the airway has been thoroughly examined, it is important to assess the esophagus as well. The standard approach is to perform an esophagoscopy to visually inspect the esophagus. In addition, the surgeon may choose to indirectly assess for TEF by insufflating the esophagus while visualizing the tracheal lumen with the telescope. In order to perform this assessment, a cuffed endotracheal tube is placed into the esophageal inlet and the cuff inflated in the esophageal inlet just behind the cricoid. Care is taken not to overinflate the cuff so as not to fracture the cricoid cartilage. The surgeon should also be cautious not to place the cuff too far into the esophagus, or it may obscure a more proximal fistula. Once the cuff is inflated, a rod telescope is placed into the trachea. If the level of the cuff is uncertain, the tube can be gently moved a few millimeters proximally and distally. The position of the inflated cuff in the esophagus can be easily visualized, as it distends the trachealis in the airway with movement. This allows for the level of the balloon cuff to be confirmed prior to insufflation. The endotracheal tube in the esophagus is connected to the anesthesiology circuit, and the esophagus is insufflated to a pressure of approximately 20 cm $H_2O$ (Pearl 6.1). With the surgeon observing the tracheal lumen via telescope, small areas of bubbling can be noted and interrogated as possible fistula sites. This technique may be particularly effective in identifying TEFs that are small or collapsed and difficult to visualize directly.

**PEARL 6.1**

In patients with esophageal continuity, it is important to decompress the stomach by removing the circuit and allowing for egress of insufflated air, prior to removing the tube. This reduces the risk of abrupt reflux of gastric contents and associated sequelae. If the child has a gastrostomy tube, the alternative approach is to vent the tube.

## Operative Approach

### Patient Selection

Tracheoesophageal fistulae most amenable to endoscopic repair have a long, narrow tract, ideally running at an angle from superior on the tracheal end to inferior on the esophageal end (Fig. 6.3). Large, short, straight posterior fistula tracts are less likely to respond to endoscopic intervention (Pearl 6.2).

**PEARL 6.2**

Recurrent TEFs, particularly those that have undergone thoracoscopic repair, frequently have a tract more amendable to endoscopic intervention. Nevertheless, some congenital fistulae are equally amenable to endoscopic repair. The low-risk profile of the endoscopic intervention makes it a worthy first alternative to an open repair, and it does not preclude open repair if it is not successful.

### Key Aspects of the Consent Process

Same as diagnostic airway endoscopy, with additional risks including:

- Airway fire if cautery is used
- Airway or esophageal mucosal injury and scarring with cautery or chemical de-epithelialization
- Failure to close the fistula
- Need for postoperative intubation for several days
- Injury to recurrent laryngeal nerve(s) and associated vocal fold weakness or paralysis if cautery is used in a proximal fistula
- A second surgeon should be present to operate the esophagoscope

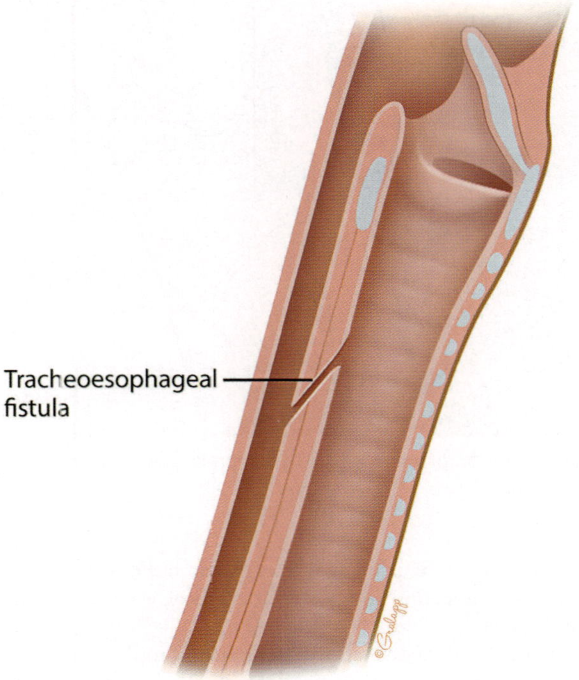


• **Fig. 6.3** Optimal anatomy of TEF for endoscopic repair: a long, narrow tract extending proximally to distally between trachea and esophagus. *TEF*, Tracheoesophageal fistula. (© 2024 Chris Gralapp.)

## Equipment

As with endoscopic laryngeal cleft repair in Chapter 4. Additional equipment includes:

- Endoscopic needle driver and knot pusher (optional)
- Tissue glue (e.g., fibrin glue—optional)
- Injectable inert filler and flexible esophageal injection device with appropriate needle (optional)
- Flexible endoscopic cautery (e.g., Bugbee urologic cautery wire—optional)
- Trichloroacetic acid (optional)
- Flexible esophagoscope with second surgeon/proceduralist—required. For portions of the procedure, endoscopic esophageal visualization is performed simultaneously with airway endoscopy. A second endoscopy tower or monitor is therefore also required
- Fluoroscopy (optional)

## Steps

1. Patient positioning: As with laryngeal cleft repair.
2. Laryngeal exposure: As above. The surgeon must obtain an adequate view of the entire larynx including epiglottis, aryepiglottic folds, arytenoids, interarytenoid space, and postcricoid. Laryngeal spreaders are not required.
3. Visualization: Simultaneous dual endoscopy is the authors' preferred method. With the patient breathing spontaneously, the assisting surgeon passes the flexible esophagoscope adjacent to the suspension laryngoscope and into the esophagus to the approximate level of the fistula. The primary surgeon then visualizes the tracheal aspect of the fistula with a rigid telescope. As noted above, a flexible suction catheter or guidewire can be passed through the fistula to facilitate localization in the esophagus.

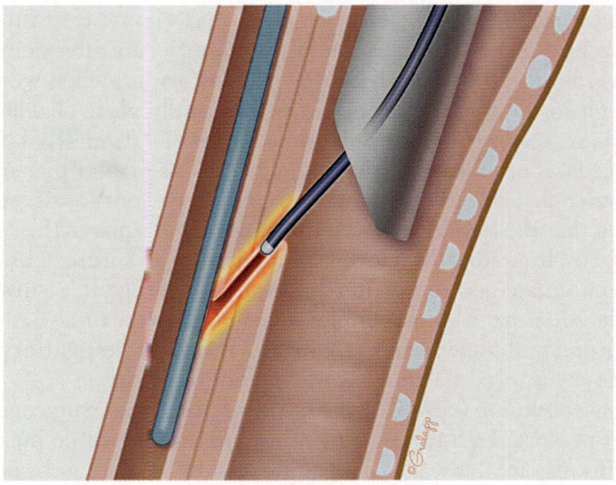

• **Fig. 6.4** Bugbee cautery wire demucosalizing tract of TEF. *TEF*, Tracheoesophageal fistula. (© 2024 Chris Gralapp.)

If the surgeon prefers to use fluoroscopy for localization, a radiopaque catheter may be passed through the fistula either directly or over a guidewire and confirmed with fluoroscopy and contrast injection.

Whether visualization is achieved with dual endoscopy or a combination of endoscopy and fluoroscopy, frequent image documentation during the procedure is important.

4. Demucosalization: The fistula tract must be demucosalized to promote scarring and closure of the tract. The authors typically use a flexible cautery wire, such as the Bugbee urologic monopolar cautery (Pearl 6.3). This is grasped gently in endoscopic alligator forceps and guided through the laryngoscope to the tracheal aspect of the fistula. With esophageal visualization occurring simultaneously, the team observes the cautery passing into the esophagus. After confirming fraction of inspired oxygen ($FiO_2$) less than 30%, the cautery is pulled back so its working tip is just at the esophageal opening of the fistula. The cautery is activated while pulling it back slowly until the entire length of the tract has been treated (Fig. 6.4). The surgeon may wish to make more than one pass with cautery, especially if the tip of the Bugbee requires cleaning.

**PEARL 6.3**

If Bugbee cautery (frequently used in urologic procedures) is not available at your institution, other flexible monopolar probes exist, including those used in the neurosurgical arena.

Some surgeons prefer to use a chemical treatment to demucosalize the TEF tract. Trichloroacetic acid is the most commonly used agent. This is typically applied to the mucosa on pledgets, which limits the ability to abate the mucosa along the entire length of the TEF tract (Pearl 6.4). For this reason, the authors do not prefer this approach.

**PEARL 6.4**

Trichloroacetic acid must be used cautiously. Collateral injury is possible even when using the chemical on a pledget or applicator.

5. Suturing (optional): Some surgeons may choose to suture the tracheal aspect of the fistula to promote closure after demucosalization. This step is relatively straightforward when working high in the trachea but becomes technically more challenging when treating more distal fistulae. 4-0 Vicryl on RB-1 taper needle is often used, though other surgeons prefer other suture materials or needle shapes. We typically tie four knots, ensuring that the knots are placed down tight and square. The suture is cut immediately above the knot; longer suture tails may accumulate secretions and promote coughing. If a suture is placed, either a single simple interrupted suture or a "figure 8" suture is sufficient and technically the most straightforward; more complex mattress sutures are not necessary.
6. Glue occlusion (optional): instead of suturing, some surgeons prefer to block the fistula tract by placing fibrin glue within the tract. This may inhibit scar closure of the tract by separating the demucosalized sides of the TEF, so an alternative is simply to place the glue in the proximal portion of the fistula. To do so, the surgeon passes a long flexible catheter into the fistula using endoscopic guidance from the airway side and then applies the glue through the catheter, allowing it to set before further instrumenting the area. Care must be taken not to spill glue into the airway, where it can become a foreign body. The authors strongly recommend against using cyanoacrylate glue, which is difficult to remove from the airway or esophagus if it spills out of the fistula.
7. Injection: suturing of the esophageal end of the fistula is very challenging and not necessary. Instead, the esophageal aspect can be closed indirectly by injecting filler material through a flexible injection device passed through the working channel of the flexible esophagoscope (Fig. 6.5). The injection is performed into the esophageal wall immediately above the fistula to compress the fistula closed at its esophageal end. Short-acting fillers lasting a few weeks are preferred; options include carboxymethylcellulose and hyaluronic acid. The intent is that one demucosalized raw surface is pushed against the other demucosalized raw surface, promoting scar union and fistula closure (Pearl 6.5). This may also be done utilizing a transglottic rather than esophageal technique, injecting the posterior tracheal wall underneath the fistula tract.

**PEARL 6.5**

This is easy to perform and also reduces the passage of air and secretions through the demucosalized fistula tract.

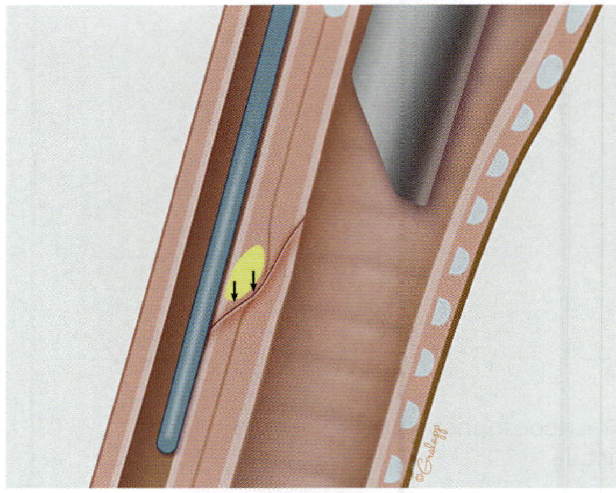

• **Fig. 6.5** Injection of filler material to compress the fistula tract. (© 2024 Chris Gralapp.)

8. Intubation: after the above steps are complete, the surgeon should suction the airways clear and place an endotracheal tube. Ideally, the cuff sits on or just below the fistula to prevent insufflation of the healing TEF. If the patient does not already have a gastrostomy tube, a nasogastric tube can also be placed under endoscopic guidance. The patient kept intubated and nil per os (NPO) with nutrition via a tube for 7 to 10 days (Pearl 6.6).

**PEARL 6.6**

Under some circumstances, and in patients without a positive pressure requirement, successful closure can be achieved without this period of intubation. However, if an attempt at closure is not successful, the second attempt should include this period of intubation if not performed initially.

# SECTION III

# Surgery for Airway Obstruction and Vocal Fold Immobility

# 7 Supraglottoplasty

TAHER VALIKA AND DANA MARA THOMPSON

## Background

Congenital laryngomalacia is the most common cause of noisy breathing in infants.[1] The stridor is caused by the collapse of supraglottic tissue into the glottic inlet during the phase of inspiration and is typically present within the first 2 weeks of life. The stridor symptoms may be present at rest and may worsen with activities such as crying, agitation, excitement, or feeding. Stridor is often worse in the supine position and with sleep and improves when infant is upright. Patients may also have symptoms of dysphagia. The diagnosis is suspected by this typical symptom presentation; however, it is established by awake flexible laryngoscopy, which shows typical findings of an omega-shaped epiglottis, collapse of the supra-arytenoid tissue, or short aryepiglottic folds. A retrodisplaced epiglottis may also be present; if so, consider underlying neurological disease as a cofactor. A definitive diagnosis of laryngomalacia requires the presence of symptoms in addition to the visual findings, as infants may have this infantile-appearing larynx without symptoms. The natural history is that symptoms peak between 4 and 6 months of age and improve between 8 and 12 months of age. Most patients outgrow stridor by 12 and 18 months of age. There are other variants of laryngomalacia that present later in life such as persistent laryngomalacia beyond infancy: sleep variant, feeding variant, and exercise variant laryngomalacia, all beyond the scope of discussion in this chapter.[2] The etiology of laryngomalacia is not fully understood and is likely due to a combination of anatomic, neurologic, and inflammatory causes leading to diminished tone of the supraglottic tissue and supporting musculature, leading to upper airway obstruction. The literature best supports neurological and inflammatory conditions in the causation.[3] Respiration, swallowing, and neuromuscular tone of the larynx are vagally mediated through the laryngeal adductor reflex. Abnormal sensorimotor integration between the peripheral vagal nerve chemoreceptors and the central nuclei related to respiration and swallowing through the laryngeal adductor reflex is thought to lead to diminished tone and play a role in the respiratory and swallowing symptoms present in infants with laryngomalacia.[3]

Gastroesophageal reflux (GERD) is the most common inflammatory condition associated with laryngomalacia. Infants are more prone to GERD due to the immature tone of the upper and lower esophageal sphincters, which can allow stomach contents to flow back into the esophagus. Gastroesophageal reflux can cause swelling of the supraglottic tissue in patients with laryngomalacia, which can lead to a large negative intrathoracic pressure during inhalation due to the supraglottic obstruction. This can promote the flow of gastric contents into the esophagus and up to the level of the larynx, further increasing edema of the supraglottic mucosa and exacerbating symptoms of both GERD and laryngomalacia (Pearl 7.1). Acid reflux may cause a neuroinflammatory response as demonstrated by altered laryngeal sensation and tone, in infants with laryngomalacia independent of other neurologic etiologies. Prolonged acid exposure can lead to a wet quality of respirations and feeding difficulty due to altered sensation and challenges swallowing to clear secretions. Because acid-suppressing medications have been shown to improve swallow function and reduce the duration of symptoms, they have become a mainstay in the treatment of infants with laryngomalacia[4] (Pearl 7.2).

**PEARL 7.1**

Infants with laryngomalacia may also experience aerophagia, which can further worsen reflux and feeding difficulty.

**PEARL 7.2**

Thickening of feeds may be used as well.

## Operative Assessment

While most infants with laryngomalacia will have mild and inconsequential inspiratory stridor and outgrow their symptoms, it is important to differentiate those with moderate and severe feeding and respiratory complications as they may require surgical intervention to improve the patency of the airway. The presence of secondary airway lesions, reflux, syndromic conditions, congenital heart disease, and neurological disease all influence disease severity and the outcome.[3,5–7]

Respiratory difficulty with significant obstruction is an absolute indication for surgical intervention. The clinical presentation of severe obstruction may include awake apnea, sleep apnea, recurrent cyanosis, pectus excavatum, stridor with respiratory compromise or severe neck or chest retractions, pulmonary hypertension, and cor pulmonale. Relative indications in the context of shared decision-making include repeated visits to an emergency department for stridor, parental anxiety, and difficulty obtaining child care due to stridor.[4] Preoperative testing is considered if helpful in disease management. Airway films may help identify secondary airway lesions. Sleep study may aid in understanding the severity of apnea or if central apnea is present. Chest imaging may be useful to screen for aspiration and chronic lung disease. Central nervous system imaging is helpful if a Chiari malformation is suspected.

Feeding problems are common in children with laryngomalacia. The high position of the infant larynx in the nasopharynx allows for the infant to coordinate suck, swallow, and breathe. Airway obstruction due to laryngomalacia leads to alteration in this coordination, swallowing difficulty leading to dysphagia, prolonged feeding times, and the need for frequent breaks to breathe. This cycle can lead to poor weight gain, aspiration, and failure to thrive due to the inability to consume enough nutrition or increased caloric expenditure due to increased work of breathing. Those who present with feeding difficulty and who develop failure to thrive usually do so within 2 months of the diagnosis.[8,9] Failure to thrive is an absolute indication for surgical intervention. Aspiration is not a contraindication to intervention and generally improves after intervention if the infant does not have a significant underlying neurological disease or severe reflux. Poor weight gain and parental difficulty feeding with altered quality of life are relative indications to consider surgical intervention after shared decision-making and risk-benefit discussion.[10,11]

Certain patients with comorbidities may be at higher risk of complications after undergoing supraglottoplasty, and it is important to carefully consider these risks before proceeding with surgery. For example, children with neurologic disease may be at a higher risk of complications after surgery. Those with Down syndrome generally have a good outcome, unless they have subglottic stenosis, significant tracheomalacia, and/or cardiac and neurologic disease. Patients with micrognathia, such as in CHARGE syndrome and Pierre Robin sequence, may have a lower success rate after supraglottoplasty due to the unique airway dynamics and laryngeal positioning in these conditions (Pearl 7.3).[7,12,13] In general, patients with syndromic conditions have a lower success rate and a higher rate of revision surgery after supraglottoplasty.[13–15] Additive comorbidities are not an absolute contraindication to supraglottoplasty; however, parents should be counseled about the higher risk of surgical failure and the potential need for revision surgery or the need for tracheostomy.

**PEARL 7.3**

This is an important point, and the clinician must recognize endoscopically the difference between isolated laryngomalacia and laryngeal obstruction in the setting of micrognathia and retrognathia. The presence of glossoptosis and epiglottic retroflection in these conditions may coexist with typical laryngomalacia, but residual airway obstruction often persists following supraglottoplasty due to posterior lingual and supraglottic displacement.

Older children with laryngomalacia variants may require intervention dependent on symptoms and degree of obstruction. While beyond the scope of this chapter, the surgical approach is similar to that for congenital laryngomalacia described later.

## Operative Approach

Historically, tracheostomy was performed to bypass the upper airway obstruction, though with advancements in endoscopic techniques, this has become reserved for refractory disease. In patients with severe disease requiring surgery, informed consent should include the risks but are not limited to airway obstruction requiring intubation or further surgery, pneumothorax, croup-like symptoms postoperatively, bleeding, supraglottic stenosis, nonresolution of dysphagia or stridor, need for tracheotomy, damage to lips, teeth, or gums, and continued sleep symptoms.

The first endoscopic procedure was described by Igular who amputated the epiglottis in the 1930s. In 1944, Schwartz was the first to describe removal of "v"-shaped wedges from the lateral borders of the epiglottis. While not published, Dr. Robin Cotton in 1976 performed unilateral removal of supraglottic tissue for a child with severe stridor with severe right ventricular hypertrophy at Cincinnati Children's Medical Center. In 1984, Lane published a case report of the modern endoscopic description of supraglottoplasty, which was then shortly followed by a case series and refined techniques by Zalzal, Seid, and others.[1,16–18] A variety of tools have been utilized. Thermal tools include $CO_2$ laser and coblation. Cold knife instrumentation includes microlaryngeal instruments or the microdebrider. As described later, we prefer cold knife microlaryngeal instrumentation for precision and avoidance of thermal injury to the supraglottic mucosa (Pearl 7.4).

**PEARL 7.4**

Cold instrumentation is often faster and requires less setup, as well as lower cost.

**PEARL 7.5**

Supraglottoplasty can be performed in an intubated patient; this may allow the surgeon more time to operate but makes visualization more challenging.

### Operative Steps for Supraglottoplasty

1. Clear communication with the anesthesiology team about the anesthetic plan completed prior to patient coming into the operating room
   A. Spontaneous ventilation via inhalational anesthesia (Pearl 7.5)
   B. Ensuring no paralytic will be given
   C. Dexamethasone 0.5 mg/kg one time dose
   D. Determining the role of premedication if performing drug-induced sleep endoscopy

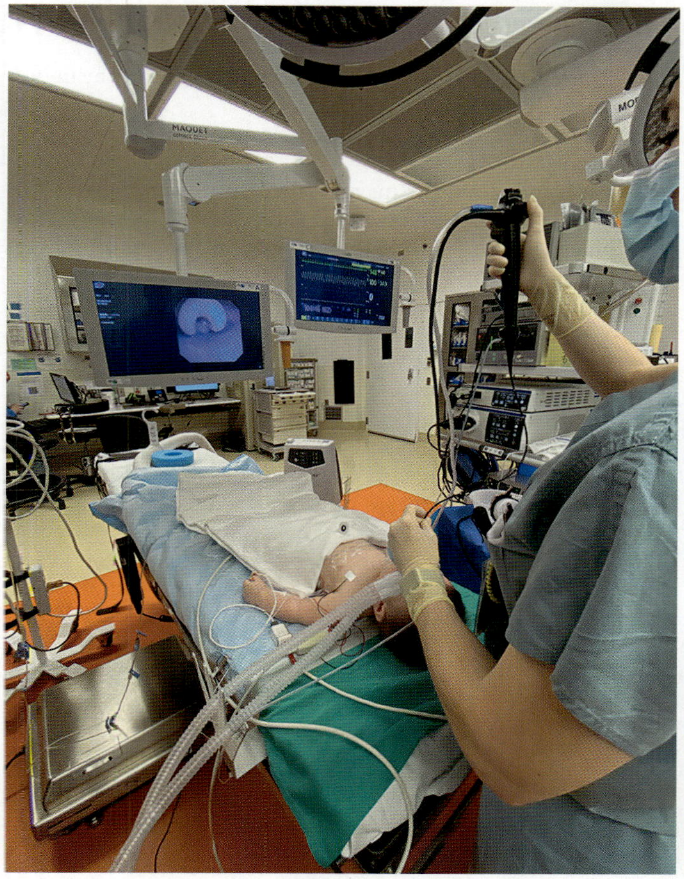

• Fig. 7.1

2. The patient is brought to the operating room and intravenous access is obtained. The patient is turned over to the Otolaryngology service for the remainder of the procedure
3. Sleep endoscopy may be performed at time to visualize the extent of collapse and rule out synchronous airway obstruction
   A. The authors prefer mask insufflation with utilization of Sevoflourane for their sleep endoscopy protocol
   B. Proper positioning of the monitors to visualize the airway as well as the vitals allows for safe and effective endoscopy (Fig. 7.1)
4. With the patient in supine position, a moist gauze is placed over the upper lips and gums, and direct laryngoscopy is performed
   A. Endotracheal tube is placed in the corner of the mouth for insufflation
   B. Vocal cords are sprayed topically with lidocaine solution and the larynx is visualized (Pearl 7.6)

**PEARL 7.6**

The impact of topical lidocaine on supraglottic prolapse is unclear; given this uncertainty, it is probably best to perform sleep endoscopy and assessment of obstruction before applying topical anesthetic.

5. Bronchoscopy is then performed by passing the telescope and visualizing the subglottis, trachea, and bilateral bronchi, ruling out any secondary airway lesions. The telescope is then removed
6. A Benjamin-Lindholm laryngoscope is inserted and the patient is placed in suspension. This is placed down the midline of the oral cavity (Fig. 7.2)
   A. Spontaneous respiration with gas and oxygen. Insufflation occurs via the sideport. Intubation may be required for infants with poor pulmonary reserve or who do not tolerate spontaneous respiration (Pearl 7.7)

**PEARL 7.7**

Under many circumstances, appropriately balanced intravenous anesthetic will obviate the need for continued inhalant anesthetic insufflation, and only oxygen is required.

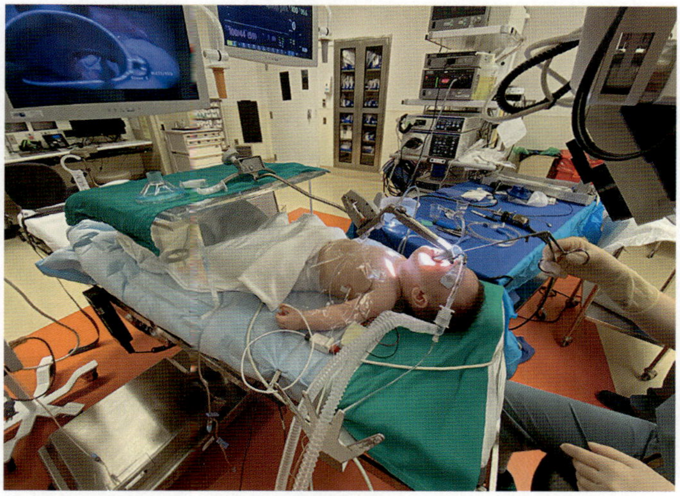

• Fig. 7.2

   B. In some patients with an anterior larynx, glossoptosis, or micrognathia, a Parsons laryngoscope can provide better visualization of the larynx due to its design
      i. This is usually placed down the right glossotonsillar sulcus into the vallecula
7. Once visualization of the supraglottis is obtained, the operative microscope is brought into the field
   A. A working distance of 400 mm is utilized to ensure the surgical instruments do not interfere with the microscope
   B. If the view is suboptimal, anterior pressure on the larynx can be provided. Tape can be used to hold pressure on gauze that has been placed over the neck by attaching the tape to the lateral edges of the bed and crossing it over the neck
8. The right supraarytenoid tissue is gently grasped with a right-sided endoscopic triangle or microlaryngeal forceps retracted to the 7 o'clock position (Figs. 7.3 and 7.4). An incision is

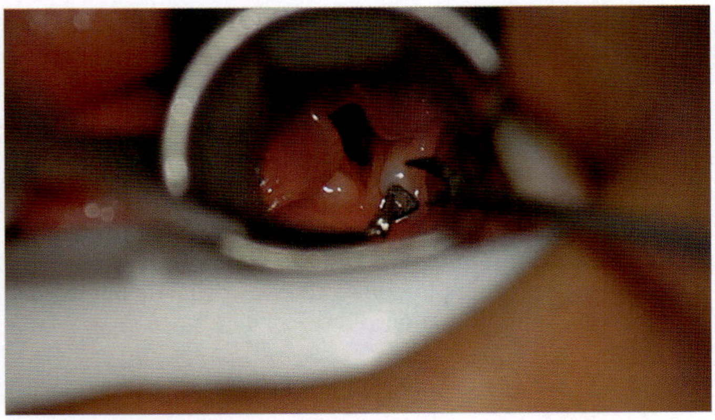

• **Fig. 7.3**

made in the right aryepiglottic fold using left-curved endoscopic scissors (Figs. 7.5 and 7.6)

   A. The scissors hug the epiglottis, ensuring to release the shortened aryepiglottic fold, and not incise the pharyngoepiglottic fold (Fig. 7.7)
   B. The grasper should be in left hand and scissors in right

9. The right supraarytenoid tissue is reflected forward now rotated to the 11 o'clock position (Figs. 7.8 and 7.9)
   A. The left-curved scissors can be utilized to palpate the underlying arytenoid cartilage
   B. The beveled scissors are then used to excise the redundant supraglottic tissue
   C. An island of mucosa may remain between the excised tissue and incised aryepiglottic fold tissue (Pearl 7.8)
10. Epinephrine (1:1000) is then applied to the site of excision for hemostasis
   A. This is a personal preference of the authors. In our experience, this works quickly and helps minimize postoperative edema
   B. No cardiac side effects have been reported with this concentration
   C. Topical Afrin can also be utilized
11. The opposing side is then completed in similar fashion
   A. Left-sided sweetheart utilized in tandem with a right-curved endoscopic scissor
   B. Grasper position at 2 o'clock for aryepiglottic fold release
   C. Grasper position at 5 o'clock for redundant tissue excision
   D. The grasper should be in right hand and scissors in left

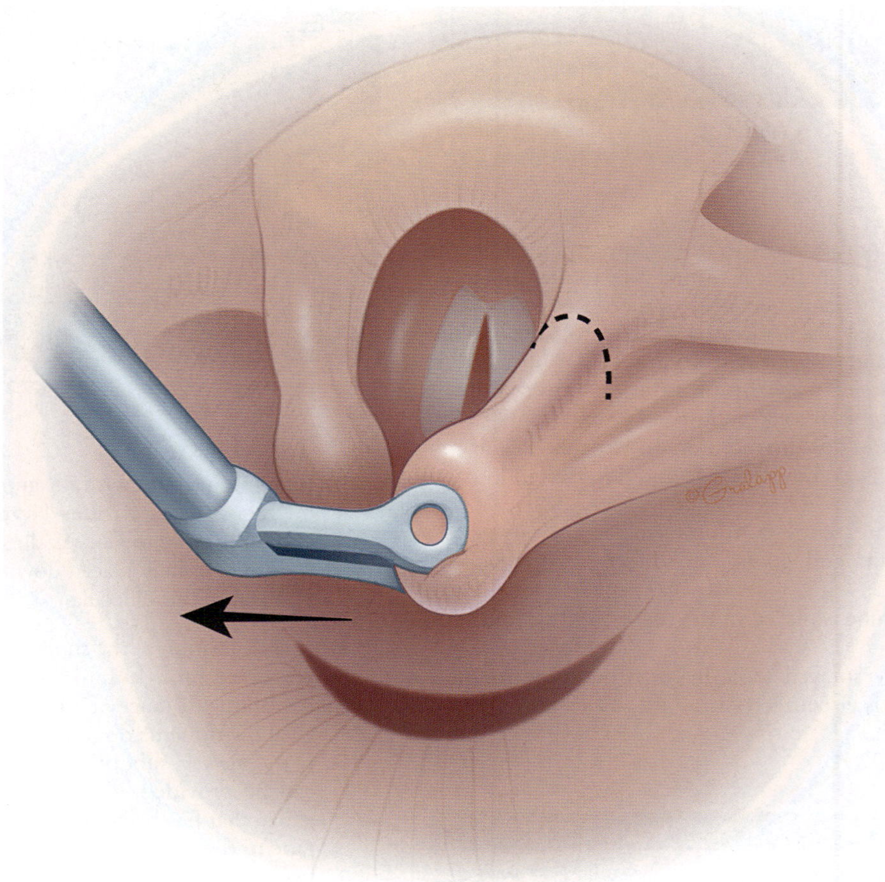

• **Fig. 7.4** (© 2024 Chris Gralapp.)

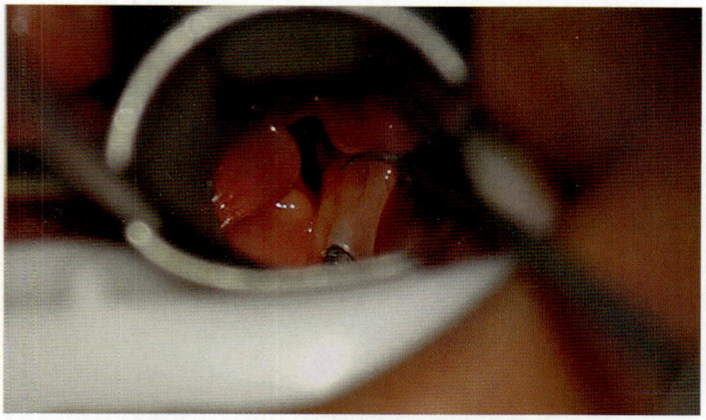

• **Fig. 7.5**

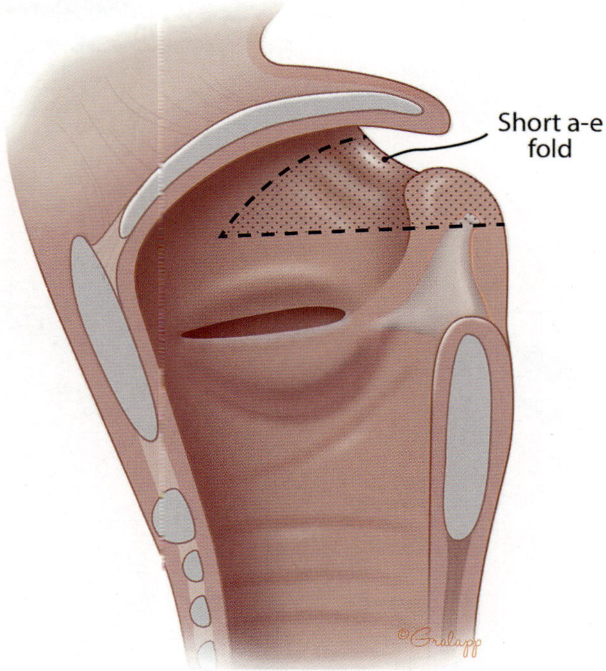


• **Fig. 7.7** (© 2024 Chris Gralapp.)

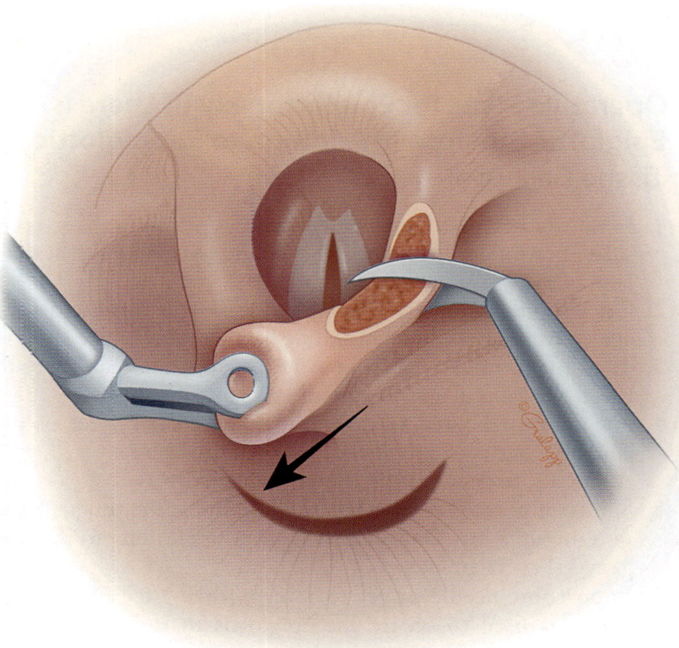

• **Fig. 7.6** (© 2024 Chris Gralapp.)

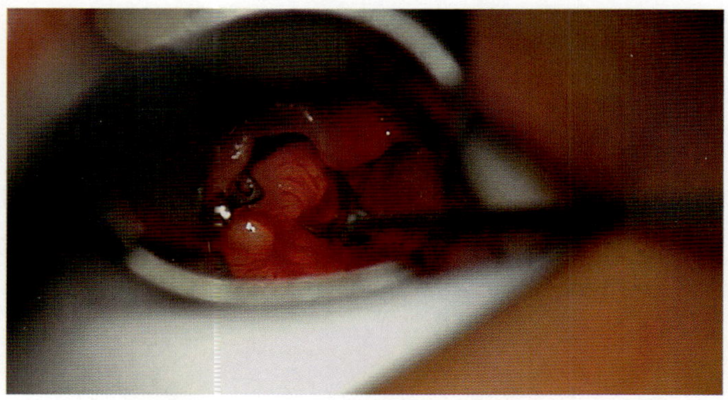

• **Fig. 7.8**

**PEARL 7.8**

This island of tissue, when maintained, may reduce the risk of adhesion formation between the two incisions.

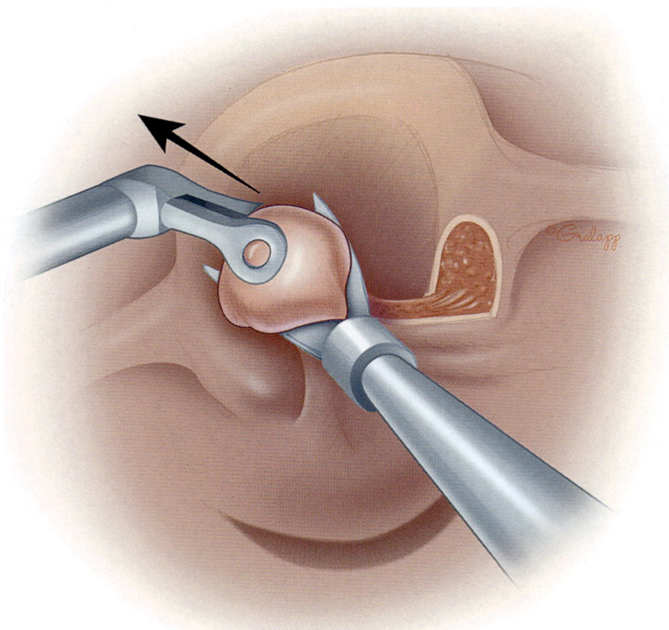


• **Fig. 7.9** (© 2024 Chris Gralapp.)

12. Distal airway should then be suctioned to clear any residual secretions or blood trapped (Pearl 7.9)

**PEARL 7.9**

Some surgeons may inject steroid into the laryngeal incisions to decrease the risk of adhesion formation, but as noted above, maintaining an intervening island of mucosa may also help with this objective.

13. The patient is then taken out of suspension and the laryngoscope removed
    A. If significant risk factors or postoperative airway edema or scarring concerns, recommend nasotracheal intubation overnight
    B. If healthy and no postoperative airway concerns, allow the patient to awaken from general anesthesia and consider administration of racemic epinephrine (not usually necessary if applying topical epinephrine during the case)
14. Most children (without underlying comorbidities, syndromes) can be discharged either the same day (author preference) or the day following surgery
    A. Antibiotics or steroids upon discharge are given at the discretion of the surgeon and based on comorbidities and other factors
    B. Continue acid suppression medications until follow-up

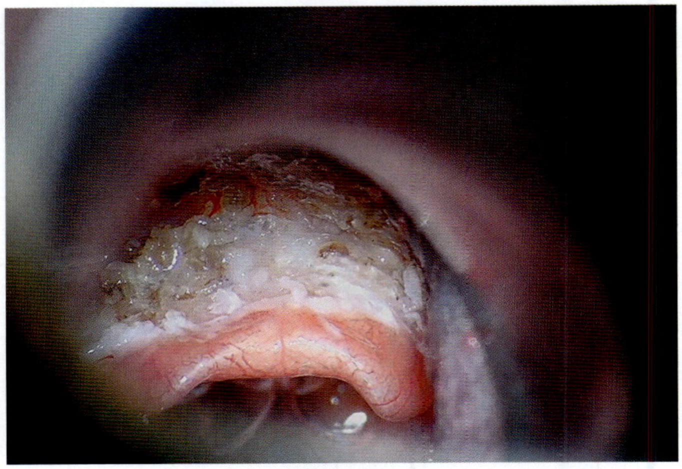

• **Fig. 7.10**

    C. If significant feeding issue and aspiration history, an appropriate assessment of swallowing and airway protection should be considered
        i. Most children continue their preoperative feeding regimen

## Operative Steps for Epiglottopexy (If There Is Epiglottic Prolapse in Addition to Supraglottic Tissue Collapse)

1. Is usually completed in tandem with supraglottoplasty, consider if retroflexed epiglottis is encountered on awake flexible laryngoscopy or sleep endoscopy
2. Once supraglottoplasty is complete, patient is intubated with age-appropriate endotracheal tube (oral or nasal)
3. The suspension laryngoscope is retracted in the oral cavity to reveal the vallecular space and the prolapsed epiglottis
4. The coblator is used to denude the vallecular surface of the epiglottis in the region of the hyoepiglottic ligament
    A. A $CO_2$ laser or suction cautery can also be used
5. Similar mucosa is removed in the midline at the tongue base, resulting in a diamond-shaped surgical site leading to the epiglottis (Fig. 7.10)
6. Endoscopic needle driver (3 mm) with a 5-0 PDS (RB-2) suture is used to secure the epiglottis to the tongue base (Fig. 7.11).
    A. First knot secured is surgeon's knot
    B. A total of six knots are thrown
    C. In neonates, a P-3 needle facilitates the ability to complete the suture as the RB-2 is often too large
7. Overnight intubation is considered if concern for significant epiglottic edema from intervention or if surgeon desires pressure on the epiglottis to aid scarring of the surgical site at the tongue base

Supraglottoplasty has favorable outcomes and low risk in the management of severe laryngomalacia. Overall, there is a success rate of greater than 90% in relieving the upper airway obstruction.[1] It is generally regarded as a safe procedure, with the most frequently cited complication being dysphagia.

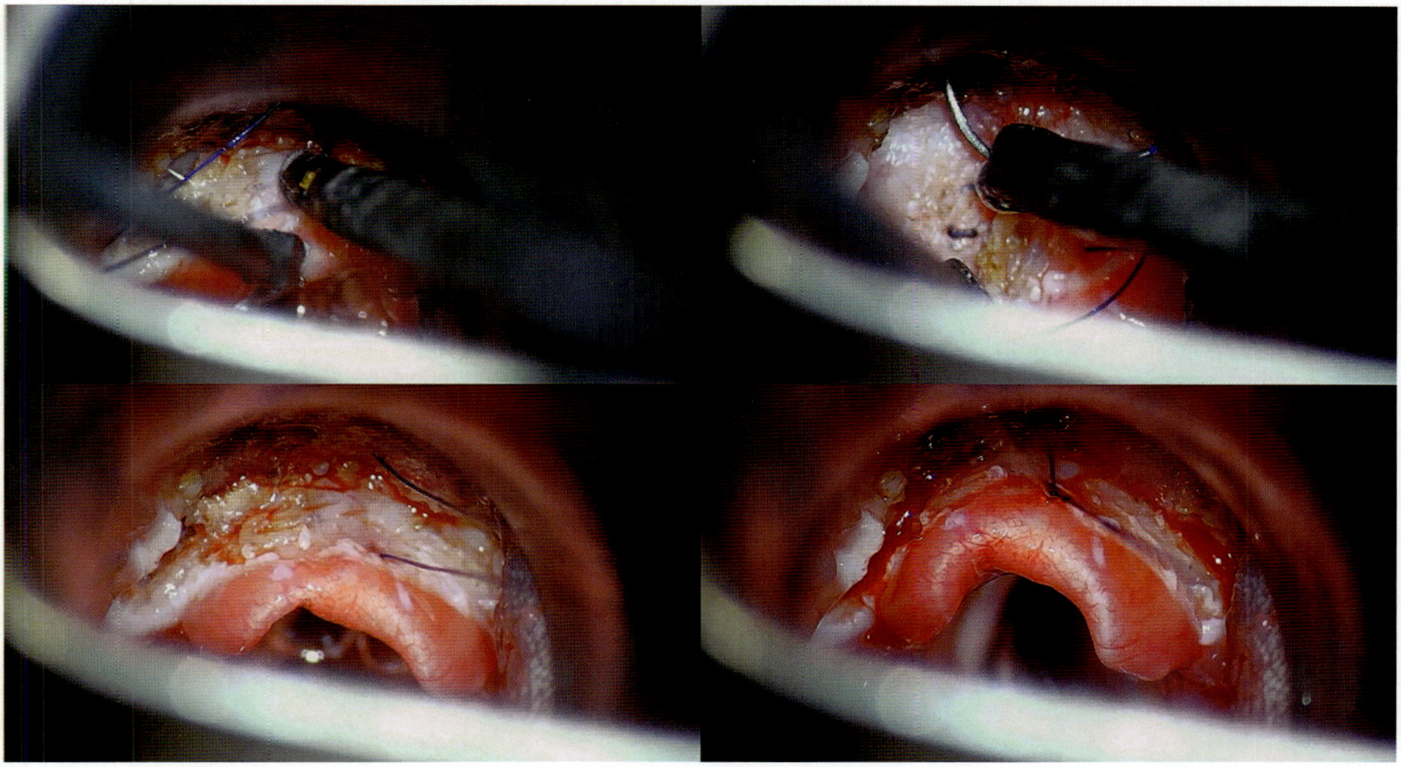

• **Fig. 7.11**

These complications are noted to be transient, and most children return to their preoperative swallow physiology.[19–21] Other rare complications include persistent aspiration, supraglottic stenosis, and granulation tissue formation. The need for a revision operation after initial supraglottoplasty can occur in up to 5–10% of patients and depends in part on comorbidities or if a unilateral procedure was done at the initial surgery.[15] If revision surgery is required, consider other underlying comorbidities as risk factors. A follow-up outpatient flexible laryngoscopy performed at 2 to 3 weeks can confirm complete healing. Nebulized ciprofloxacin-dexamethasone otic drops (20 drops in 5 mL of saline, BID, × 7–14 days) can be utilized to manage inflammation or granulation at the surgical site (Pearl 7.10). Acid suppression should be continued in the post operative healing phase. On average, patients may be on acid suppression medications for up to 8 months.

**PEARL 7.10**

Note that topical application of otic drops to the airway is considered off-label in the United States. In small infants, there is some risk of adrenal suppression with extended use of topical steroids in the airway.

## References


1. Richter GT, Thompson DM. The surgical management of laryngomalacia. *Otolaryngol Clin North Am.* 2008;41(5):837–864, vii. doi:10.1016/j.otc.2008.04.011.
2. Richter GT, Rutter MJ, deAlarcon A, Orvidas LJ, Thompson DM. Late-onset laryngomalacia: a variant of disease. *Arch Otolaryngol Head Neck Surg.* 2008;134(1):75–80. doi:10.1001/archoto.2007.17.
3. Thompson DM. Laryngomalacia: factors that influence disease severity and outcomes of management. *Curr Opin Otolaryngol Head Neck Surg.* 2010;18(6):564–570. doi:10.1097/MOO.0b013e3283405e48.
4. Carter J, Rahbar R, Brigger M, et al. International Pediatric ORL Group (IPOG) laryngomalacia consensus recommendations. *Int J Pediatr Otorhinolaryngol.* 2016;86:256–261. doi:10.1016/j.ijporl.2016.04.007.
5. Shah V. Laryngomalacia: the importance of disease severity. *Otolaryngol Head Neck Surg.* 2019;5(1):1–5. doi:10.24966/OHNS-010X/100028.
6. Dickson JM, Richter GT, Meinzen-Derr J, Rutter MJ, Thompson DM. Secondary airway lesions in infants with laryngomalacia. *Ann Otol Rhinol Laryngol.* 2009;118(1):37–43. doi:10.1177/000348940911800107.
7. Liu C, Ulualp SO. Type I Chiari malformation presenting with laryngomalacia and dysphagia. *Pediatr Int Off J Jpn Pediatr Soc.* 2015;57(4):795–797. doi:10.1111/ped.12639.
8. Irace AL, Dombrowski ND, Kawai K, et al. Evaluation of aspiration in infants with laryngomalacia and recurrent respiratory and feeding difficulties. *JAMA Otolaryngol Head Neck Surg.* 2019;145(2):146–151. doi:10.1001/jamaoto.2018.3642.
9. Jaffal H, Isaac A, Johannsen W, Campbell S, El-Hakim HG. The prevalence of swallowing dysfunction in children with laryngomalacia: a systematic review. *Int J Pediatr Otorhinolaryngol.* 2020;139:110464. doi:10.1016/j.ijporl.2020.110464.
10. Vandjelovic ND, Brown JR, Traboulsi HT, Thottam PJ. Impact of infant supraglottoplasty on quality of life. *Otolaryngol Head Neck Surg.* 2018;159(3):564–571. doi:10.1177/0194599818775091.
11. Thottam PJ, Simons JP, Choi S, Maguire R, Mehta DK. Clinical relevance of quality of life in laryngomalacia. *Laryngoscope.* 2016;126(5):1232–1235. doi:10.1002/lary.25491.

12. Bakeman AE, Shaffer AD, Tobey ABJ, et al. Prevalence and management of laryngomalacia in patients with pierre robin sequence. *Cleft Palate Craniofac J.* 2023;60(11):1395–1403. doi:10.1177/10556656221107298.
13. Mathews F, Shaffer AD, Georg MW, Ford MD, Jabbour N, Simons JP. Laryngomalacia in patients with craniosynostosis. *Ann Otol Rhinol Laryngol.* 2018;127(8):543–550. doi:10.1177/0003489418779413.
14. Farhood Z, Ong AA, Nguyen SA, Gillespie MB, Discolo CM, White DR. Objective outcomes of supraglottoplasty for children with laryngomalacia and obstructive sleep apnea: a meta-analysis. *JAMA Otolaryngol Head Neck Surg.* 2016;142(7):665–671. doi:10.1001/jamaoto.2016.0830.
15. Day KE, Discolo CM, Meier JD, Wolf BJ, Halstead LA, White DR. Risk factors for supraglottoplasty failure. *Otolaryngol Head Neck Surg.* 2012;146(2):298–301. doi:10.1177/0194599811425652.
16. Olney DR, Greinwald JH, Smith RJ, Bauman NM. Laryngomalacia and its treatment. *Laryngoscope.* 1999;109(11):1770–1775. doi:10.1097/00005537-199911000-00009.
17. Faria J, Behar P. Medical and surgical management of congenital laryngomalacia: a case-control study. *Otolaryngol Head Neck Surg.* 2014;151(5):845–851. doi:10.1177/0194599814541921.
18. Holinger LD, Konior RJ. Surgical management of severe laryngomalacia. *Laryngoscope.* 1989;99(2):136–142. doi:10.1288/00005537-198902000-00004.
19. Nguyen M, Brooks L, Wetzel M, Raol N. Swallowing outcomes following supraglottoplasty: a retrospective review. *Laryngoscope.* 2021;131(12):2817–2822. doi:10.1002/lary.29704.
20. McSwiney PF, Cavanagh NP, Languth P. Outcome in congenital stridor (laryngomalacia). *Arch Dis Child.* 1977;52(3):215–218. doi:10.1136/adc.52.3.215.
21. Simons JP, Greenberg LL, Mehta DK, Fabio A, Maguire RC, Mandell DL. Laryngomalacia and swallowing function in children. *Laryngoscope.* 2016;126(2):478–484. doi:10.1002/lary.25440.

# 8

# Endoscopic Submucosal Arytenoidectomy and Lateral Arytenopexy

SCOTT RICKERT AND DOUGLAS R. SIDELL

## Background

Glottic stenosis can occur from either vocal fold paralysis or scar formation with fixation of the cricoarytenoid joint. Glottic stenosis typically presents with poor airflow but with a relatively strong voice. In order to correct glottic stenosis and improve airflow, one must enlarge the cross-sectional area of the airway, potentially adversely affecting voice and swallowing. This balance of airway, voice, and swallowing has been the primary challenge surgically, and many open and endoscopic techniques have been devised to best address this challenge. Open techniques include laryngotracheal reconstruction with grafting. Endoscopic techniques include total arytenoidectomy, posterior cordotomy, partial arytenoidectomy, arytenopexy, vocal fold suture lateralization, and endoscopic laryngotracheal posterior graft placement.

Endoscopic arytenoidectomy was first described as an approach to improve glottic stenosis in 1983.[1] Partial arytenoidectomy was first described in 1993 with the removal of the overlying mucosa and preservation of the vocal process.[2] Subsequent submucosal approaches were described in 2000,[3] which claimed improved mucosal healing and decreased granulation in the supraglottis. Further modifications to the endoscopic submucosal arytenoidectomy have been described as well and have been used not only in improving glottic airflow but also in preserving and potentially improving voice. These techniques include laser-assisted endoscopic medial arytenoidectomy,[4] superomedial partial arytenoidectomy,[5] and subtotal submucosal arytenoidectomy with lateralization sutures.[6] As there are nuances in the presentation of glottic stenosis, it is important that the surgical approach is nuanced as well. This chapter describes the general approach to performing a submucosal arytenoidectomy as well as some modifications to the approach based on the nature of the glottic stenosis and its presentation. A description of arytenopexy is also provided.

## Operative Approach

### Patient Selection

Candidates for these operations will typically present with posterior glottic stenosis, fixed supraglottic obstruction due to arytenoid prolapse, or both. While arytenopexy relies to some degree on cricoarytenoid joint mobility, arytenoidectomy does not. The surgeon should include palpation of the cricoarytenoid joint during operative endoscopy to make this determination. If an arytenopexy is performed and the joint is ankylotic, this may require lysis of adhesion at the cricoarytenoid joint prior to performing the arytenopexy.

In the basic approach of endoscopic submucosal arytenoidectomy, the patient's airway is well visualized during direct microlaryngoscopy in the operating room under general anesthesia. It is important to communicate well with the anesthesia team to ensure the optimal depth of anesthesia for microlaryngeal surgery. If the patient can tolerate apneic technique with no endotracheal tube in place during the procedure, exposure to the surgical field is ideal. If the patient is not able to be adequately sustained without desaturation with an apneic technique, intermittent intubation with a small endotracheal tube may be necessary to provide enough time to perform the endoscopic arytenoidectomy. Supplemental oxygenation via an endotracheal tube in the mouth or nose may also be considered.

With a stable and adequate airway, an appropriate amount of 1% lidocaine without epinephrine is placed on the vocal folds to prevent laryngospasm prior to intervention. The airway is examined to ensure no other airway lesions are present prior to performing the arytenoidectomy. The patient is then placed in suspension with the posterior larynx entirely in view (Fig. 8.1A). An operating microscope or Hopkins rod telescope is often used to provide a magnified view of the surgical site. Both techniques can be performed with a two-handed technique, but the Hopkins rod requires an assistant or mounting device to hold the telescope in place. This may add challenges in ease of dissection as the field of surgery is limited with an extra instrument in the surgical field. The microscope also allows for binocular vision, which is not possible when using the Hopkins rod.

When the arytenoid is adequately exposed, a small amount of 1% lidocaine with 1:100,000 epinephrine is injected into the area of the planned incision on the superior surface of the arytenoid for hemostasis and to hydrodissect the mucosa from the cartilage, using an orotracheal injection device or the surgeon's

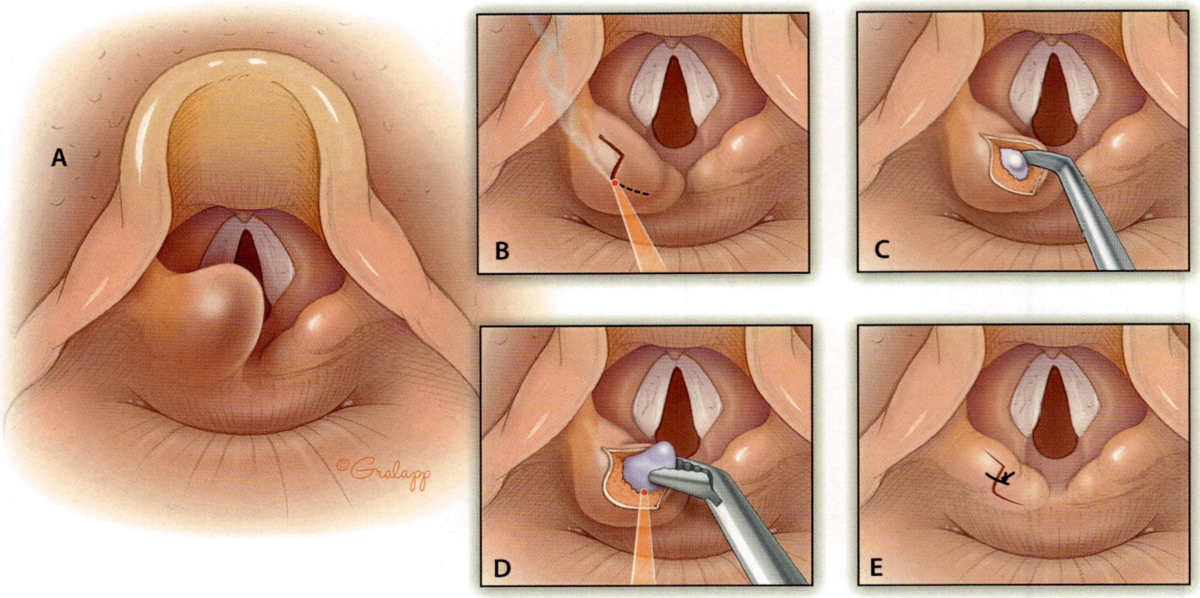


• **Fig. 8.1** (A) Illustration of the endoscopic view of posterior larynx in patient. (B) Incision marking the approach for an endoscopic medial arytenoidectomy. (C) Soft tissue dissection, freeing mucosa from the cartilaginous arytenoid. (D) The arytenoid is grasped with a forceps and elevated out of the mucosa. Laser or micro-laryngeal scissors can be used to divide the arytenoid at the base of dissection. (E) Closure of the incision is then performed endoscopically. (© 2024 Chris Gralapp.)

preferred substitute. The incision should be placed on the most superior surface of the arytenoid and can be either a linear or an S- or Z-shaped incision (Fig. 8.1B). An S- or Z-shaped incision can improve exposure of the arytenoid cartilage and result in an easier dissection of the medial aspect of the arytenoid body. Although dissection of the mucosa from the medial arytenoid is performed through the superior incision, it is important to avoid carrying the incision itself to the medial aspect of the arytenoid. An incision placed near the interarytenoid space may lead to interarytenoid scarring during the healing process. Once the medial aspect of the arytenoid is exposed, one can carefully dissect the surrounding soft tissue from the arytenoid cartilage itself.

The soft tissue is typically dissected from the cartilaginous arytenoid using a small endoscopic spatula (Fig. 8.1C). Because the cartilage has a firm surface, one can use the spatula with a one-handed technique. To gain better countertraction, Bouchayer forceps or an equivalent instrument can be used to retract the soft tissue laterally during dissection. The spatula can then dissect the medial arytenoid more efficiently.

Once the medial dissection of the arytenoid is complete, a similar technique is used on the lateral aspect of the arytenoid cartilage. After the arytenoid cartilage is sufficiently separated from the underlying soft tissue, the cartilage is brought out through the incision site with the grasping forceps and removed using endoscopic scissors to divide the arytenoid at the base of the dissection (Fig. 8.1D). Depending on the goal of the arytenoidectomy surgery, the surgeon can remove anywhere from a small portion of the medial arytenoid to a near-complete arytenoidectomy, leaving only a small portion of the lateral arytenoid. Hemostasis should be easily controlled with placement of oxymetazoline cottonoid pledgets in the area of dissection as needed (Pearl 8.1). If bleeding is not controlled adequately and enters the airway, it may cause laryngospasm and require intubation for a brief period before continuing with the procedure.

**PEARL 8.1**

Dilute Epinephrine (E.g., 1:20,000) May Also Be Used Instead Of Oxymetazoline.
Once the arytenoid is carefully removed and hemostasis is achieved, the incision site can be closed with 2 to 3 endoscopic absorbable sutures, which are oriented laterally on the arytenoid surface. Careful attention must be paid to not place them medially as they can potentially interfere with the patency of the airway or cause irritation leading to coughing or gagging postoperatively (Pearl 8.2).

**PEARL 8.2**

Long suture tails may also irritate the posterior pharyngeal wall, causing granulation and synechiae.

Once the arytenoid is carefully removed and hemostasis is achieved, the incision site can be closed with 2–3 endoscopic absorbable sutures (Fig. 8.1E; Pearl 8.2).

## Adjuncts to Arytenoidectomy

There are many modifications to the endoscopic arytenoidectomy. While a medial arytenoidectomy does remove the bulk of the arytenoid and opens the posterior laryngeal inlet, there is opportunity to improve the posterior glottic airway by supplementing with other endoscopic techniques depending on the nature of the glottic airway.

These techniques not only improve the glottic airflow but may also allow preservation and potential improvement in voice. These include laser-assisted endoscopic medial arytenoidectomy,[4] superomedial partial arytenoidectomy,[5] and subtotal submucosal arytenoidectomy with lateralization sutures.[6]

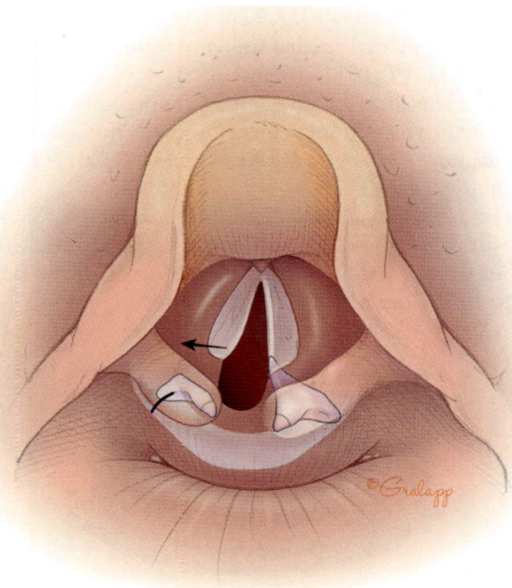

• **Fig. 8.2** Illustration of arytenoid remnant following suture arytenopexy, as viewed on direct laryngoscopy. (© 2024 Chris Gralapp.)

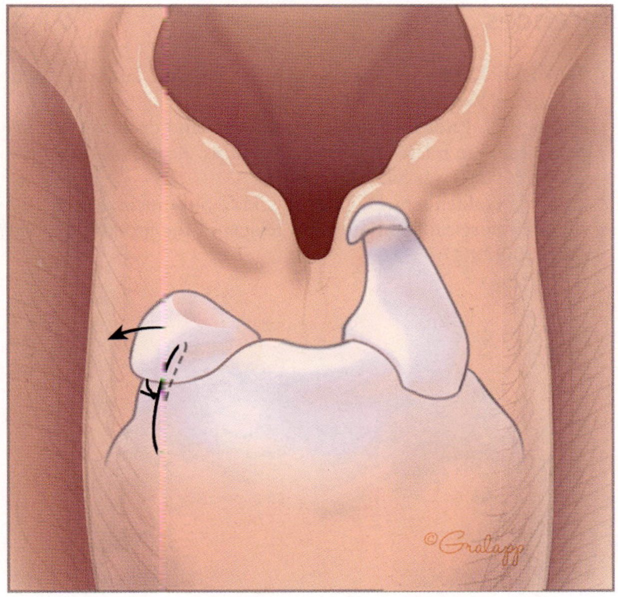

• **Fig. 8.3** Illustration (viewed from the posterior larynx) of arytenoid remnant, following suture arytenopexy to the cricoid cartilage. (© 2024 Chris Gralapp.)

## Endoscopic Arytenopexy

Arytenopexy performed in conjunction with an endoscopic medial arytenoidectomy allows for further expansion of the glottic airway. In general, widening the glottic airway with any technique allows for greater airflow but may compromise the ability to provide adequate voice and increase the risk of aspiration. As such, arytenopexy may impact voice more than arytenoidectomy alone, as the arytenoid body vocal process remnants are further lateralized. Careful attention must be paid to ensure that opening the glottic airway through these techniques does not adversely affect voice and swallowing to a greater detriment than the improvement in the airway.

Description of procedure:

If a submucosal flap has not been elevated, an incision can be made extending from the arytenoidectomy defect posteriorly and laterally over the body of the arytenoid toward the superior aspect of the cricoid cartilage.

Blunt dissection is then performed to expose the arytenoid remnant adjacent to the muscular process. Additional exposure can be performed beyond the cricoarytenoid joint, but it is not necessary under all circumstances.

After adequate exposure is achieved, a monofilament or absorbable braided suture with a tapered needle can then be used to perform the arytenopexy. A suture such as a 3-0 double-armed Prolene is often used.

The needle is first passed through the posterolateral arytenoid adjacent to the muscular process.

The second pass of the needle is directed at the exposed aspect of the superior cricoid. It is important to consider the vector of suture placement, as the suture is intended, when on tension, to both abduct (rotate) and directly lateralize the arytenoid body remnant. Adequate perichondrium must be captured with the needle pass to ensure suture stability.

The suture is then manually placed on tension to ensure that the arytenoid body remnant is rotated in abduction and maintained in a lateralized position. Once this has been confirmed and the desired degree of patency achieved, the suture can be tied (Fig. 8.2–8.3). If needed, a second suture can be used to achieve the desired effect. If a submucosal flap has been elevated, it can then be closed loosely.

The balance between airway patency, voice quality, and safe swallow function leads to the use of a multitude of different endoscopic approaches to arytenoidectomy with or without arytenopexy. The nuance of whether one performs a superomedial partial arytenoidectomy or a subtotal arytenoidectomy depends greatly on the degree to which airflow is limited and the location of airflow restriction. The preservation of healthy mucosa is an important aspect of the endoscopic approach, as it prevents interarytenoid scarring and preserves sensation. As these endoscopic approaches advance, the basic principles of mucosal preservation and judicious tissue removal continue to be the guiding principles for successful interventions of the posterior glottic airway.

### ADDITIONAL CLINICAL PEARLS

In cases of limited mobility of the arytenoid complex, performing balloon dilation of the posterior glottis at the beginning of the procedure can gently distract the prolapsed and medialized arytenoid into a more favorable position. This can facilitate arytenopexy procedures by loosening any adhesive fixation at the cricoarytenoid joint and by establishing a potential vector for suture placement. Lastly, this simple maneuver can provide visual guidance on the anticipated result one is hoping to achieve.

In select older children and adolescents with concurrent vocal fold immobility and an adequate glottic airway, consideration of concurrent vocal fold injection to overcome vocalis atrophy can be helpful in balancing airway obstruction with glottic incompetence.

If the surgeon feels that endoscopic arytenopexy is not providing the desired improvement in airway patency, they should consider conversion to a combined open and endoscopic approach. When performing a combined endoscopic and open approach, such as arytenoid abduction lateropexy, the use of a metal button or titanium miniplate can be used to provide a scaffold upon which to tie the pexy suture for stability.

## References


1. Ossoff RH, Karlan MS, Sisson GA. Endoscopic laser arytenoidectomy. *Lasers Surg Med.* 1983;2(4):293–299.
2. Crumley RL. Endoscopic laser medial arytenoidectomy for airway manage-ment in bilateral laryngeal paralysis. *Ann Otol Rhinol Laryngol.* 1993;102(2):81–84.
3. Danino J, Goldenberg D, Joachims HZ. Submucosal arytenoidectomy: new surgical technique and review of the literature. *J Otolaryngol.* 2000;29(1):13–16.
4. Kim HM, Kwon SK, Hah JH, Kim KH, Sung MW. Laser-assisted endoscopic submucosal medial arytenoidectomy (LESMA). *Laryngoscope.* 2007;117(9):1611–1614.
5. Mahieu R, Heuveling D, Mahieu H. Superomedial partial arytenoidectomy for voice improvement by correction of posterior glottic insufficiency. *Eur Arch Otorhinolaryngol.* 2020;277:1417–1426. https://doi.org/10.1007/s00405-020-05859-2.
6. Shoffel-Havakuk H, Lahav Y, Reuven Y, Shopen Y, Shapira-Galitz Y, Hamzany Y. Subtotal Submucosal Arytenoidectomy with Lateralization Sutures (SMALS) covered by a Mucosal Flap. *Laryngoscope.* 2023. https://doi.org/10.1002/lary.30940.

# 9

# Cordotomy/Arytenoidectomy/Vocal Fold Suture Lateralization

DINESH KHATRI CHHETRI

## Background

Bilateral vocal fold immobility (BVFI) is one of the most challenging conditions treated by the otolaryngologist. Bilateral vocal fold immobility generally presents in two forms: (1) neurogenic bilateral vocal fold paralysis (BVFP) or (2) posterior glottic stenosis (PGS). The latter is more common and more prevalent in females. The glottis functions in airway maintenance, airway protection, and phonation. The most significant functional consequence of BVFI is airway obstruction manifesting as inspiratory stridor. The severity of airway distress at presentation depends on the amount of glottal opening present, timeline of development of the disorder, baseline functional reserve of the patient, and presence of paradoxical vocal fold motion during inspiration. Greater glottal opening, especially with some residual vocal fold motion, chronic development of immobility, high functional reserve, and absence of concurrent paradoxical vocal fold motion, results in lesser severity of airway symptoms. The voice consequence depends on the degree of glottal closure achieved during adduction and presence of concurrent pathology of the membranous vocal folds such as lesions or scarring. Generally, patients who need airway intervention have a normal to near-normal voice. If the voice is poor due to a large glottal gap, then airway intervention is likely not indicated. Dysphagia is less common in the setting of BVFI, except in cases such as progressive neurodegenerative disease or a history of radiation therapy for head and neck cancer.

## Operative Assessment and Planning

### Patient Selection

Surgical intervention in BVFI can be challenging and should be pursued only if (1) the patient is symptomatic; (2) the patient desires improvement of the symptoms; and (3) the intervention is expected to improve the quality of life and not lead to further harm (e.g., dysphagia). The most important consideration for surgical intervention is symptomatic airway obstruction (dyspnea or stridor). Some patients may present with seemingly small glottic airway on laryngoscopy and yet have minimal stridor or airway obstruction symptoms. If airway symptoms are tolerated, then there is no urgency for intervention, as surgery for BVFI can be technically challenging and will have some negative voice consequences. Conversely, airway obstruction leading to significant functional deficit such as difficulty walking, breathing, speaking, or swallowing requires intervention, at some cost to voice quality. Patients with PGS often have medical comorbidities (e.g., cardiovascular, pulmonary, metabolic, gastrointestinal) that need to be addressed in the perioperative period.

### Key Aspects of Informed Consent

***What is to be done*:** The primary surgical goal in BVFI is to expand the glottic airway to the degree needed to relieve symptomatic airway obstruction. The secondary goal is to maintain voice as much as possible, which is antagonistic to the primary goal. A balance can be achieved by focusing on expanding the cartilaginous glottis for airway expansion while preserving the membranous glottis for maintenance of phonation. Adequate phonatory ability for communication is nearly always possible after posterior glottic expansion surgery. However, patients have to be informed that although a balance between airway and voice is sought, improved airway patency is the primary goal and phonation may be adversely affected in unpredictable ways. A less desired approach is to perform a conservative and limited airway expansion, for example in professional voice users, if there is an understanding and agreement that a subsequent procedure may be needed should the initial procedure result in inadequate relief of airway symptoms. For symptomatic patients unwilling to compromise on losing any voice, a tracheostomy is the most optimal treatment.

***Approach*:** The primary approach to treating BVFI is transoral endoscopic surgery under microsuspension direct laryngoscopy. While many surgical techniques have been proposed the most common are transverse cordotomy, arytenoidectomy, and vocal fold lateralization. A significant concern is whether to perform a concurrent tracheostomy if not already present. This depends on various factors, including (1) adequacy of glottal expansion achieved intraoperatively; (2) status of the opposite vocal fold motion (presence of some motion lessens the need for concurrent tracheostomy); (3) assessment of the expected difficulty of reintubation postoperatively (if there is concern for difficult intubation, then a tracheostomy should be performed concurrently); and (4) if there is adequate space for the operative procedures with concurrent presence of endotracheal tube for ventilation, if required.

## Major Equipment

A variety of large- and small-bore rigid laryngoscopes are needed to adequately treat the airway. A Dedo or similar-caliber laryngoscope that allows binocular vision for microlaryngoscopy is adequate for performing the glottic procedures (Pearl 9.1). A laryngoscope holder tray attached to the bed is most convenient to hold the suspension arm of the laryngoscope. Ventilation during the operation can be performed via a small microlaryngeal or laser tube, or via concurrent tracheostomy. Jet ventilation is not convenient, as the laryngoscope may need frequent readjustments to obtain the lateral angles needed for surgery. A 0-degree Hopkins rod rigid endoscope is useful for close-up assessment of the larynx and the subglottis for intraoperative assessment of progress (Pearl 9.2). A high-powered binocular microscope is critical for freeing both hands for the surgical maneuvers. Flexible bronchoscope is useful for concurrent assessment of the entire airway as needed. A $CO_2$ laser, preferably with a micromanipulator and pattern generator, is indispensable to perform the surgeries.

**PEARL 9.1**

In pediatric patients, a Lindholm or Parsons laryngoscope will often provide excellent exposure of the entire glottis without frequent readjustment. This in turn may allow oxygenation and ventilation via the laryngoscope side port, or with high-flow nasal cannula.

**PEARL 9.2**

A 30- or 70-degree telescope will allow the surgeon to visualize the long axis of the vocal folds, the free edge of the vocal folds, and the anterior commissure in a way that furthers understanding of the patient's specific anatomy. However, the majority of the operation is best done with a 0 degree telescope or microscope.

# Operative Approach

## Patient Positioning and Laryngeal Exposure

Abnormal airway anatomy or a "difficult airway" is often why patients end up with PGS. Thus laryngeal exposure may be challenging. Many patients who have BVFI have body habitus or oropharyngeal anatomy that makes it difficult to expose the larynx. Several maneuvers can be performed to get optimal exposure of the larynx: (1) the upper torso of the supine patient should be ramped such that the cervicothoracic vertebrae are slightly flexed and the atlantooccipital joint is slightly extended (i.e., "sniffing position") such that the level of the external auditory canal is above the level of the sternal notch; (2) an anterior neck compression can be placed to depress the larynx and bring it to view (e.g., by using a small towel over the larynx and extending tape across the two sides of the operative table to press down on the towel); and (3) after a period of suspension, tissue creep may allow the suspension to be cranked up some more to improve exposure. Fortunately, the operative site is the posterior larynx, and adequate exposure is generally achieved. However, a full view of the larynx does provide an overall assessment of the adequacy of the final glottic aperture achieved. It cannot be overemphasized that the dentition must be protected during suspension laryngoscopy using dental guards. Aquaplast or similar thermoplastic nasal splints are one of the best materials to create a custom-fitting dental guard in patients with teeth.

## Operative Techniques

### *Transverse Cordotomy*

The vocal fold with less mobility on office laryngoscopy is chosen for the procedure. If both vocal folds have similar immobility, then the left side is chosen by convention, but this is not critical, as airway outcome is not dependent on the chosen side. The arytenoids are palpated for joint mobility in cases of PGS, and the more restricted side should be selected. After adequate exposure of the vocal fold, the posterior 30% to 50% of the membranous vocal fold is ablated with $CO_2$ laser.[1] The key to success is to extend the cordotomy laterally flush with the subglottis and to extend the ablation onto the false vocal fold (Fig. 9.1A). Otherwise, regrowth of tissue at the cordotomy site with recurrence of glottic stenosis and airway symptoms may occur. Despite this precaution, some patients may heal unpredictably and should be informed at preoperative counseling that repeat surgery is occasionally necessary. A small amount (0.1–0.2 ml) of Kenalog steroid (40 mg/ml) is injected into the cordotomy site to prevent scar formation. Ideal outcomes should result in posterior glottic expansion with adequately lateralized vocal fold with significant relief of airway obstruction symptoms (Fig. 9.1B, C). Voice outcomes are variable and depend on the condition of the contralateral vocal fold. Although transverse cordotomy is still quite common, especially in recalcitrant cases, voice-sparing surgeries such as arytenoidectomy are preferable.

### *Arytenoidectomy*

Arytenoidectomy procedures focus on expanding the cartilaginous glottis while avoiding ablation of the membranous vocal fold in order to preserve voice. There are three iterations of this procedure. The simplest version is the medial arytenoidectomy, which is similar to transverse cordotomy but with the ablation occurring from the tip of the vocal process toward posterior and lateral glottis. The lateral excision also needs to extend flush to subglottis to achieve an adequate airway. Medial arytenoidectomy can be extended to a transverse cordotomy to achieve the necessary glottic expansion (Fig. 9.1A).

The second iteration of the procedure is a *partial* arytenoidectomy, which ablates anterior half of the arytenoid including the vocal process.[2] To perform this procedure, the laryngoscope is adjusted to expose the anterior wall of the arytenoid. Mucosal ablation of a small area using laser is performed to expose the superior arytenoid, then the laser ablation is focused entirely on the cartilage including the vocal process, sparing as much of the remaining mucosa overlying medial arytenoid and vocal fold mucosa as possible. After partial ablation of the anterior arytenoid to the vocal process, a transverse incision of the width of the vocal fold is made at the level of the vocal process. The posteromedially based mucosa remaining after the arytenoidectomy is then draped posterolaterally and sutured to lateral mucosa using a 5-0 vicryl suture (Fig. 9.2B1). The vocal fold is sutured posterolaterally to laryngeal wall tissue using a 5-0 vicryl suture. This procedure works especially well in

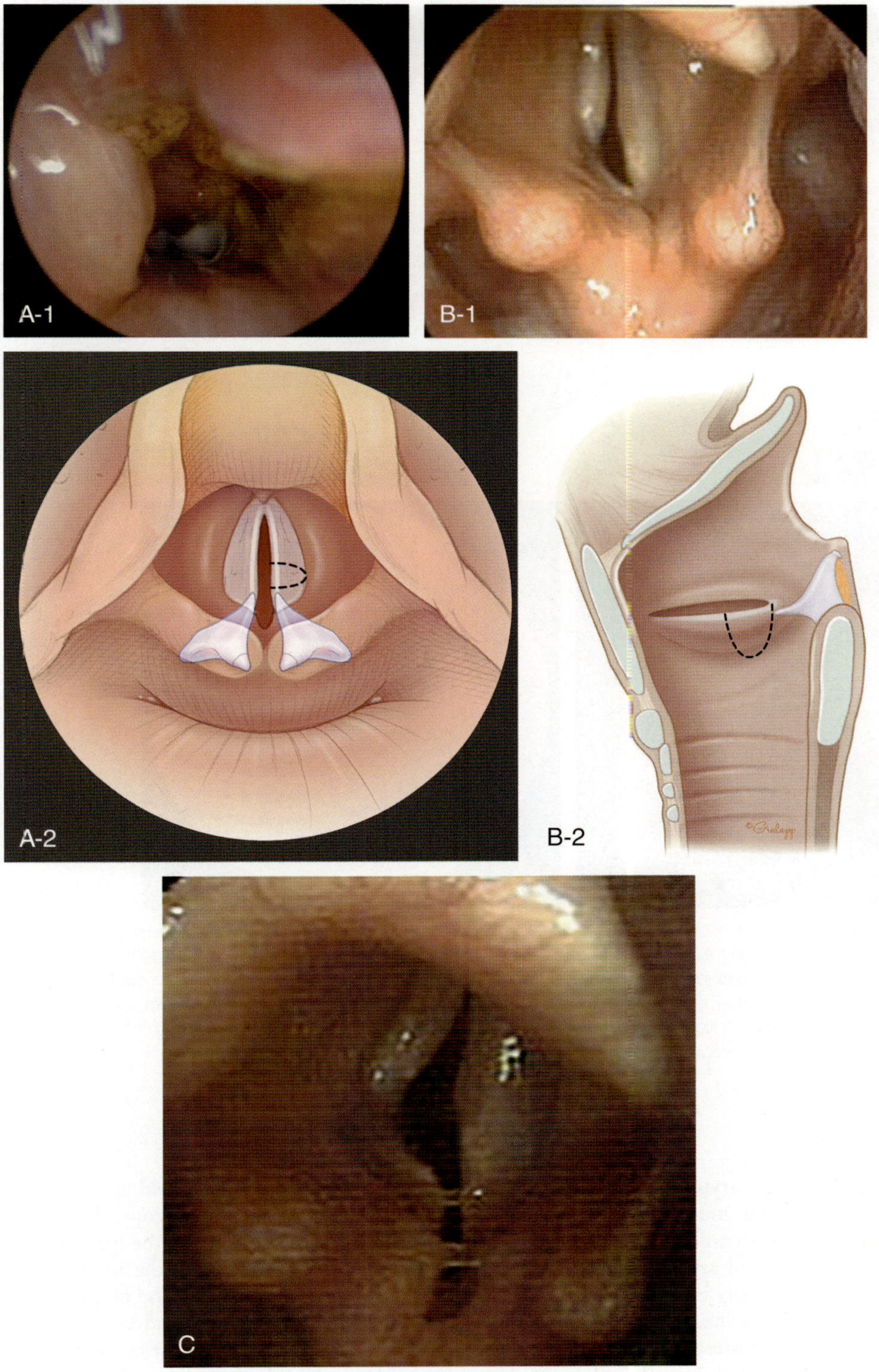


• **Fig. 9.1** (A-1) An intraoperative view of a transverse cordotomy of the *right* vocal fold. The posterior 30% of the membranous vocal fold has been ablated along with medial arytenoidectomy in a patient with posterior glottic stenosis. (A-2) Illustration of the endoscopic view of cordotomy location, anterior to the vocal process. (B-1) Office laryngoscopy after *left* transverse cordotomy without arytenoidectomy in a different patient resulting in a moderately open airway. (B-2) Illustration of the sagittal view of a transverse cordotomy, anterior to the vocal process. (C) Another example of *left* transverse cordotomy without arytenoidectomy resulting in a wide open airway. (Illustrations © 2024 Chris Gralapp.)

cases of BVFP and is an elegant way to expand the glottis and facilitate proper wound healing by covering raw surfaces.

The third arytenoidectomy procedure is an endoscopic *total* arytenoidectomy.[3] This is needed in cases of PGS, as it is quite difficult to mobilize the mucosa and obtain adequate glottic expansion with partial arytenoidectomy alone. As with the partial arytenoidectomy described earlier, the mucosa overlying the anterior superior face of the arytenoid is ablated until the tip of the

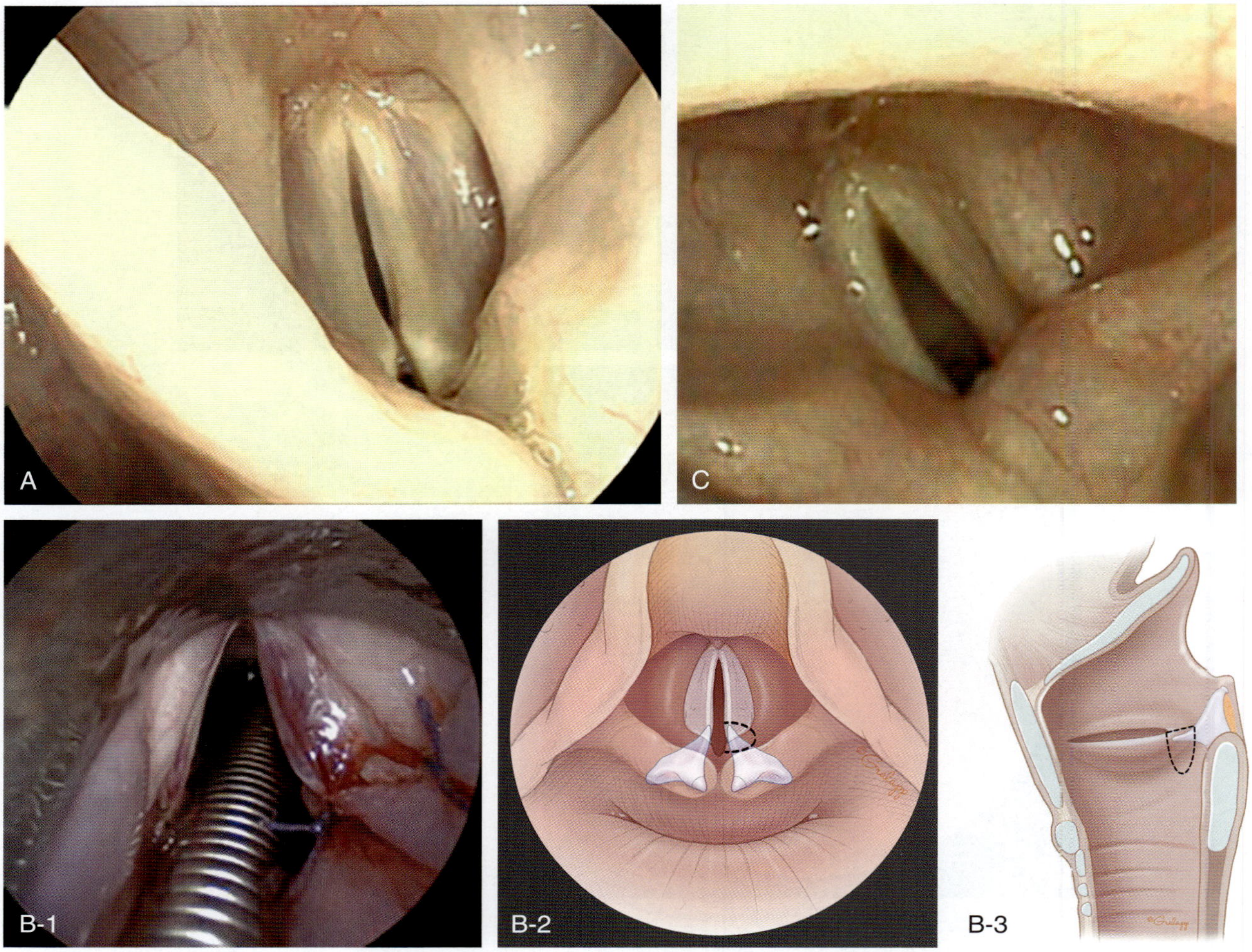


• **Fig. 9.2** A 79-year-old female with bilateral vocal fold paralysis after total thyroidectomy. (A) Preoperative office laryngoscopy view of glottal gap. (B-1) Intraoperative view after partial arytenoidectomy, suturing of posteromedially based mucosal flap, and endoscopic suture lateralization of the *right* vocal fold. Tracheostomy was not performed. (B-2) Illustration of the endoscopic view of partial arytenoidedectomy, incorporating vocal process. (B-3) Illustration of partial arytenodiectomy, sagittal view. (C) Postoperative office laryngoscopy showing improved airway and resolution of stridor. (Illustrations © 2024 Chris Gralapp.)

arytenoid is encountered. Then the arytenoid cartilage is ablated completely with laser while saving as much of the mucosa as possible. Soft tissue attached to the arytenoid is peeled off as the arytenoid is vaporized. Total removal of arytenoid down to cricoid cartilage can be a tedious process. Any bleeding is managed with endoscopic cautery device. As with the partial arytenoidectomy procedure discussed earlier, the posteromedially based mucosa is draped and sutured laterally and the vocal fold is lateralized with endoscopic suturing to the lateral wall (Figs. 9.3 and 9.4). Another perspective on this operation is provided in Chapter 8. If inadequate lateralization of the vocal fold is observed with internal endoscopic suturing, external endoscopic suture lateralization may be performed as outlined in the next section (Fig. 9.4).

### *Vocal Fold Suture Lateralization*

Glottic expansion in BVFI may also be performed with suture lateralization of the vocal fold. As this procedure can be performed without ablation of laryngeal tissue, it can also be considered in acute BVFP. The vocal fold to be lateralized is exposed under microsuspension laryngoscopy. The neck is prepped and a 1- to 2-cm incision is made on the ipsilateral neck just above the level of the inferior border of the thyroid cartilage and just anterior to the vertical portion of the oblique line. Subplatysmal flaps are elevated superiorly just above the halfway point of the thyroid cartilage and inferiorly just below the inferior border of the thyroid cartilage. A 16-gauge angiocatheter is inserted just below the thyroid cartilage and visualized appearing endoscopically into the subglottis about the level of the vocal process. The needle is removed, leaving the hollow catheter in place through which a 3-0 prolene is passed externally to internally. The suture is grasped with alligator forceps and brought outside the bore of the laryngoscope while the other end remains outside the neck. A second angiocatheter is passed through the thyroid cartilage to enter the posterior ventricle about the level of the vocal process, the angiocatheter needle is removed leaving the hollow catheter in place (Figs. 9.5A and 9.6A), and a 4-0 prolene is passed through the

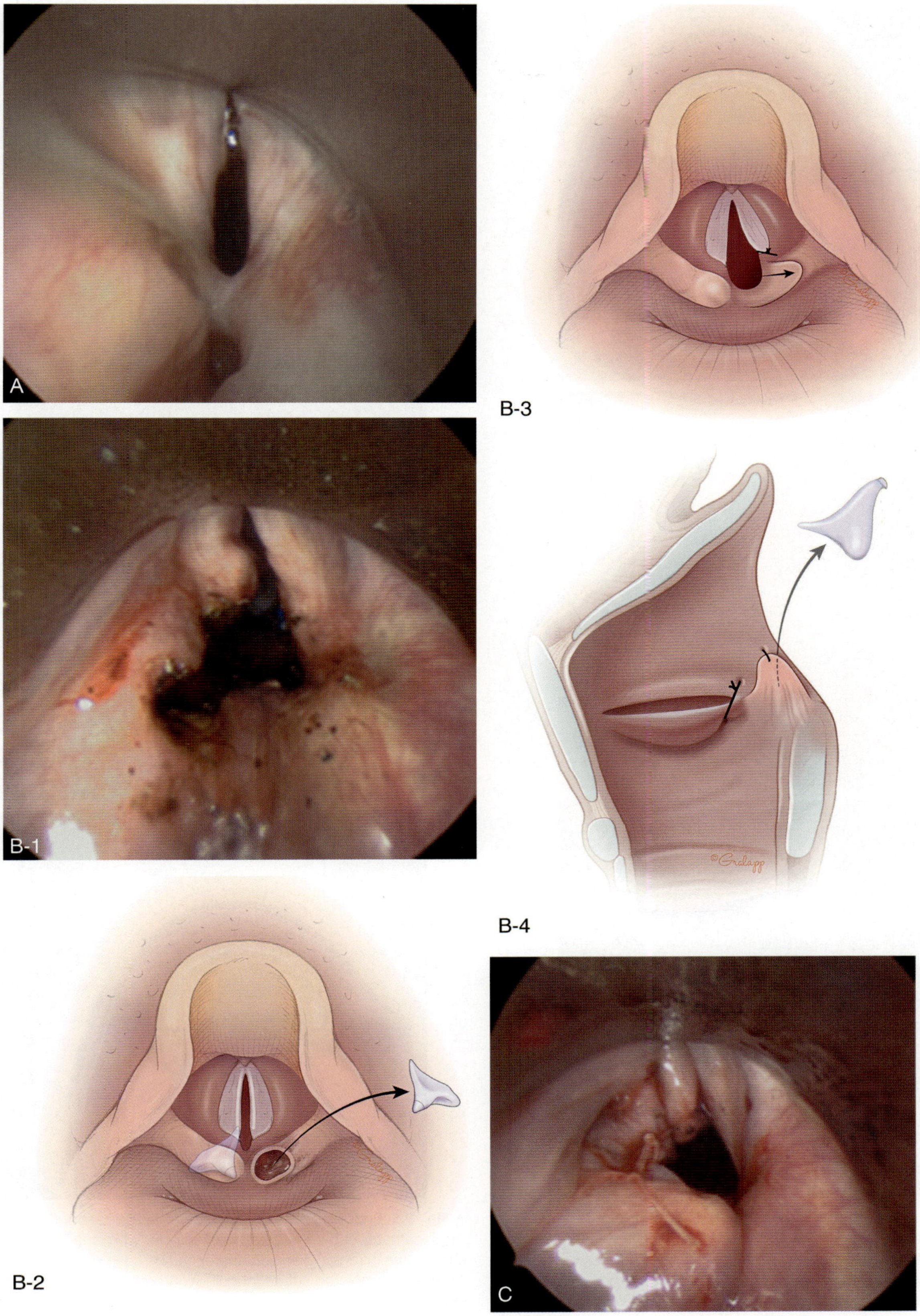


• **Fig. 9.3** Intraoperative views of a posterior glottic stenosis in a 68-year-old female after prolonged intubation for heart failure. (A) Intraoperative exposure of *left* arytenoid for total arytenoidectomy. (B-1) Total arytenoidectomy has been performed preserving all mucosa and a cordotomy at the level of the vocal process has been performed. (B-2) Illustrated rendition of *right* arytenoidectomy; (B-3) Endoscopic view and (B-4) sagittal view of closure. (C) After suturing laterally of a posteromedially based mucosal flap and endoscopic suture lateralization of the *left* vocal fold. (Illustrations © 2024 Chris Gralapp.

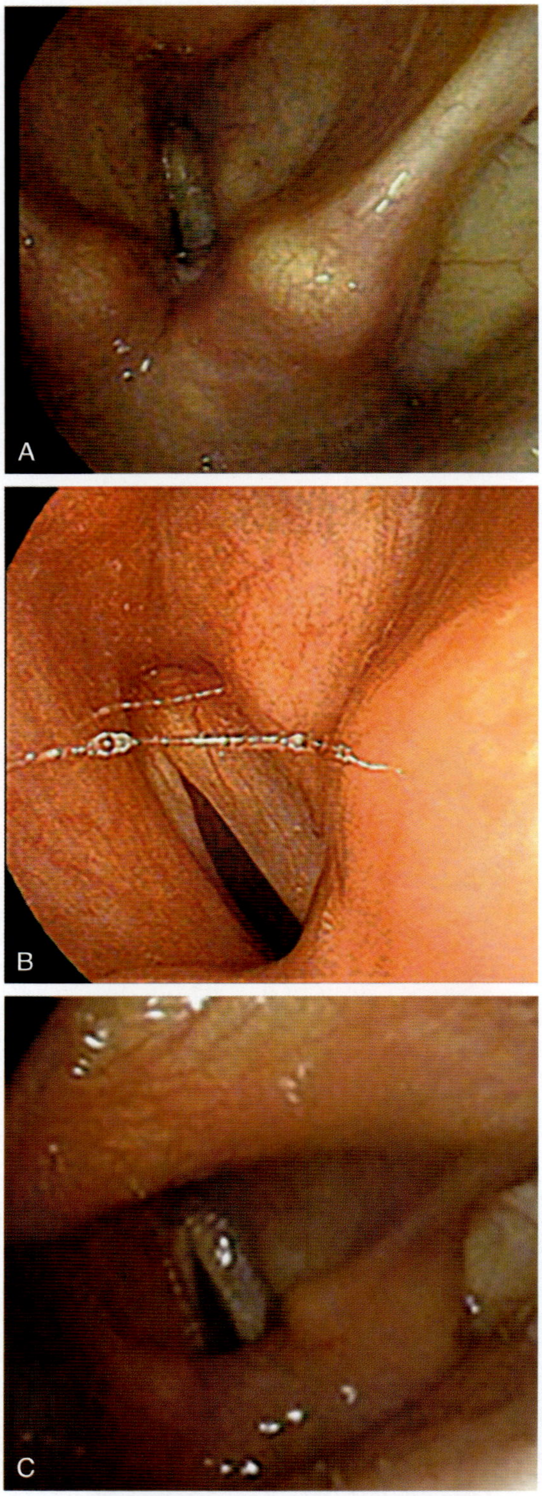


• **Fig. 9.4** Office laryngoscopy in the same patient from Fig. 9.3 (A) Preoperative office laryngoscopy view. (B) Postoperative office laryngoscopy view after *left-sided* surgery as shown in Fig. 9.3. Although her symptoms were significantly improved and she could tolerate capping, she still felt some shortness of breath with capping, and a right arytenoidectomy was performed. (C) Postoperative office laryngoscopy view after the *bilateral* procedures and decannulation.

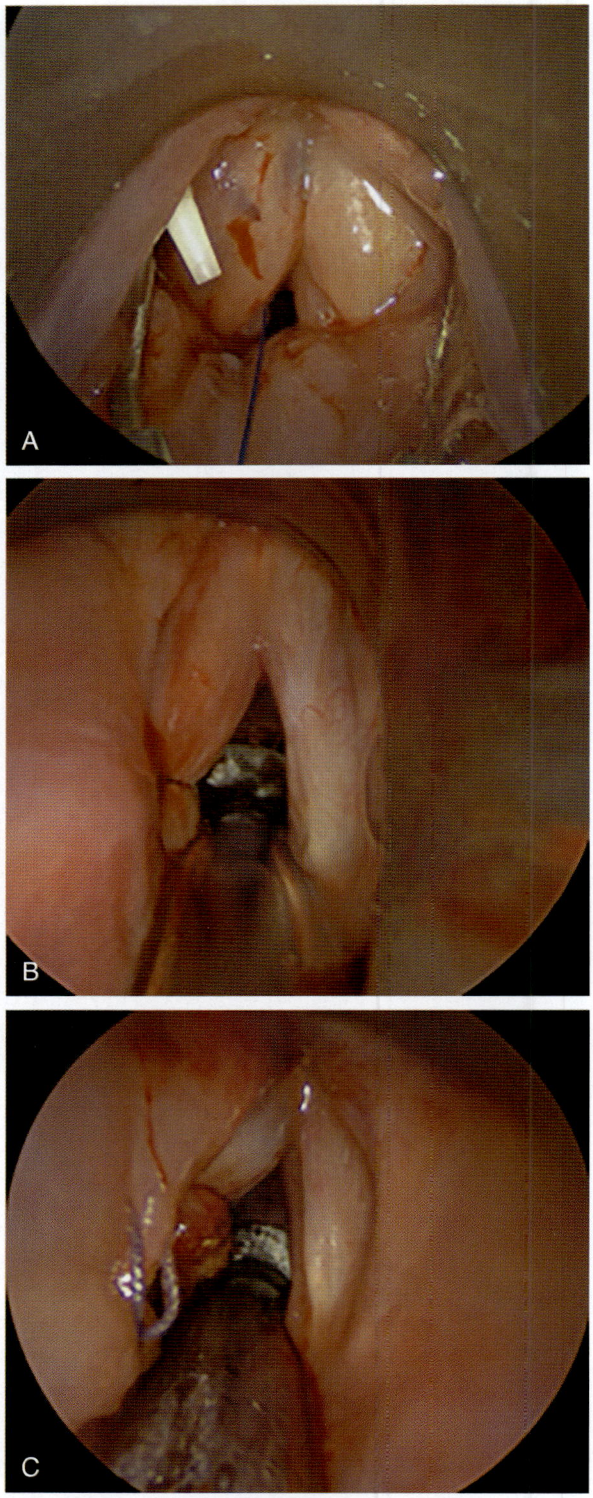


• **Fig. 9.5** Endoscopic external suture lateralization. (A) The superior angiocatheter can be seen at the ventricle, while the 3-0 prolene passed through an infraglottic angiocatheter can be seen at the posterior commissure. (B) Completed suture lateralization performed in a patient with bilateral vocal fold paralysis after thyroidectomy. (C) Suture lateralization was performed in a patient with posterior glottic stenosis after total arytenoidectomy when endoscopic internal suture lateralization was inadequate due to tissue scarring and inability to lateralize sufficiently.

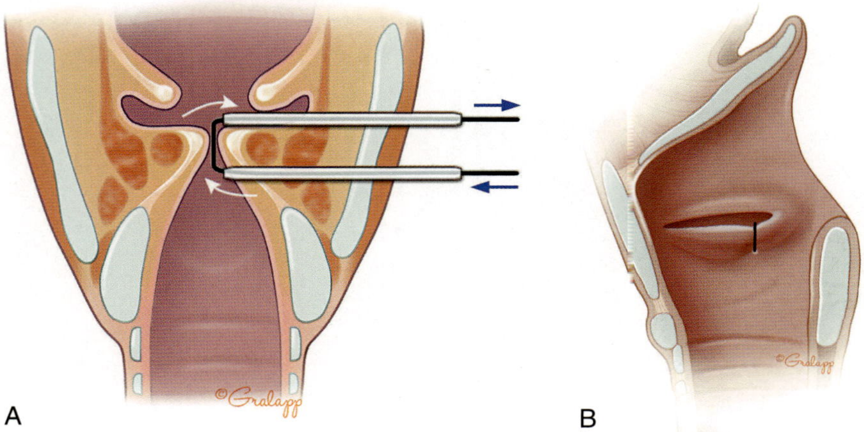


• **Fig. 9.6** Endoscopic suture lateralization with coronal (A) and sagittal (B) illustrations depicting suture placement. (Illustrations © 2024 Chris Gralapp.)

catheter, grasped with the alligator forceps, and brought outside the laryngoscope. The 3-0 and 4-0 sutures are tied at their ends outside the laryngoscope into a tight knot and the 4-0 suture is pulled from externally along with the angiocatheter, pulling the end of the 3-0 prolene outside the neck. The two ends of the 3-0 prolene are then tied over the thyroid cartilage or strap muscles while visualizing and adjusting the vocal fold lateralization endoscopically (Figs. 9.5B and 9.6B). While suture lateralization can be performed in BVFP without tissue ablation, as vocal fold tissue is compliant, in PSG some ablation of laryngeal tissue is necessary for airway expansion. Tissue ablation includes partial lateral thyroarytenoid muscle resection to create room for the vocal fold to move laterally during suture lateralization, while saving the medial vocal fold wall mucosa intact to promote healing. After ablation of tissue, the lateralized tissue can heal in place with decreased risk of vocal fold medialization that can sometimes occur over time. Suture lateralization may also be performed in cases of total arytenoidectomy when internal endoscopic suture lateralization does not lead to adequate glottic expansion and there is a concern for inadequate airway for extubation (Fig. 9.5C).

## Summary

Glottic expansion surgery in BVFI should be personalized to the individual larynx and etiology. Voice-preserving partial and total arytenoidectomy procedures with internal or external suture lateralization procedures are initially preferred over more destructive procedures such as transverse cordotomy. Patients should be counseled regarding potential reduction in voice quality and loudness after any glottic expansion surgery.

## References

1. Kashima HK. Bilateral vocal fold motion impairment: pathophysiology and management by transverse cordotomy. *Ann Otol Rhinol Laryngol.* 1991;100(9 Pt 1):717–721.
2. Yilmaz T. Endoscopic partial arytenoidectomy for bilateral vocal fold paralysis: medially based mucosal flap technique. *J Voice.* 2019;33(5):751–758.
3. Yilmaz T. Endoscopic total arytenoidectomy for bilateral abductor vocal fold paralysis: a new flap technique and personal experience with 50 cases. *Laryngoscope.* 2012;122(10):2219–2226.

# 10

# Endoscopic Anterior/Posterior (A/P) Cricoid Split

MICHAEL J. RUTTER AND DOUGLAS R. SIDELL

## Background

Although applied for other purposes since its inception, the endoscopic anterior/posterior (A/P) cricoid split was first described in 2017 as an intervention for children with bilateral true vocal fold immobility (BTVFI).[1] Due to the relatively high proportion of children with spontaneous recovery of vocal fold immobility in the first 12 months of life, any intervention performed to manage BTVFI should have minimal impact on the native larynx and its function. Historically, tracheostomy is performed for patients with airway obstruction in the setting of BTVFI; however, due to potential morbidity and social impacts of this procedure, efforts have been made to avoid tracheostomy when possible. In the first description of the endoscopic A/P split, 19 patients were evaluated across four institutions, with an overall success rate of 74% in avoiding tracheostomy or other laryngeal framework surgery.[1] Since that time, several other publications have been produced describing the technique, and we encourage the reader to perform an up-to-date evaluation of the literature prior to embarking on this procedure. It is important to note that while endoscopic A/P cricoid split is not universally successful, it is a rapid procedure that has allowed patients to avoid tracheostomy under many circumstances, and it does not preclude future tracheostomy if unsuccessful. As such, a detailed discussion of the goals of the procedure, including the potential for success and failure, and the potential for future tracheostomy, should all be performed prior to embarking on endoscopic A/P split.

## Patient Selection

1. *Younger/smaller children (infants):* Although a set age criterion for this procedure does not exist, the goal of the A/P cricoid split is to increase the diameter of the posterior larynx, thus creating an exponential increase in airflow across the glottis and subglottis. Because a very small increase in the patency of the airway in younger/smaller children creates a proportionally large increase in the overall percentage of the cross-sectional area of the glottis available for airflow, this intervention is thought to be most effective during infancy.
2. *Able to maintain spontaneous ventilation while sedated in the OR:* Although a small breathing tube can be inserted and removed at intervals during the procedure, exposure of the larynx requires the patient to be extubated while performing the anterior and posterior cricoid incisions.
3. *Tracheostomy candidates*: Typically, this procedure is performed with the goal of avoiding tracheostomy in patients who would otherwise require it to bypass dynamic obstruction at the level of the glottis and subglottis. For this reason, patients with bilateral vocal fold paralysis requiring intubation or positive airway pressure (PAP) to adequately ventilate are optimal candidates for the A/P cricoid split. Patients who ventilate adequately without pressure support and without requiring intubation are thus NOT ideal candidates for this procedure. Additionally, patients who have fixed and/or severe glottic or subglottic narrowing, those with pulmonary disease that requires mechanical ventilatory support, and infants with neurologic dysfunction leading to central apnea, are poor candidates.

## Key Aspects of the Consent Process

- Risks typically associated with endoscopic airway procedures during infancy also apply to this operation and are not repeated in detail here.
- Endoscopic A/P cricoid split does NOT preclude the ability to perform tracheostomy in the future, and parents should be counseled thoroughly that A/P cricoid split is not universally effective. A future tracheostomy or other airway intervention may be required.
- Laryngeal stenosis at the incision site is thought to be a very rare occurrence when this procedure is performed appropriately but should still be discussed preoperatively.
- Because postoperative intubation is required, all risks associated with intubation should be discussed (not limited to airway management risks, laryngeal sequelae of intubation, infectious risks such as pneumonia, and possible sedation requirements).
- Temporary dysphagia related to the procedure, or ongoing dysphagia (often unrelated to the procedure) are possible.

## Operative Approach

### Equipment

- Suspension laryngoscopy equipment (Lindholm or Parson's laryngoscope, suspension arm, and table)
- Operating microscope

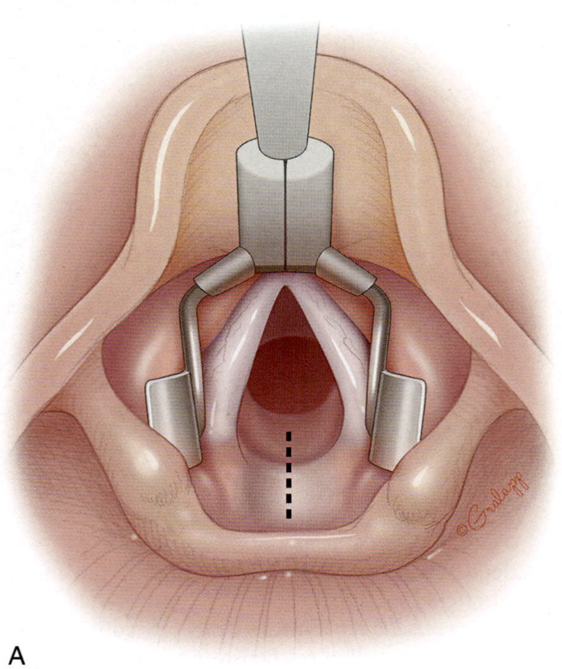


• **Fig. 10.1A** Exposure of the posterior cricoid plate with vocal fold spreaders reversed. (©2024 Chris Gralapp.)

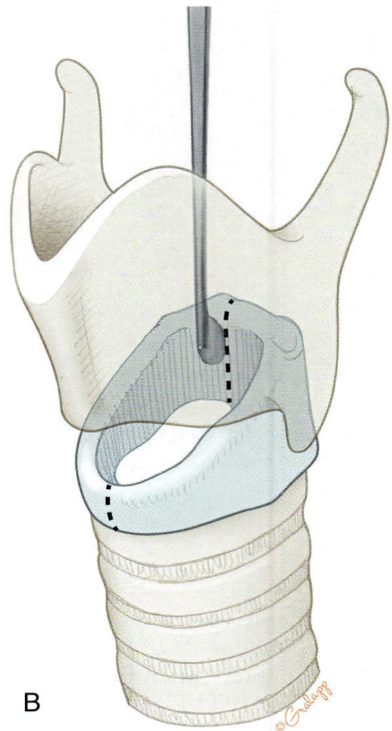


• **Fig. 10.1B** Illustration of D-knife being used to create the posterior cricoid incision. This can also be performed using a Sickle knife or Blitzer knife, and laryngeal scissors may be helpful to complete the incision. (©2024 Chris Gralapp.)

- Laryngeal spreaders
- Orotracheal injection device
- Microlaryngeal instruments:
  - Sickle Knife or Blitzer Knife
  - Microlaryngeal scissors (straight and upbiting)
  - Laryngeal spatula
- Laryngeal suction (variety of sizes)
- Laryngeal balloons
- Endotracheal tube(s)

**PEARL 10.1**

The procedure may be done with telescope visualization, particularly with a narrow-angled (30-degree) glass rod telescope. However, this is more challenging and removes the option of bimanual operation.

## Steps

1. Patient positioning: The patient is positioned supine with head at the top of the table. The table is turned 90 degrees with the patient's left side towards the anesthesiology provider. No shoulder roll is used. With young infants and patients with trisomy 21, take particular care not to overextend the neck. When properly exposed, the glottis and posterior supraglottis should be readily visible and accessible surgically.
2. Laryngeal exposure: A Lindholm laryngoscope is inserted, and the larynx is suspended. Oxygen flow is provided via a nasal cannula or entrained through an endotracheal tube sitting in the posterior pharynx or hypopharynx. Laryngeal spreaders are placed to allow for unobstructed visualization of the cricoid. Initially, the laryngeal spreader should be placed in an inverted fashion. A rubber band can be used to maintain the laryngeal spreaders in position, allowing for visualization of the posterior cricoid plate (Fig. 10.1A).
3. Operating Microscope: The operating microscope is brought in to allow for hands-free visualization and depth perception. Focal length is set to approximately 400 mm (Pearl 10.1).
4. The mucosa overlying the posterior cricoid plate is injected with a small volume (e.g., 0.1–0.2 mL) of 1% lidocaine with 1:100,000 parts epinephrine.
5. Creating the posterior incision (Fig. 10.1B): A D-knife, Sickle Knife or Blitzer Knife (disposable sickle knife, preferred for its ability to provide tactile feedback and extremely sharp cutting edge) is used to first make an incision in the posterior aspect of the cricoid plate (Pearl 10.2). Hemostasis can be achieved with oxymetazoline-soaked pledgets. The incision is carried through the entire length of the cricoid, ideally terminating at the level of the posterior cricoid perichondrium. Straight or upbiting scissors can be used to complete this incision at the inferior apex if needed. Unlike older patients or those with posterior glottic and subglottic stenosis, the posterior incision in infants is very easy to create, taking approximately 1 or 2 minutes to achieve. Caution must be exercised to avoid making the incision too deep. This is accomplished by using the instrument to constantly palpate along the length of the incision, feeling for islands of remaining cartilage prior to continuing the incision. When a complete excision is created, the posterior cricoid incision margins are visibly separate and mobile on palpation. If the separation of the posterior halves of the cricoid is not obvious, the incision is unlikely to be complete (Pearl 10.3).
6. Creating the anterior incision (Fig. 10.2A): After creating the posterior incision, the orientation of the laryngeal spreaders can be reversed to allow for visualization of the anterior

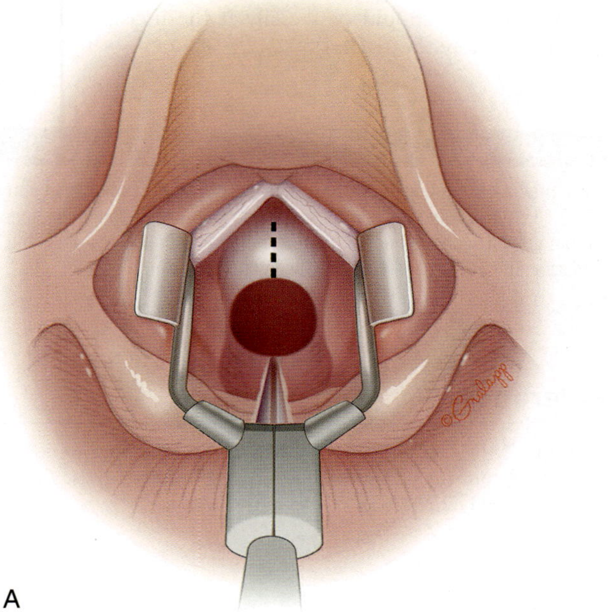


• **Fig. 10.2A** Exposure of the anterior cricoid plate with the vocal fold spreaders in normal position. Anterior pressure on the cricoid with the nondominant hand can help bring the anterior cricoid into view, if needed. (©2024 Chris Gralapp.)

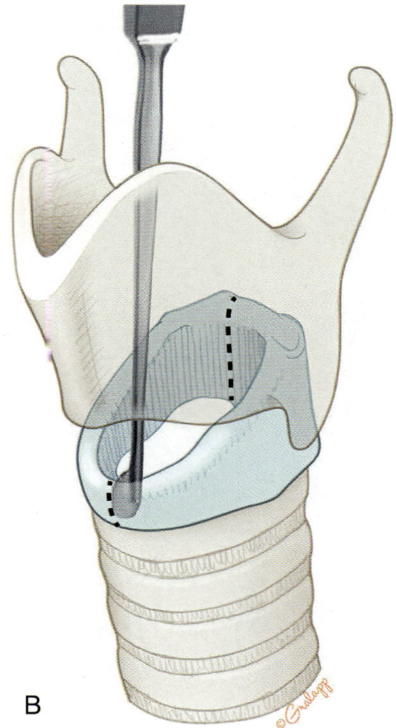


• **Fig. 10.2B** Visualization of the anterior cricoid incision being created with a D-knife. This can also be performed using a Sickle knife or Blitzer knife. (©2024 Chris Gralapp.)

**PEARL 10.2**

If needed, the Blitzer knife may be bent slightly toward the cutting edge using a heavy needle driver. This creates more "springiness" in the shaft of the instrument and allows the application of increased force against the cartilage. The surgeon must be even more careful about excessively deep incisions in this case.

**PEARL 10.3**

Ideally, the surgeon should see the posterior perichondrium intact behind the divided cartilage, as a smooth white layer. A blunt right-angle probe can be based into the esophageal inlet and used to palpate the split from behind to confirm no through-and-through defect has been created.

cricoid. If the anterior cricoid is not readily visible, gentle external pressure can be applied with the nondominant hand. Using the D-knife, Blitzer knife, or a sharp Sickle blade, the anterior cricoid ring is incised (Fig. 10.2B). This incision relieves the natural memory of the cricoid ring, which will otherwise push the margins of the posterior cricoid incision together.

7. Balloon Expansion (Fig. 10.3A): After completion of the cricoid incisions, a noncompliant airway balloon is placed across the subglottis, spanning the anterior and posterior incision sites. The balloon should be chosen by considering an airway diameter that is 0.5-size larger than an endotracheal tube that is age-appropriate for the child. For example, an infant with an age-appropriate 3.5 endotracheal tube airway should have a balloon chosen that approximates the outer diameter of a 4.0 Endotracheal tube (a 6 mm balloon would be used). The balloon is inflated and deflated, with the purpose of relieving any additional tissue bands creating tension on the incision sites (Fig. 10.3B). The balloon does not need to remain inflated as one would do in the setting of stenosis management.
8. After balloon dilation, the airway is visualized with a Hopkins rod, secretions are suctioned from the airway, and the patient is intubated with an endotracheal tube that is half a size larger

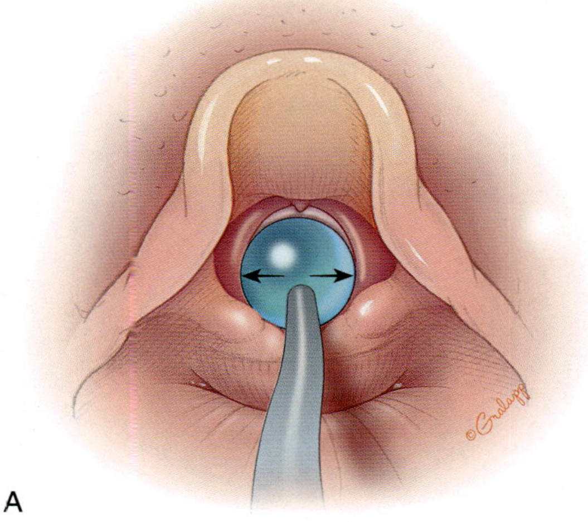


• **Fig. 10.3A** Laryngeal view of a noncompliant airway balloon used to expand the airway and relieve any remaining tension at the incision sites. (©2024 Chris Gralapp.)

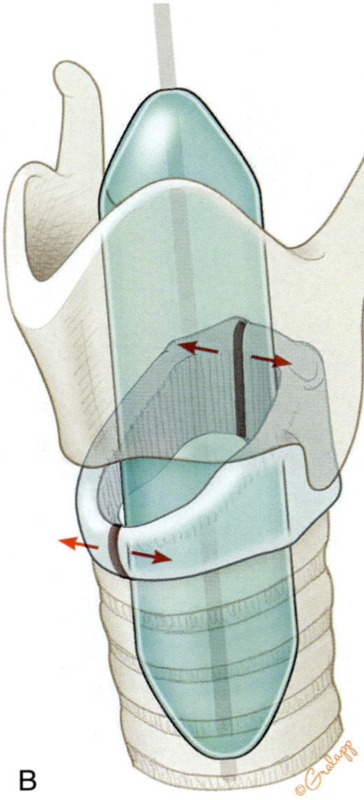

B

• **Fig. 10.3B** Illustration of the noncompliant airway balloon, traversing the cricoid incisions and providing lateral expansion at the incision sites. (©2024 Chris Gralapp.)

than an age-appropriate airway for that patient. The endotracheal tube should pass easily if the incisions were created appropriately (Pearl 10.4).

**PEARL 10.4**

The preferred duration of postoperative intubation varies between surgeons 7 to 10 days is common. It is reasonable to plan extubation in the operating room to allow debridement of granulation, further balloon dilation, and assessment of the healing of the divided portions of the cricoid.

## Reference

1. Rutter MJ, Hart CK, Alarcon A, et al. Endoscopic anterior-posterior **cricoid** split for pediatric bilateral vocal fold paralysis. *Laryngoscope.* 2018;128(1):257–263.

# 11

# Endoscopic Posterior Cricoid Split With Rib Graft

JOHN DAHL AND ANDY INGLIS

## Background

Subglottic stenosis (SGS), posterior glottic stenosis (PGS), and bilateral vocal fold immobility (BVFI) represent three distinct but potentially coexisting pathophysiologic processes that frequently require expansion augmentation of the posterior cricoid cartilage to relieve airway obstruction and improve airflow. Each of these processes presents surgeons with the challenge of creating an adequate airway while maintaining the patient's ability to protect their airway, swallowing function, and vocalization. Traditional approaches to address posterior glottic and subglottic narrowing are performed through an open transcervical approach, which has a significant number of risks, including, but not limited to, external scarring, negative impact of laryngofissure (if performed) on voice and swallowing, and the need for postoperative intubation or stenting.

The endoscopic posterior cricoid split with rib graft (EPCS/RG) procedure addresses SGS, PGS, and BVFI while reducing some of the potential complications associated with transcervical cricoid expansion procedures. The technique involves dividing the posterior cricoid cartilage using a $CO_2$ laser, endoscopic scissor, or knife and placing a costal cartilage graft under microscopic or endoscopic visualization. The EPCS/RG approach does not require a laryngofissure and allows for accurate placement of the posterior cricoid costal cartilage graft. Controversy exists in the literature regarding the need for a tracheostomy to be in place prior to performing the EPCS/RG procedure (Pearl 11.1); because a graft could become dislodged with catastrophic airway consequences in the early postoperative period, the vast majority of cases reported were performed with a tracheostomy in place (Pearl 11.2). Available data from multiple centers indicate that the EPCS/RG procedure has the best outcomes, determined by decannulation rates, for patients with SGS and PGS compared to those with BVFI.

**PEARL 11.1**

Notably, the presence (or absence) of a tracheostomy tube will not preclude graft dislodgement; a subset of patients who do not have a stent (or endotracheal tube) in place during the initial 7 to 10 days following surgery will experience displacement of the graft. While rare, graft dislodgement with a stent in place has also been described.

**PEARL 11.2**

In our practice, many patients have had preexisting tracheostomy due to the airway obstruction for which the graft is being placed. However, the operation can certainly be done with spontaneous ventilation and without tracheostomy in patients with adequate pulmonary reserve; in that case, patients are usually kept intubated for 7 to 10 days postoperatively to support the graft during initial healing.

## Operative Approach

### Patient Selection

Patients with SGS, PGS, or BVFI who are tracheostomy dependent or have significant respiratory symptoms secondary to airway pathology may be candidates. In contrast, patients with high grade 3 (pinhole airway) or grade 4 SGS, or those with an anterior stenosis, are not usually appropriate candidates for the EPCS/RG procedure. For patients without a tracheostomy in place, the attending surgeon must determine, in conjunction with the patient/family, if a tracheostomy should be placed at the time of EPCS/RG procedure.

Before proceeding with the EPCS/RG procedure, patients should have:

- Full assessment of voice and swallowing, neurologic limitations, cardiac and pulmonary function, esophageal pathology (eosinophilic esophagitis [EOE], gastroesophageal reflux disease [GERD]), and obstructive sleep apnea.
- Detailed awake fiberoptic laryngeal endoscopy, including detailed assessment of vocal fold mobility, with video documentation.
- Detailed laryngoscopy under anesthesia documenting ability to achieve adequate exposure, active and passive vocal fold mobility (Pearl 11.3), subglottic or other laryngeal stenosis, posterior glottic anatomy including presence of cleft, and sizing of subglottic airway with uncuffed endotracheal tubes per Myer and Cotton, with photo/video documentation.

**PEARL 11.3**

Palpation of the cricoarytenoid joints is the standard method to assess passive motion; active motion may not be accurately reflected under general anesthesia.

- Full endoscopic assessment of the tracheobronchial tree looking for concurrent pathologies such as suprastomal granulomas, tracheomalacia, etc.

## Key Aspects of the Consent Process

- Risks of general anesthesia
- Risks of injury to oral, pharyngeal, and airway structures
- Laser risks including airway fire
- Risks of costal graft harvest including pain, hematoma, and pneumothorax
- Graft dislodgement which could result in acute, severe airway obstruction, especially in patients who do not have a tracheostomy in place
- Graft failure (resorption, infection, etc.)
- Aspiration
- Dysphonia
- Inadequate expansion of the posterior cricoid cartilage

## Equipment

- Appropriately sized Lindholm or other wide-field laryngoscope. Laryngoscopes designed to have their tips placed in the vallecula generally provide the best exposure
- Hopkins rod telescope (0 degree, 40 degree), 4 mm and 2.8 mm
- Equipment to spray medications on larynx
- Self-retaining ratcheting laryngeal retraction forceps, aka "laryngeal spreaders" or "Lindholm laryngeal distending forceps" (required) (Fig. 11.1)
- Uncuffed endotracheal tubes of varying diameters for airway sizing
- Operating microscope with laser micromanipulator, laryngeal D-knife, or beaver blade on an extra-long handle
- $CO_2$ laser and associated laser safety equipment (required if using laser)
- Microlaryngeal instruments, including right angled probe and heavyweight microlaryngeal alligator forceps (required)
- Instrument set for harvesting and carving costal cartilage graft (required)
- Suture and dressing for closing costal cartilage donor site (surgeon preference) (required)
- Penrose drain for costal cartilage donor site
- 15- and 11-blades and teflon block for carving costal cartilage graft
- 5-0 prolene suture for use as a safety suture during graft placement
- 2% lidocaine without epinephrine
- 0.5% Marcaine without epinephrine
- 1% lidocaine with epinephrine
- Laryngeal injection needle

## Steps

### *Repeat Diagnostic Endoscopy*

- Perform microdirect laryngoscopy, arytenoid palpation, airway sizing as described earlier
- Obtain photo documentation of the airway subsites prior to any interventions
- At this point, some may prefer to remove the laryngoscope and harvest the rib graft before performing the cricoidotomy. Because difficulties may be encountered performing the cricoidotomy via the endoscopic approach, the authors generally perform the cricoidotomy first.

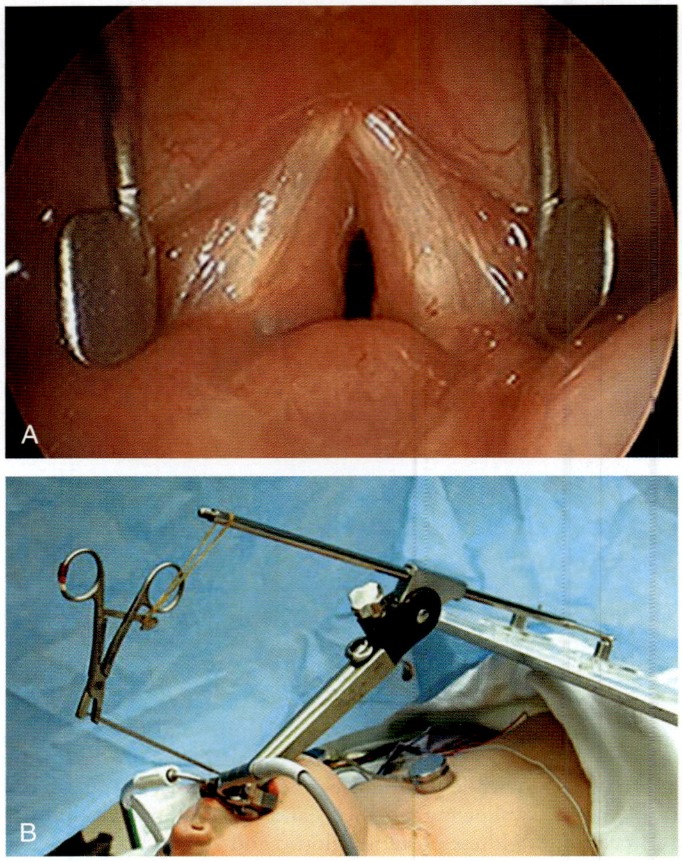


• **Fig. 11.1** Inverted laryngeal distending forceps. Distending forceps are inverted; blades are placed in the posterior laryngeal ventricles: handle is gently suspended with rubber band.

- The cricoidotomy can be performed either with a $CO_2$ laser/micromanipulator or endoscopically with "cold steel." The surgeon's choice may depend on personal comfort with the different techniques, as well as equipment/staffing availability and patient factors.

## Endoscopic Cricoid Split Using $CO_2$ Laser

- 1% lidocaine with 1:100,000 epinephrine is infiltrated submucosally into the interarytenoid region and over the posterior cricoid plate to minimize bleeding.
- If a tracheostomy tube is present, a metal tracheotomy tube (Pearl 11.4) is placed into the stoma and the insufflation channel on the laryngoscope is set to suction. Other standard laser precautions are set in place.

**PEARL 11.4**

A laser-safe endotracheal tube may also be used through the tracheostoma, if the patient's airway is large enough.

- A $CO_2$ laser in a continuous high-energy, "thermal relaxation" pulse mode with settings of 150 mJ/pulse at 10 pulses/sec through a micromanipulator with a 0.4 mm spot size is used to divide the anterior fibers of the interarytenoid musculature.

When setting up the laser, the goal is to produce the smallest spot size and minimal char to the cartilage.

- The remaining interarytenoid muscle fibers are then retracted posteriorly using a "stout" microlaryngeal alligator forceps or straight suction, exposing as much of the superior rim of the posterior cricoid as possible.
- The $CO_2$ laser is then used to divide the posterior lamina of the cricoid cartilage, working anterosuperiorly to posteroinferiorly. Exposure is best achieved using one hand to gently lift the distal airway by picking up the tracheotomy tube and the other hand using a suction or alligator forceps to retract the superior portion of the posterior lamina of the cricoid posteroinferiorly. This has the effect of rotating the cricoid cartilage at a more *en face* angle and allows the surgeon to better align the incision straight down the airway. This maneuver requires setting the laser spot in a convenient location and releasing the joystick.
- As the cricoidotomy continues inferiorly, the cartilage is distracted by increasing the spread on the distending forceps and by spreading the cut surfaces with alligator forceps.

## Endoscopic Cricoid Split Using "Cold Steel"

- Local anesthetic containing epinephrine is infiltrated submucosally into the interarytenoid region and over the posterior cricoid plate to minimize bleeding.
- Some surgeons may prefer to perform the cricoidotomy with a laryngeal D-knife or other sharp instrument (Pearl 11.5). Visualization during cricoidotomy may be enhanced with an angled telescope.

**PEARL 11.5**

A combination of available instruments is often desirable, as each patient differs in the degree of laryngeal scarring, thickness of the cricoid plate, and laryngeal exposure, among other factors. The use of laryngeal scissors is often helpful, due to their ability to provide tactile feedback, precisely engage the remaining posterior cricoid attachments, and be used within the cricoid defect to assess for cricoid expansion. Of note, when the cricoid plate is completely incised posteriorly, the change (ability to expand the cricoid in the defect) is not subtle. If this is not the case, then there is likely a residual bridge of posterior cricoid remaining.

- Finding a suitable knife for dividing the posterior lamina of the cricoid can be problematic: the blade must be sharp enough to easily cut the cricoid, the handle long enough to reach the bottom of the cricoid, the shaft thin enough to see around either with the microscope or telescope, and the shaft stiff enough to allow adequate downward pressure on the blade of the knife (Pearls 11.6 and 11.7).

**PEARL 11.6**

A bent Blitzer knife can be useful in this setting. The Blitzer knife is a disposable sickle knife that is extremely sharp and provides excellent tactile feedback to the surgeon.

**PEARL 11.7**

The inferiormost portion of the cricoid is often left undivided by less experienced surgeons. It is important to palpate this area with a right-angled probe to ensure complete division of the posterior cricoid.

## Laryngeal Assessment Following Completion of Cridoidotomy

- Distract the cut edges of the cricoid and assess the stiffness of the cricoid. Examine the esophageal mucosa for injury from the laryngeal side directly, and from the esophageal side by passing a blunt probe into the esophageal introitus and gently tenting the mucosa anteriorly between the edges of the cricoidotomy.
- Estimate the degree of cricoid expansion required in millimeters. This can be facilitated by holding a right-angled probe horizontally in the cricoidotomy and comparing desired expansion to the known length of the end of the probe (Fig. 11.2). In general, the maximal graft width that can be inserted is roughly equal to the length of the membranous vocal folds (Pearl 11.8).
- Obtain photo documentation.

**PEARL 11.8**

At this point, some surgeons use an otologic round knife or other instrument to create "pockets" between each of the divided halves of the posterior lamina and the perichondium on its posterior aspect. This creates space for the graft flanges behind the cricoid cartilage and makes graft insertion easier in some cases.

## Harvest Costal Cartilage Graft

- The costal cartilage donor site is prepped and draped in a sterile manner.
- An incision is made along the lower costal margin of the sixth rib on the right side in the presumed location of the inframammary fold.
- The entire segment of cartilaginous sixth rib is harvested (Fig. 11.3). This will be adequate for two grafts, which provides redundancy should there be a problem with the carving of the first graft.
- The wound is closed in layers. A Penrose drain can be placed per surgeon preference.
- An intercostal nerve block is then performed by injecting 0.5% Marcaine without epinephrine to the inferior aspect of the eighth and ninth ribs.

## Carve the Costal Cartilage Graft

- The goal is to produce a piece of cartilage that is wide enough to provide adequate expansion (Pearl 11.9), will be shaped such that it will seat securely and not migrate, and will be successfully incorporated into the laryngeal framework. Ideally, the graft will have stout posterior flanges to prevent it from migrating anteriorly and at least a lip or anterior flange

**PEARL 11.9**

As with the creation of all costal grafts in laryngeal framework surgery, one can expect the loss of a small percentage of width of the graft following surgery. While this must be considered, the consequences of overexpansion, namely pulmonary aspiration and breathy dysphonia, should not be underappreciated. A balance must be achieved between improving airway patency and maintaining pulmonary health and a serviceable voice.

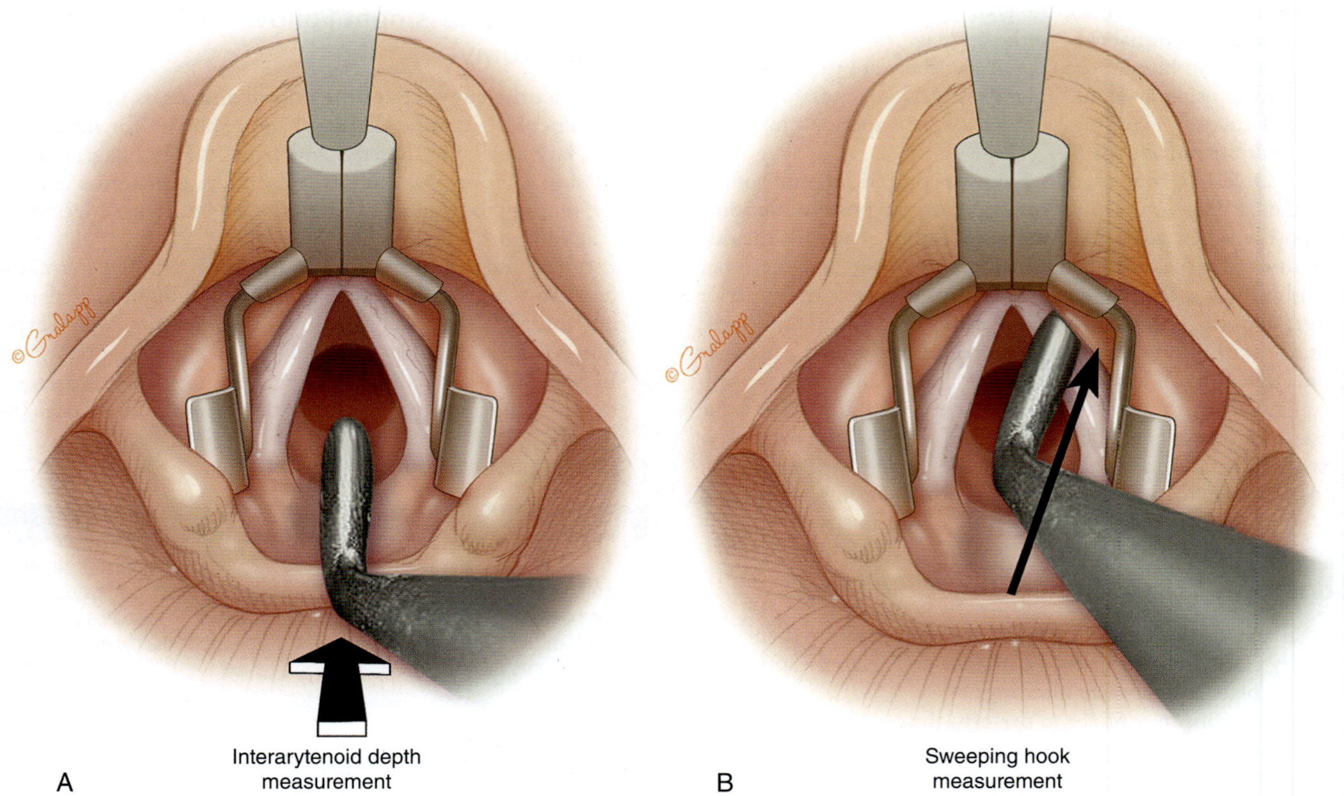


• **Fig. 11.2** Assessing the degree of distraction with a right-angle probe. Following completion of the cricoidotomy, the larynx is examined with an angled telescope, the esophageal mucosa inspected, and the desired distraction is estimated by comparing to the length of a tip of an angled forceps. (©2024 Chris Gralapp.)

to prevent it from slipping posteriorly (Fig. 11.4). To accomplish this, the rib must be thicker than the posterior lamina of the cricoid.

- Traditionally, the cartilage is carved with the long axis of the rib running vertically in the larynx. This severely limits the amount of expansion possible, especially if both a posterior flange and anterior lip are present (Pearl 11.10).

**PEARL 11.10**

If the graft is to be placed vertically, some surgeons cut the cranial end of the graft into a point or "house" shape to allow the graft to wedge into the remaining interarytenoid muscle, if present.

- An alternative is to fashion the graft so it is placed with the long axis horizontally (Fig. 11.4). With this approach, there is no practical limit to the degree of expansion one can achieve, and more secure flanges can be produced. The downside, which is of unclear significance, is that the graft will not be long enough to contact the entire length of the cricoidotomy. Steps for this latter style of graft are as follows:
- When maximal distraction is desired, the graft is trimmed to a width slightly less than the length of the vocal cords (as estimated using the right-angle probe). Graft length ranges from 6 to 10 mm in total length depending on the size of the patient.

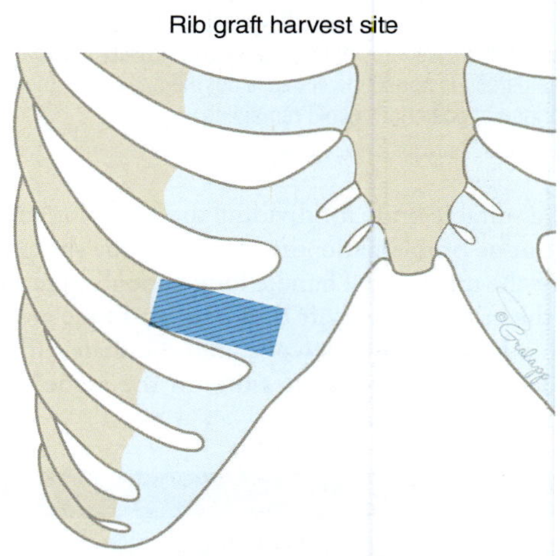


• **Fig. 11.3** Site of rib graft harvest. (©2024 Chris Gralapp.)

- An 11-blade is used to carve precise grooves on both sides of the graft, producing posterior flanges in a "keystone" shape. The distance from the anterior face of the posterior flange to the anterior face of the graft should be greater than the thickness of the cricoid lamina.

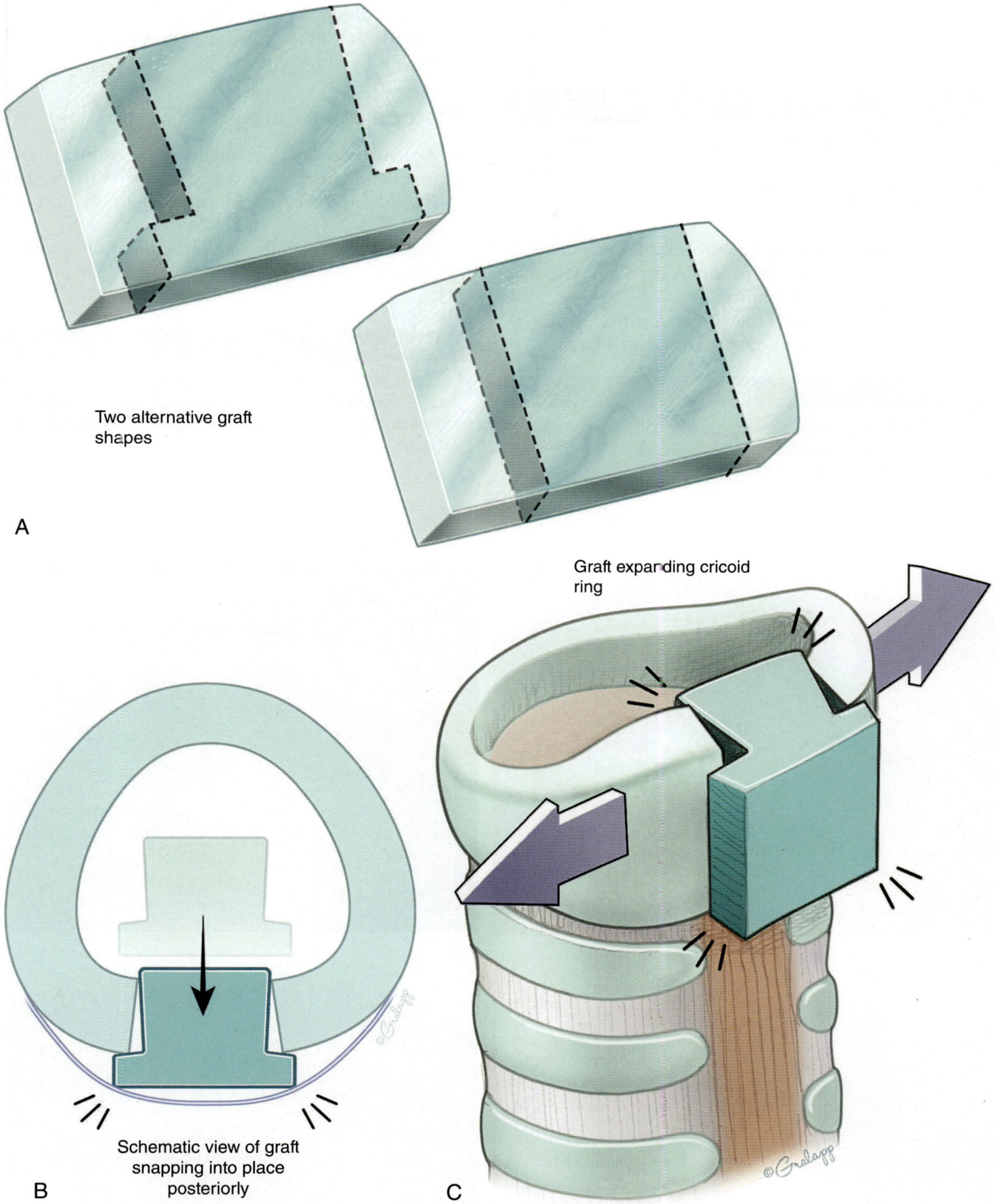


• **Fig. 11.4** Graft flange geometry: The graft (*blue*) needs to snap securely in place in the gap in the cricoid (*gray*). Total thickness of the graft must be equal to the thickness of the cricoid plus the thickness of the posterior flange and the anterior lip of the graft. (©2024 Chris Gralapp.)

- A 5-0 prolene "safety suture" is placed through the superior part of the graft and secured with a loose loop. This is used to retrieve the graft should it fall below the larynx during graft placement.
- Obtain photo documentation.

## Costal Cartilage Graft Placement

- This step is performed under microscopic visualization.
- The graft is grasped with "heavyweight" microlaryngeal forceps (e.g., Benjamin microlaryngeal forceps, Karl Storz), and one flange of the graft is inserted posterior to the cricoid cartilage (Fig. 11.5).

- The forceps are then used to apply pressure on the endolaryngeal surface of the graft to insert the second flange posterior to the cricoid cartilage (Pearl 11.11).

**PEARL 11.11**

If the graft is not fully seated, once the flanges are engaged behind the cricoid, an airway dilation balloon catheter may be used to place even, firm pressure on the graft to seat it more posteriorly.

- Distending forceps are removed; degree of expansion is assessed: stability of graft confirmed via palpation. A laryngeal stent may be placed when graft stability is uncertain.
- The loop on the safety suture is then divided with microlaryngeal scissors and removed from the patient (Pearl 11.12).

**PEARL 11.12**

Some surgeons place an endoscopic suture in the interarytenoid mucosa to help secure the graft; it is unclear whether this adds value.

- Obtain photo documentation.
- Metal trach tube replaced with appropriately sized standard trach tube (if present).

## Postoperative Care

- Patients with mature tracheotomy stomas may be observed in a ward bed for a few days prior to discharge. Others should be observed in intensive care unit (ICU) (Pearl 11.13).
- Patients eating orally should be place on a soft or full liquid diet.

**PEARL 11.13**

If a patient does not have a tracheostomy and instead has a "single stage" operation with postoperative intubation, they should be returned to the operating room for endoscopy and possible extubation in 7 to 10 days.

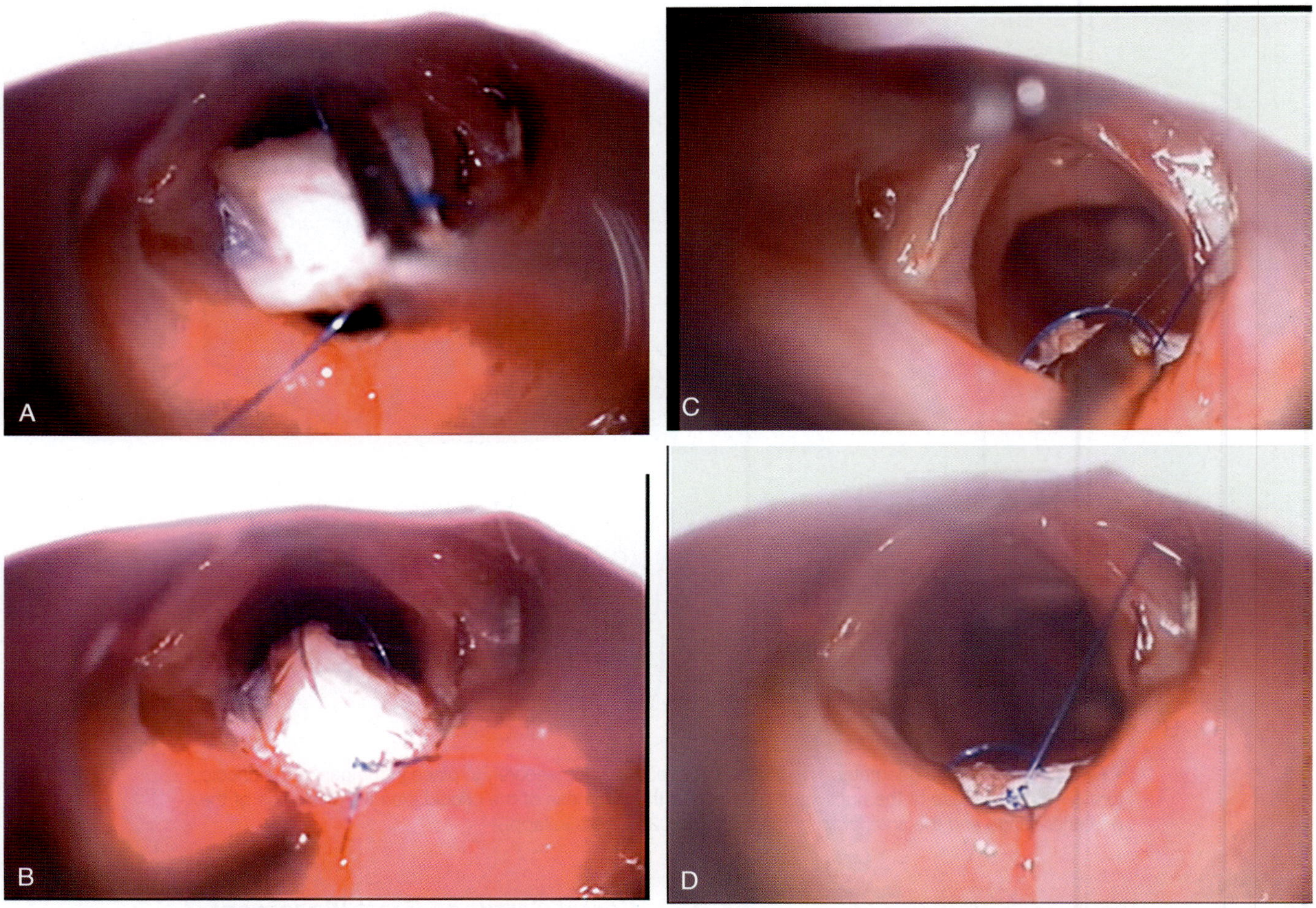


• **Fig. 11.5** Graft insertion. (A) Graft with safety suture is inserted through glottis. (B) The right posterior flange is engaged behind cricoid lamina. (C) Alligator forceps, with jaws splayed, push and rotate the left side of graft in place. (D) Appearance of graft prior to releasing the distending forceps and removal of safety suture.

# 12

# Endoscopic Management of Subglottic Cysts

NICHOLAS JAMES SMITH

## Background

Pediatric subglottic cysts are an uncommon but increasingly known cause of airway obstruction in infants.[1] While congenital cysts have been reported, subglottic cysts occur almost exclusively in premature infants with a history of endotracheal intubation.[2] It is hypothesized that cyst formation results from fibrosis and trauma following intubation, leading to obstruction of submucosal mucus gland ducts. Symptoms of subglottic airway obstruction include inspiratory or biphasic stridor, apnea, recurrent croup, and feeding problems. Although a diagnosis can be made with flexible laryngoscopy in an office setting, the gold standard for diagnosis and management is microlaryngoscopy and bronchoscopy with intervention.[3]

The current treatment of choice for symptomatic subglottic cysts is endoscopic marsupialization with cold steel instruments, lasers, or monopolar cautery with the Bugbee fulgurating electrode. This chapter focuses on endoscopic operative management of subglottic cysts (Video 12.1).

## Operative Endoscopic Assessment and Approach

### Patient Selection

Patients with clinical suspicion of subglottic airway obstruction based on clinical history will benefit from formal endoscopic assessment.

### Key Aspects of the Consent Process

Standard risks of operative airway endoscopy should be discussed, including:

- Risks of general anesthesia
- Risks of injury to oral, pharyngeal, and airway structures
- Airway fire if cautery or laser is used
- Postoperative stridor usually resolving in 12 to 24 hours; may last longer in patients with hypotonia or other neurologic problems

### Equipment

- Appropriately sized laryngoscope (Miller or Wisconsin)
- Appropriately sized rigid pediatric ventilating bronchoscope (Storz) with Hopkins rod telescope (Fig. 12.1)
- Equipment to spray medications (lidocaine) on larynx
- Depending on method:
  - Bugbee fulgurating electrode (cautery) (Pearl 12.1)
  - $CO_2$ laser fiber
  - Optical forceps

**PEARL 12.1**

If Bugbee is not available at your institution, there are a variety of neurosurgical electrodes that function similarly and are highly effective.

### Steps

The reference standard for diagnosis of subglottic cysts is rigid airway endoscopy performed under general anesthesia. Steps for this assessment and management are as follows:

1. Patient positioning: The patient is positioned supine with the head at the top of the operating table. The table is turned 90 degrees with the patient's left side toward the anesthesiology provider. A shoulder roll may be used. If the patient's head tends to roll to one side or the other, a rolled towel or gel donut can be placed around the head. With young infants and patients with trisomy 21, take particular care not to overextend the neck (Pearl 12.2). When properly exposed, the glottis and subglottis should be readily visible and accessible surgically.

**PEARL 12.2**

This is a salient point, as patients with trisomy 21 often have mild laryngeal narrowing when compared to age-matched controls, and are thus at higher risk for intubation with an endotracheal tube that is too large for the larynx. As such, cysts may be more common in this population.

2. Laser: If laser is to be used, the appropriate generator and fiber should be attached to the bronchoscope and correct function confirmed. Laser safety precautions should include protecting the patient with wet eye pads and wet

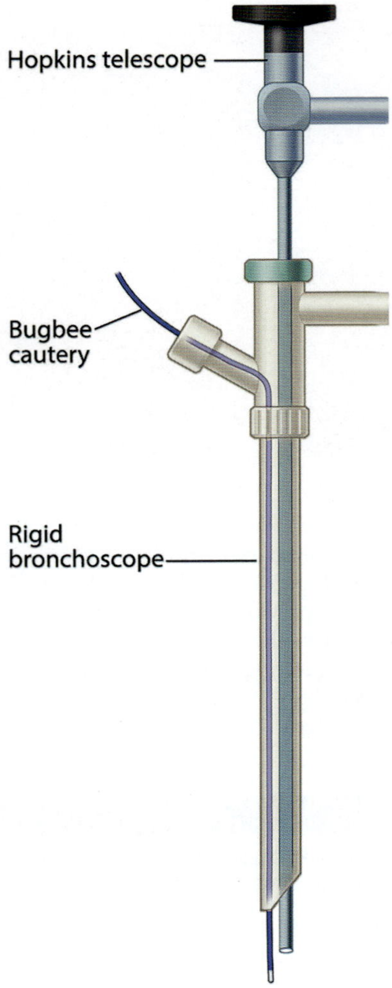


• **Fig. 12.1** Pediatric ventilating bronchoscope. (© 2024 Chris Gralapp.)

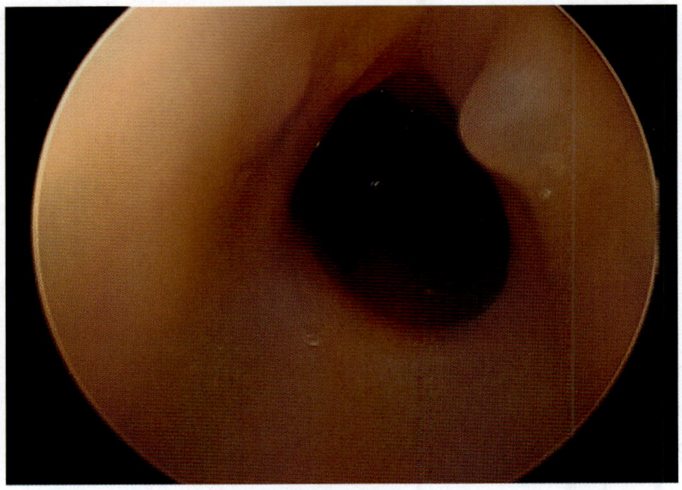

• **Fig. 12.2** Subglottic cyst visualized using 4-mm Hopkins rod telescope.

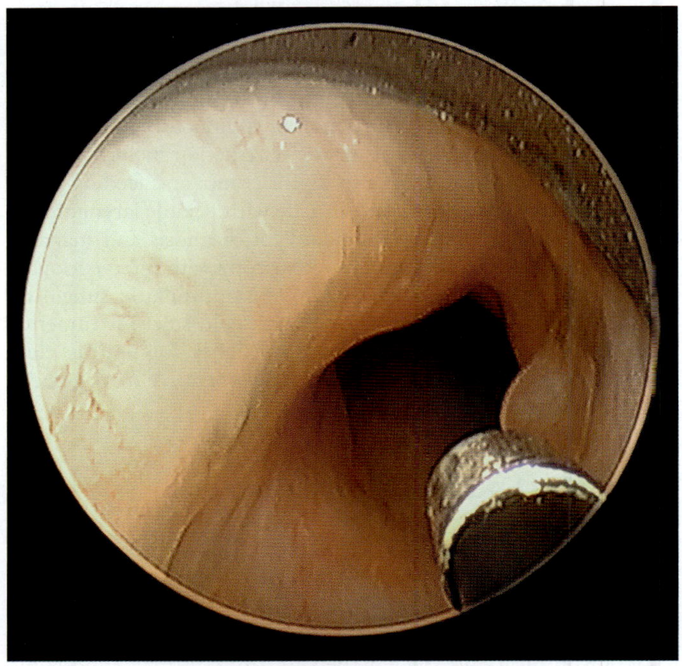

• **Fig. 12.3** Bugbee cautery of subglottic cyst using a 3.5-mm rigid bronchoscope.

towels to minimize the risk of laser scatter and burns. Any exposed tissue can be damaged by the laser, including the teeth. Inspired oxygen fraction should be confirmed 30% or less. The laser should be tested to confirm correct function and good alignment with the visible aiming beam, and good function of any protective shutter. All personnel in the operating room should wear appropriate eye protection. An appropriate laser filter should be placed between the camera head and telescope.

3. Under telescopic visualization with Hopkins rod and after application of topical laryngeal anesthetic, the airway is systematically examined in detail while the patient's respirations remain spontaneous. Photodocumentation is taken of the supraglottis, glottis, subglottis, and trachea. The subglottic cyst is visualized as shown in Fig. 12.2 and Video 12.1.
4. The appropriately sized pediatric rigid bronchoscope is then attached to the telescope and inserted to the level of the glottis. The anesthesia circuit is connected to the bronchoscope for ventilation. The fraction of inspired oxygen ($FiO_2$) is lowered to less than 30% if laser or Bugbee cautery is utilized. The cyst is identified. The $CO_2$ laser fiber or Bugbee cautery is threaded through the suction port of the bronchoscope (Figs. 12.3 and 12.4). If using cautery, the cautery is set to 8 watts (Pearls 12.3 and 12.4). The cyst wall is blanched and perforated to marsupialize the cyst(s) (Fig. 12.5; Video 12.2). Mucoid fluid is expressed from the cyst. For patients with multiple subglottic cysts, nonobstructing cysts can be left unruptured to decrease the risk of scar formation (Pearl 12.5). If rigid

**PEARL 12.3**

An alternative setup, if rigid bronchoscopes or tracheoscopes are not available, is to use a suspension laryngoscope, such as the Lindholm, and grasp the Bugbee cautery electrode in an endoscopic forcep to manipulate it within the airway lumen.

**PEARL 12.4**

Alternatively, the Bugbee cautery can be passed through a large laryngeal suction (providing tip guidance/control) during the procedure.

**PEARL 12.5**

Some surgeons also inject steroid into the base of the cauterized cysts to decrease risk of scar formation; balloon dilation may also be used to express mucus from the treated cysts and flatten remaining nonobstructive cysts.

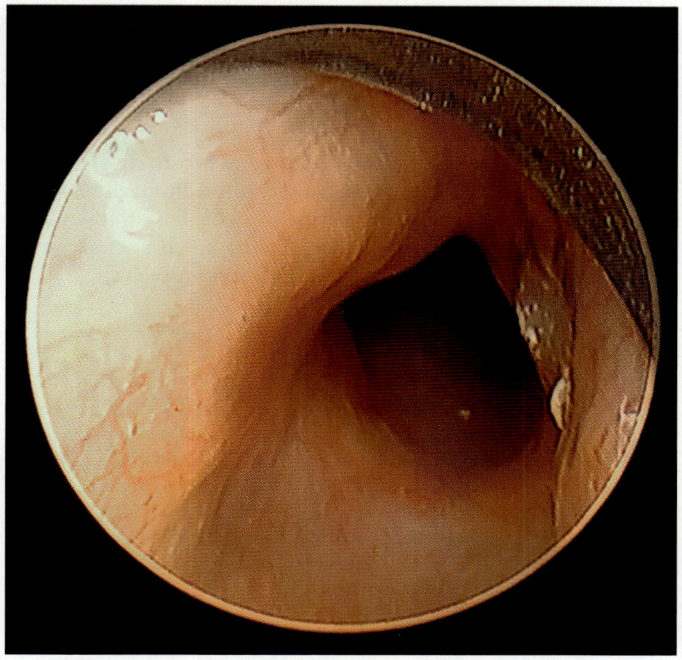

• **Fig. 12.5** Immediate postoperative photo after Bugbee cautery.

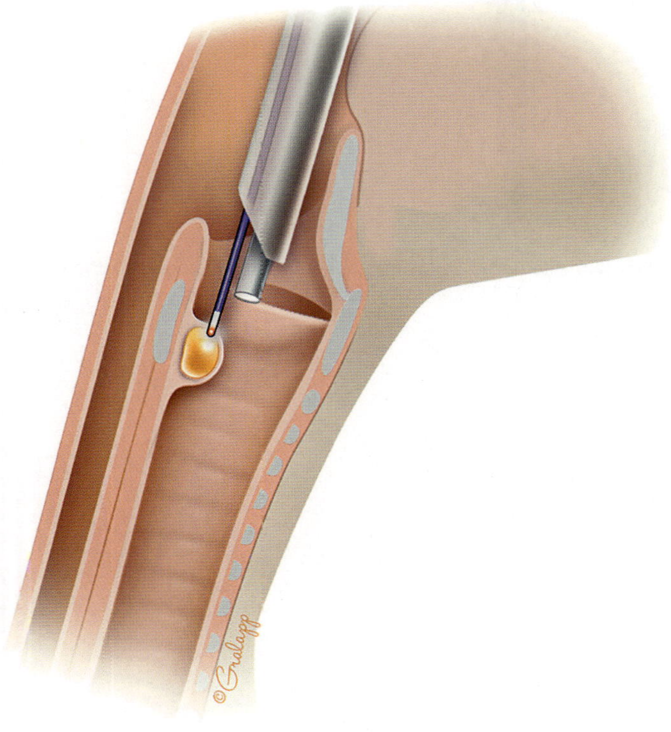

• **Fig. 12.4** Bugbee cautery of subglottic cyst. (© 2024 Chris Gralapp.)

bronchoscopes or tracheoscopes are not available, a suspension laryngoscope, such as a Lindholm laryngoscope, along with an alligator forceps or large laryngeal suction can be used to introduce the cautery electrode to the cyst within the airway lumen (Fig. 12.6).

5. Postoperative care: Patients without a tracheostomy are admitted postoperatively for airway observation, intravenous corticosteroids, and nebulizer treatments (corticosteroids and/or racemic epinephrine) as needed. Follow-up bronchoscopy is performed on an as-needed basis if symptoms recur.

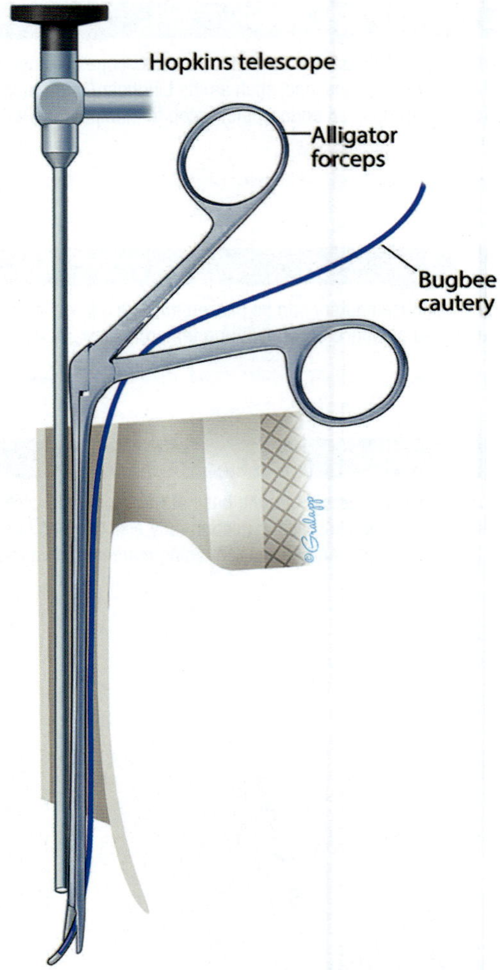


• **Fig. 12.6** Alternative setup for cautery of subglottic cyst without bronchoscope. (© 2024 Chris Gralapp.)

## References

1. Richardson MA, Winford TW, Norris BK, Reed JM. Management of pediatric subglottic cysts using the bugbee fulgurating electrode. *JAMA Otolaryngol Head Neck Surg*. 2014;140(2):164–168.
2. Couriel JM, Phelan PD. Subglottic cysts: a complication of neonatal endotracheal intubation? *Pediatrics*. 1981;68(1):103–105.
3. Steehler MK, Groblewski JC, Milmoe GJ, Harley EH. Management of subglottic cysts with mitomycin-C: a case series and literature review. *Int J Pediatr Otorhinolaryngol*. 2011;75(3):360–363.

# 13 Endoscopic Radial Incision, Dilation, and Injection for Stenosis

CATHERINE K. HART

## Background

In the early days of airway surgery, dilation was a primary means of management of airway stenosis. A variety of instruments were employed with variable results. As advances were made in open airway surgery in the late 20th century, dilation fell out of favor.[1,2] However, when balloon dilators were developed in the late 21st century, dilation experienced a resurgence and is now considered a mainstay for primary stenosis management as well as an adjuvant to open airway procedures.

## Operative Approach

### Patient Selection

Dilation is not effective for all types of stenosis. It is most useful for the management of intraluminal scarring, particularly thin, immature areas of scarring. Dilation can also be useful following open airway procedures to manage recurrent stenosis during the healing process. Areas of dense, mature scar are not as amenable to dilation. Similarly, dilation is not useful in cases where the airway framework or the exoskeleton of the airway is inadequate (e.g., lateral subglottic shelving, tracheal A-frame deformity, complete tracheal rings, or absence of tracheal cartilage) (Pearl 13.1). These cases require a more definitive expansion or resection procedure to correct the stenosis.

**PEARL 13.1**

In many cases, soft edematous stenosis is also not responsive to dilation; the edema simply recurs shortly after dilation.

### Key Aspects of the Consent Process

Standard risks of operative airway endoscopy should be discussed, including:

- Risks of general anesthesia
- Risks of injury to oral, pharyngeal, and airway structures.

Additional benefits and risks of dilation, radial incision, steroid injection:

- Many airway conditions can be managed via an endoscopic or open approach
- Essential to explain the risks and benefits of both approaches
- Endoscopic approach is often faster but usually needs to be repeated
- Prepare patient/family (and yourself) for the possibility that endoscopic approach may not be successful

### Equipment

- Appropriately sized laryngoscope with suspension
- Hopkins rod telescope (0 degree)
- Appropriately sized ventilating bronchoscope
- Equipment to spray medications on larynx
- Appropriately sized airway balloon dilator
- Microlaryngeal instruments, including a blade for scar incision
- Injection device for steroid injection

### Additional Equipment Notes

Ideally, a balloon dilator is used, as this allows for precise radial, high-pressure dilation without shear forces. Dilation can also be performed with endotracheal tubes or rigid dilators if a balloon dilator is not available.

It is important to select the appropriate-size balloon prior to the procedure. Balloon size is determined based on the age-appropriate airway diameter. Balloon size is determined by taking the outer diameter of the age-appropriate endotracheal tube and adding 1 to 2 mm for dilation of the larynx and 2 to 3 mm for dilation of the trachea. For example, if the child's airway should be sized with a 5.0 uncuffed endotracheal tube, which has an outer diameter of 6.2 mm, one would select an 8-mm balloon to dilate the larynx and a 9-mm balloon to dilate the subglottis or trachea (Pearl 13.2).

The disposable Blitzer blade is an excellent option, as it is always sharp and has a fine point that is easy to manipulate within the airway (Pearl 13.3).

**PEARL 13.2**

The ability to recognize different forms of subglottic narrowing, including framework abnormalities, or stenosis of endoluminal origin (boggy edema, immature scarring, and mature scar tissue) is imperative. This has implications when considering management options. If the presence or absence of a laryngeal framework abnormality is uncertain, the initial dilation can be performed with a smaller balloon first, with subsequent dilations as described herein.

**PEARL 13.3**

Because this instrument is disposable, the surgeon can also bend it slightly just behind the blade itself. This allows better access beyond a stenosis and increased leverage to cut fibrotic scar tissue.

If an injection device is not available, a butterfly needle and alligator forceps can also be used.

## Steps of the Procedure (Including Tips/Tricks)

1. The patient is positioned in the standard position for airway evaluation: supine on the operating table with the head at the top of the bed. The bed is typically rotated 90 degrees with anesthesia to the left of the patient.
2. As with any airway intervention, the initial step is to perform a thorough endoscopic examination of the airway. Once the airway and stenosis have been evaluated, it is necessary to decide if balloon dilation will be undertaken alone or if additional procedures will also be performed (Fig. 13.1).
3. To perform balloon dilation, the deflated balloon is passed into the airway and positioned under telescopic visualization through the stenosis so that the balloon spans the length of the stenosis (Fig. 13.2). Once in position, the balloon is inflated (Fig. 13.3). Each balloon comes with a designated burst

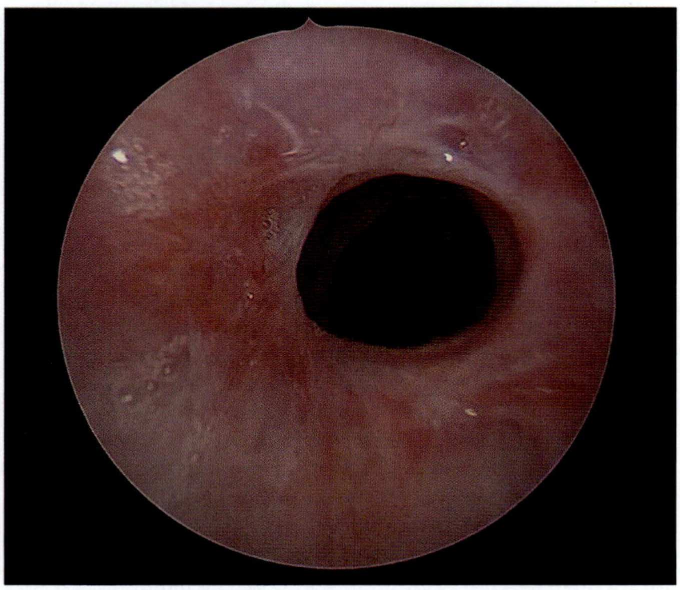

• **Fig. 13.1** Initial appearance of scar bands.

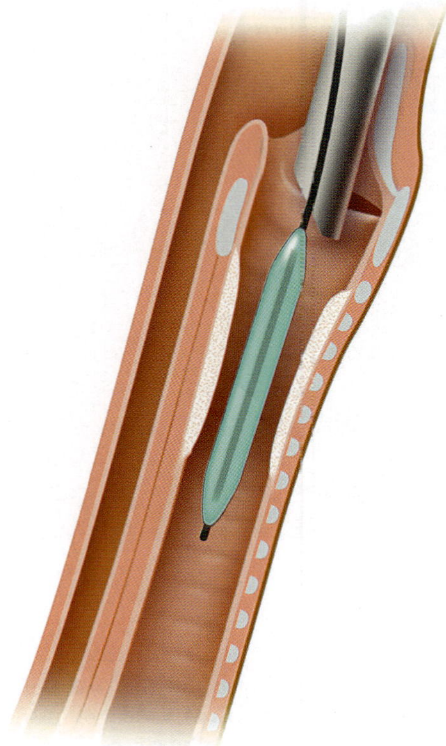

• **Fig. 13.2** Artist rendering of balloon dilator being passed into the airway with the balloon deflated. (© 2024 Chris Gralapp.)

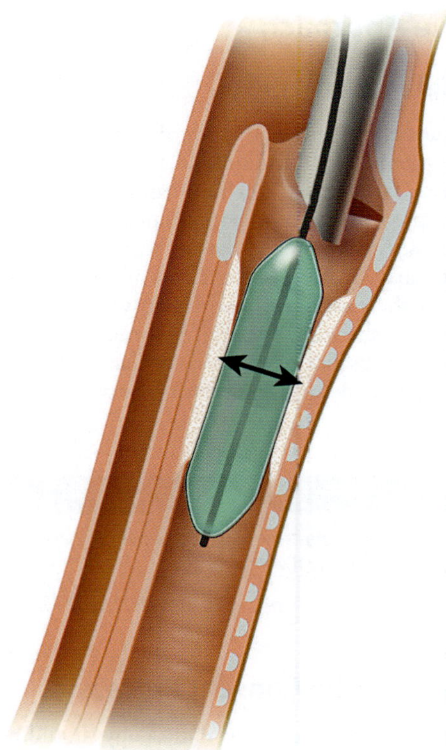

• **Fig. 13.3** Artist rendering of the balloon being inflated under direct visualization once it is in position. (© 2024 Chris Gralapp.)

## TIPS

- The surgical assistant who inflates the balloon should observe the needle on the manometer throughout the dilation. If the needle drops below the goal pressure, additional saline should be added to maintain adequate pressure (Pearl 13.4).
- If a patient cannot tolerate two minutes consecutive minutes of dilation, the balloon should be reinserted and reinflated for an additional period of time following reoxygenation of the patient.
- Although rare, in case of balloon malfunction, the surgeon should have a sharp endoscopic tool available to pop the balloon if it does not deflate properly. This can also be performed via a trans-tracheal approach if necessary (e.g., inserting a needle through the anterior neck and trachea, into the balloon).

## PEARL 13.4

An abrupt drop in pressure may suggest that either the balloon or the airway has ruptured.

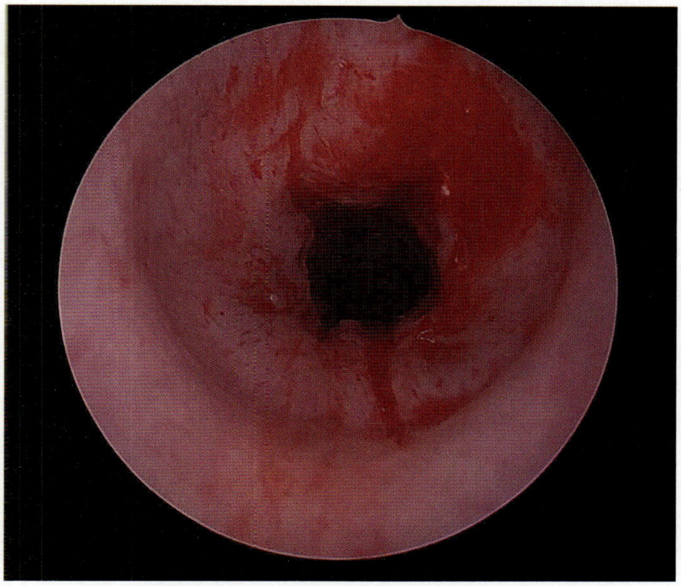

• **Fig. 13.4** Image of airway following intervention.

pressure, which determines the maximal amount of saline that should be instilled into the balloon. The duration of time for balloon dilation varies based on the patient's ability to maintain oxygenation and surgeon preference. Two minutes is the typical duration of time used for balloon dilation unless the patient desaturates prior to completing the entire duration of dilation. When dilation is complete, the balloon is deflated and removed (Video 13.1).

4. In circumstances in which steroid is to be injected, this can be performed prior to or after scar division and dilation. There is no substantial evidence to support one approach over another, and expert opinion varies. Regardless of timing, steroid is injected submucosally in a circumferential manner. This can be done using an orotracheal injection needle under direct visualization (Video 13.2). If no such device is available, a butterfly needle with the attached tubing can be used. The flanges of the needle must be trimmed to allow it to fit into the airway. Once trimmed, the edge of a flange is grasped with an alligator forceps, and this is passed into the airway under direct visualization with the telescope.
5. In circumstances where radial incision of the scar band is desired, this is usually performed prior to dilation. After completing the initial assessment of the airway, the patient can be placed into suspension to allow the surgeon to hold both the telescope and a blade. If there is a skilled assistant available, the assistant can hold the intubating laryngoscope in position to allow the surgeon to have two free hands.
6. Under endoscopic visualization, a blade is introduced and radial incisions are made through the scar band. Typically, three to four incisions are made in a circumferential manner to allow the scar to release more easily when dilated (Video 13.3) (Pearls 13.5 and 13.6).

## PEARL 13.5

It is important to remember that the purpose of the radial incisions, when coupled with dilation, is to provide a guided release of the scar tissue. Through-and-through incisions or resection of tissue are not necessary under most circumstances. If an incision is made that is not adequate, a deeper incision can always be made. On the contrary, if the lumen of the airway is violated, this may be a more difficult sequela to manage

## PEARL 13.6

It may be best to avoid incisions directed toward the posterior midline of the trachea, as this directs some of the dilation forces toward the membranous trachea, which is more prone to tear during dilation.

7. Balloon dilation is now performed using the steps described earlier (Video 13.4) (Pearl 13.7).

## PEARL 13.7

The precise order of operations (incision, injection, dilation) is not absolute. However, dilation after incision is logical, and dilation after injection has two benefits: (1) the dilation spreads the injected steroid further through the tissues; and (2) injection tends to bulk the tissues temporarily; dilation reverses this effect.

8. Upon completion of interventions, the airway is reassessed via endoscopy with photodocumentation, and sizing of the airway is repeated (Fig. 13.4).
9. In most cases, serial dilation with or without incision and injection is planned. These are typically spaced 1 to 3 weeks apart. It is important to recognize that if four or five dilations have been performed and the stenosis remains, a different treatment strategy should be considered.

## TIPS

- If there are multiple scar bands that need to be divided, it is best to divide the distal scar band first to avoid having bleeding that interferes with visualization during division of the proximal scar band. This is not always possible, however, if proximal stenosis is severe.
- If persistent bleeding occurs, pledgets soaked in oxymetazoline or dilute epinephrine can be held over the incisions to help achieve hemostasis.

## References


1. Santos D, Mitchell R. The history of pediatric airway reconstruction. *Laryngoscope*. 2010;120:815–820.
2. Cotton RT, Evans JN. Laryngotracheal reconstruction in children. Five-year follow-up. *Ann Otol Rhinol Laryngol*. 1981;90:516–520.

# 14

# Endoluminal Airway Stents

JUAN L. ANTON-PACHECO

## Background

Endoluminal airway stents are manufactured artificial hollow devices that are placed in the trachea or bronchi of patients in order to maintain lumen patency. In children, they are mainly used for treating tracheobronchial obstruction due to stenosis or malacia (Figs. 14.1 and 14.2). As a general rule, stenting is not a first-line treatment and is mostly used in very sick children when other surgical or endoscopic procedures have failed or are not indicated. Endoluminal airway stents are typically categorized by the material from which they are constructed. Accordingly, stents are divided into four major groups: (1) metallic stents; (2) plastic or silicone stents; (3) hybrid devices; and (4) biodegradable stents.

This chapter focuses on the endoscopic insertion technique of endoluminal airway stents, pointing out the differences in the procedures depending on the type of stent used.

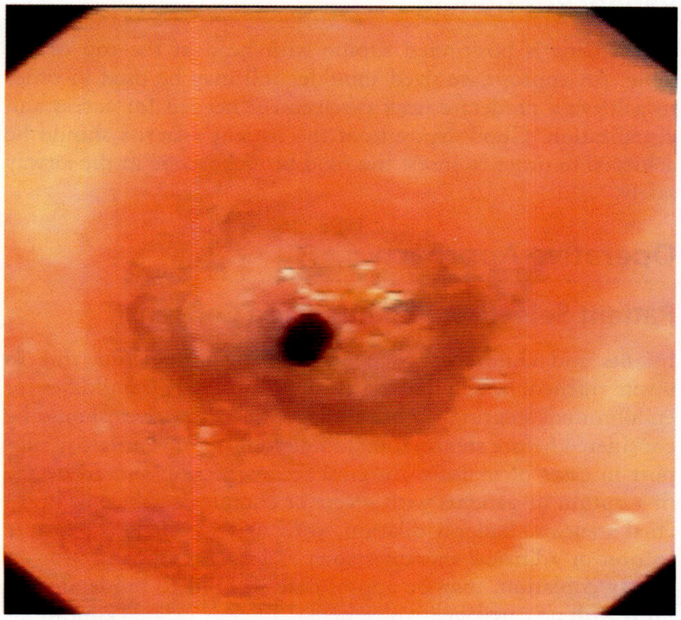

• **Fig. 14.1** Bronchoscopic image showing a tracheal stenosis.

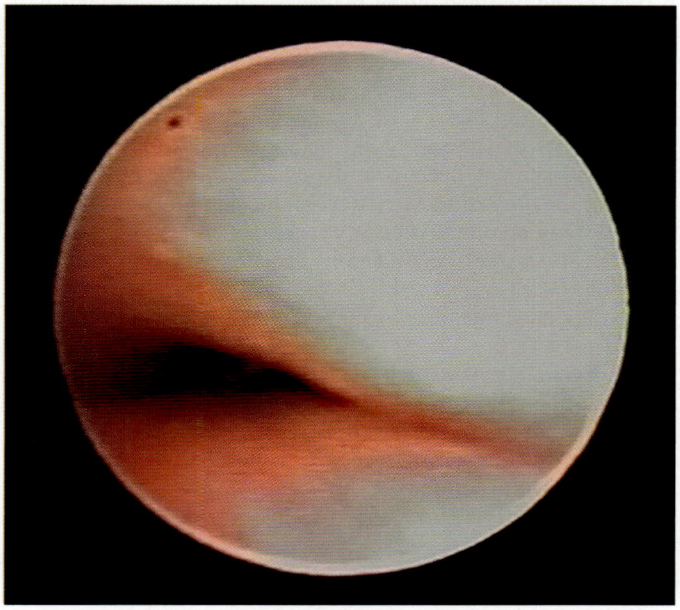

• **Fig. 14.2** Bronchoscopic image showing a case of tracheomalacia.

## Operative Endoscopic Assessment

### Patient Selection

Patients with severe central airway obstruction (trachea and/or main bronchi) in whom other therapeutic alternatives have failed may benefit from endoluminal stenting. This decision should ideally be made by a multidisciplinary team.

### Key Aspects of Informed Consent

Standard risks of interventional airway endoscopy should be addressed together with the specific stent-related potential complications, including:

- Granulation tissue formation
- Stent migration
- Mucous plugging
- Airway injury or erosion, including erosion into surrounding structures such as vessels or the esophagus
- Possibility of stent removal
- Stent degradation
- Need for additional procedures, possibly multiple

### Equipment

Operative assessment should be performed in the operating room, under general anesthesia, by an experienced team.

Endoscopic equipment should include:

- Laryngoscope (Miller and Macintosh) (Pearl 14.1)
- Appropriately sized flexible videobronchoscopes
- Pediatric set of rigid bronchoscopes and instrumentation
- Hopkins rod telescopes (0°)
- High-definition image technology
- Backup stents of other sizes and materials, if possible

**PEARL 14.1**

The editors often use suspension laryngoscopy with a Lindholm laryngoscope.

### Patient Positioning

The patient is positioned supine with head at the top of the table. An appropriate-sized shoulder roll may be used in order to achieve a moderate neck extension if needed for access and visualization. Good exposure of the patient´s larynx should be achieved in order to insert the rigid bronchoscope in the airway safely.

## Operative Approach

### Patient Selection and Informed Consent

Infants and children with central airway obstruction due to severe tracheobronchomalacia or stenosis may be candidates for endoluminal stenting. Other therapeutic alternatives should be considered before stenting, including long-term ventilatory support in cases of malacia. Surgical reconstruction should be the first option in patients with severe or complex tracheal or bronchial stenosis. Balloon dilation, with or without laser photoresection or adjuvant therapies such as local steroid injection or airway coblation, may be appropriate in mild to moderate stenosis with no cartilage involvement. Other associated conditions such as gastroesophageal reflux or recurrent tracheoesophageal fistula should be ruled out or managed adequately. Patients with syndromic airway malacia or associated cardiovascular anomalies, causing extrinsic airway compression, constitute a well defined subset of patients that may benefit from endoluminal stenting.

Parents or caregivers should be thoroughly informed about other management options and possible complications during and after the procedure. Certain complications are more prone to occur depending on the type of stent used:

- Metal mesh stents: granulation tissue formation, erosion, hazardous removal (Figs. 14.3–14.5)
- Plastic stents: mucous plugging, kinking, migration (Fig. 14.6, Video 14.1)
- Biodegradable stents: temporary relief of symptoms requiring re-stenting (Fig. 14.7).

With appropriate patient and stent selection, together with an uneventful insertion procedure, endoluminal airway stents may provide an immediate clinical improvement. However, close clinical surveillance with regular bronchoscopic explorations is mandatory.

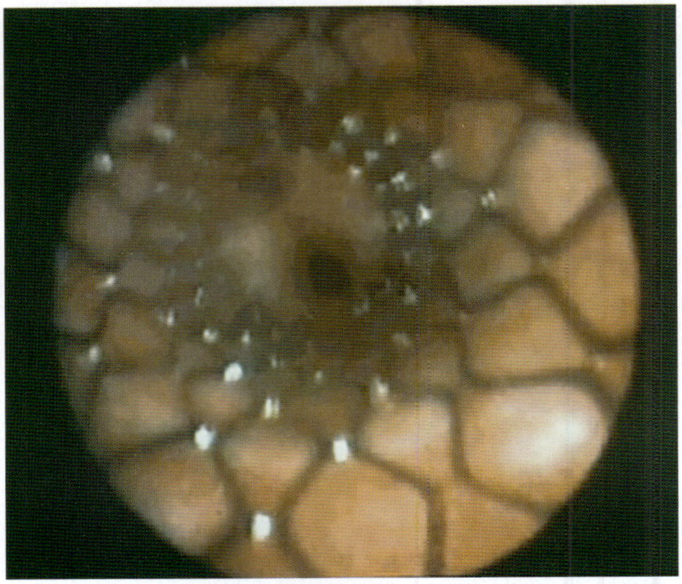

• **Fig. 14.3** Bronchoscopic view of a metallic stent in the trachea.

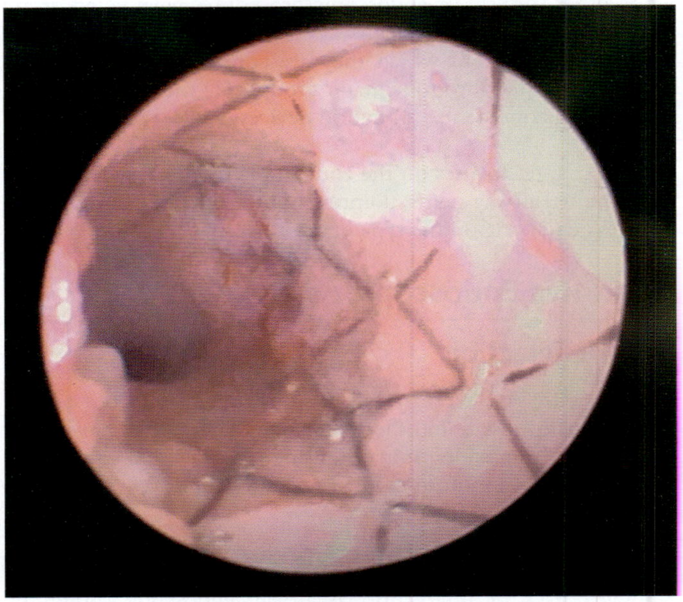

• **Fig. 14.4** Bronchoscopic view of a metallic stent in the left main bronchus.

### Equipment

As with endoscopic assessment discussed earlier, additional equipment includes:

- Rigid and semi-rigid endoscopic alligator forceps
- Suction catheters: rigid and flexible
- Fluoroscopy equipment (Pearl 14.2)
- Dedicated stent insertion devices
- Balloon dilation catheters

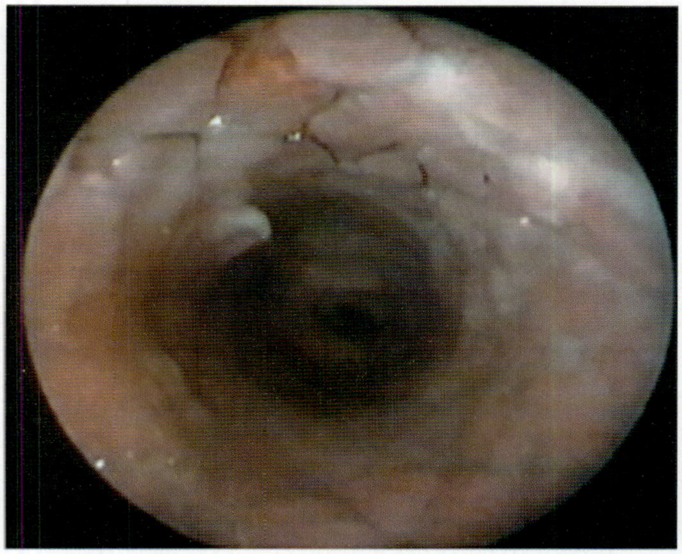

• **Fig. 14.5** Endoscopic image of mild granulation tissue caused by a metallic tracheal stent.

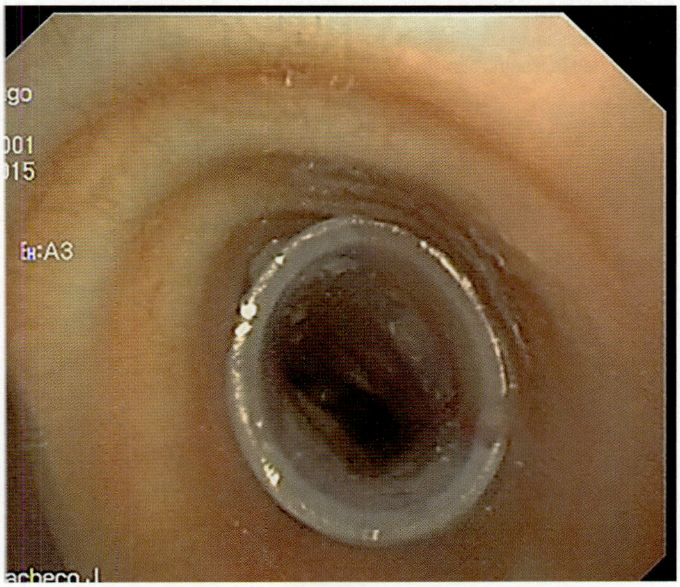

• **Fig. 14.6** Endoscopic image of a tracheal silicone stent.

**PEARL 14.2**

The use of fluoroscopy varies by surgeon; it is not a typical part of the editors' practice in stent placement.

## Operative Steps

The endoscopic technique of airway stenting may vary depending on the type of stent used. In infants and small children, metal mesh stents have been historically the most frequently used. Recently, biodegradable stents have gained popularity in some countries, and because of their advantages compared to other types of stents, they will probably have a main role in the future. Plastic stents are more frequently indicated in older children and adults, while hybrid stents usually require insertion devices that are too bulky for their use in small infants.

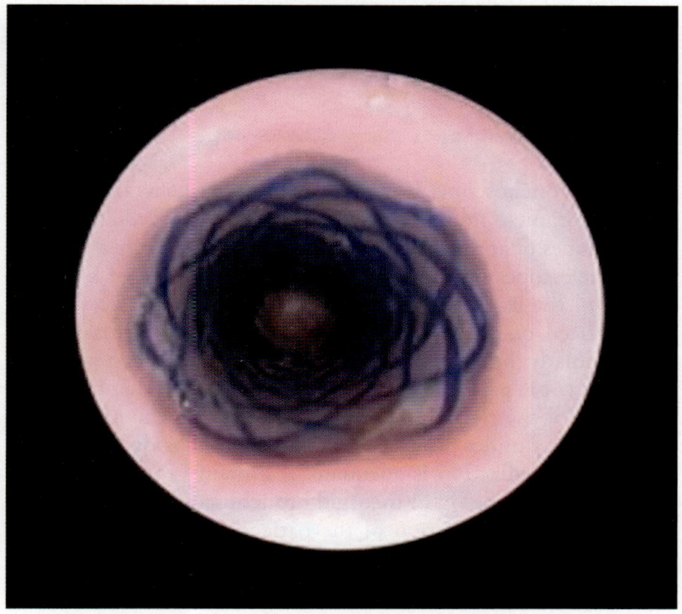

• **Fig. 14.7** Bronchoscopic view of a biodegradable stent in the trachea.

Herein, we describe the steps of the endoscopic insertion procedure for metallic and biodegradable stents.

## Metallic Stents

1. Patient positioning: Supine with a small roll under the patient's shoulders.
2. Airway exposure: The surgeon must obtain an adequate view of the larynx in order to insert the rigid bronchoscope in the trachea safely. An appropriately sized laryngoscope will help in this maneuver.
3. Visualization: Prior to rigid bronchoscopy, the entire airway should be explored under spontaneous ventilation with a flexible videobronchoscope in order to assess its dynamic behavior (this issue is crucial in cases of suspected tracheobronchomalacia). Parameters of the exam should be noted, such as the degree of positive pressure being delivered, status of spontaneous ventilation or paralysis, and status of chest cavity being open or closed (Pearl 14.3). Any signs of inflammation, ischemia, and infection should be considered with a low threshold to obtain cultures. The segment to be stented (either tracheal or bronchial) should be accurately determined (this information should be correlated with cross-sectional imaging for evaluation of the surrounding anatomy).

**PEARL 14.3**

Open versus closed chest cavity is a critical point particularly when considering vascular compression of the airway.

4. Rigid bronchoscopy: It is performed under general anesthesia with complete muscle relaxation (Pearl 14.4). Pediatric bronchoscopes of appropriate size should be used together with rod lens telescopes (0°) and a high-resolution camera. If the distal part of the trachea is to be stented, a radiopaque needle may be placed on the patient's chest marking the carina. This is particularly helpful when placing biodegradable stents with fluoroscopic guidance, as described later in the chapter. Then, the tip of the rigid bronchoscope is placed in the mid part of the trachea under fluoroscopic control or via endoscopic guidance if visualization is adequate. If a main bronchus is to be stented, then the tip of the rigid bronchoscope is placed facing its entrance. Ventilation of the patient is performed through the dedicated bronchoscope port. Patient's lips, tongue, and teeth (if present) are protected with a small gauze.
5. Stent loading: Metallic stents used in children are generally balloon expandable. The stent is loaded unexpanded on an angioplasty catheter of appropriate size (15–30 mm long) and inserted through the main port of the rigid bronchoscope (Fig. 14.8).
6. In cases when spontaneous ventilation is used, the stent and deployment devices can be inserted in parallel with the telescope or flexible bronchoscope through the open glottis, obviating the need for a rigid bronchoscope. This can enable better maneuvering of the stent but does require spontaneous ventilation with adequate anesthesia. Nebulized and topical lidocaine given just prior to manipulation of the airway can facilitate this scenario.
7. Stent placement: Under continuous fluoroscopic control, the balloon catheter is inflated with a pressure gauge syringe system to its established nominal pressure inside the trachea or main bronchi. Consequently, the metallic stent is deployed to the desired diameter (usually 5–8 mm in small infants) (Fig. 14.9). Next, the balloon is deflated completely and removed from the airway (Pearls 14.5 and 14.6). Ventilation through the rigid bronchoscope is resumed immediately after. This step of the procedure should not last more than 20 seconds (Fig. 14.10).

**PEARL 14.4**

The use of muscle relaxation varies by surgeon preference. The editors' practice is to do the procedure with spontaneous ventilation when possible.

**PEARL 14.5**

The surgeon should keep in mind that as metallic stents expand in diameter, they shorten in length.

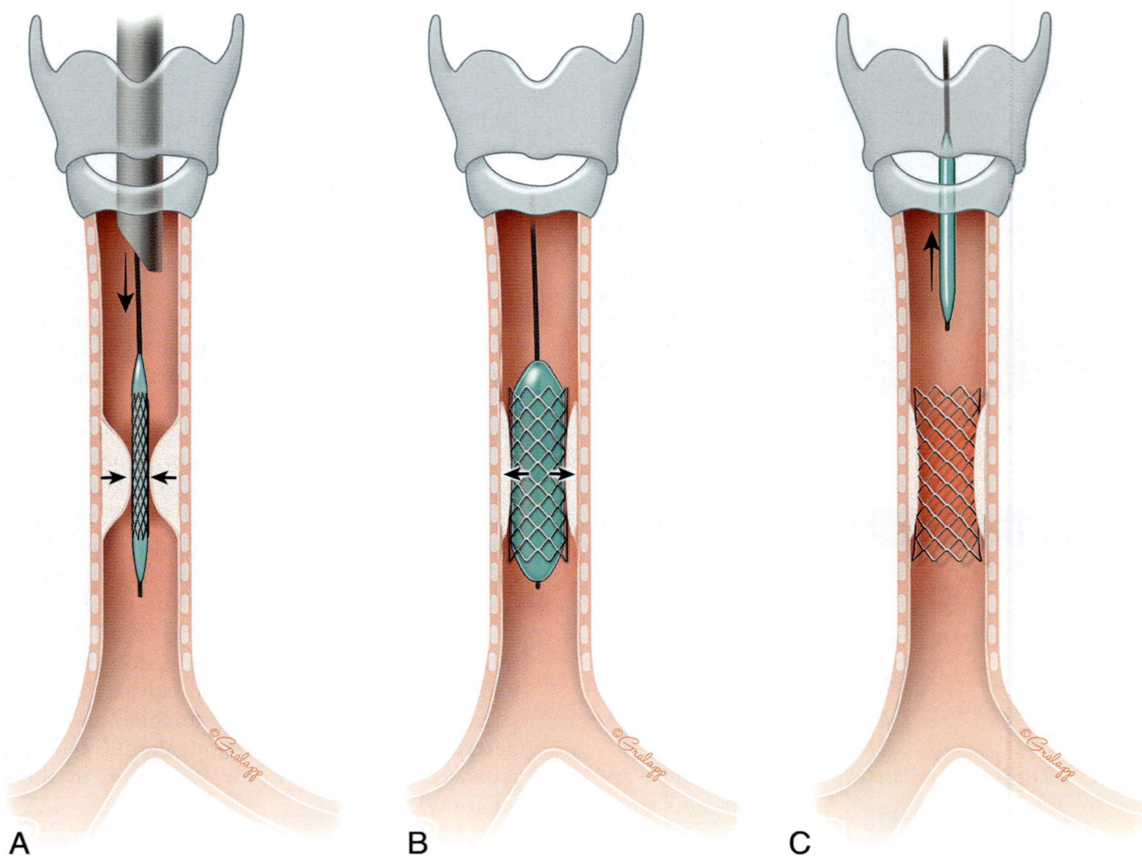


• **Fig. 14.8** Artist rendering demonstrating the placement of a metallic stent in the trachea. (© 2024 Chris Gralapp.)

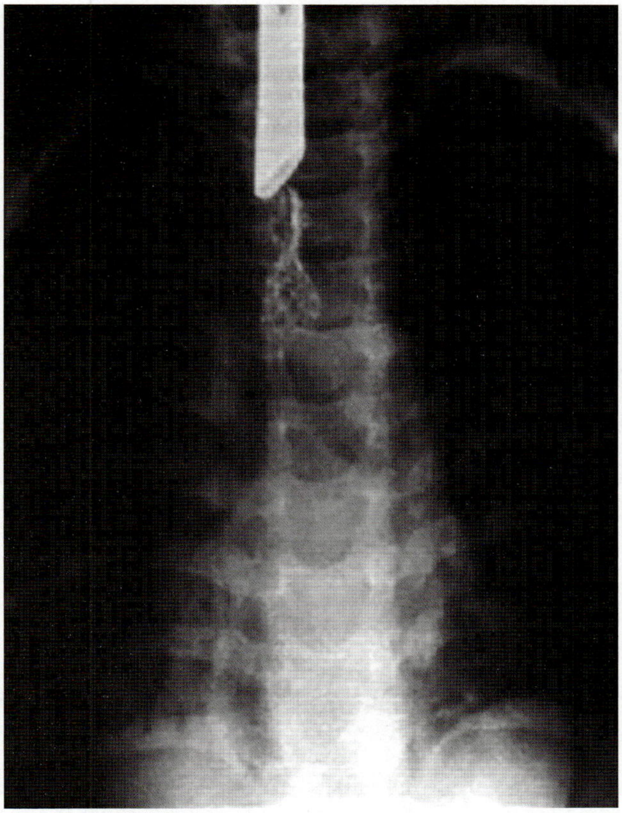

• **Fig. 14.9** Fluoroscopic image of a metallic stent being deployed in the trachea.

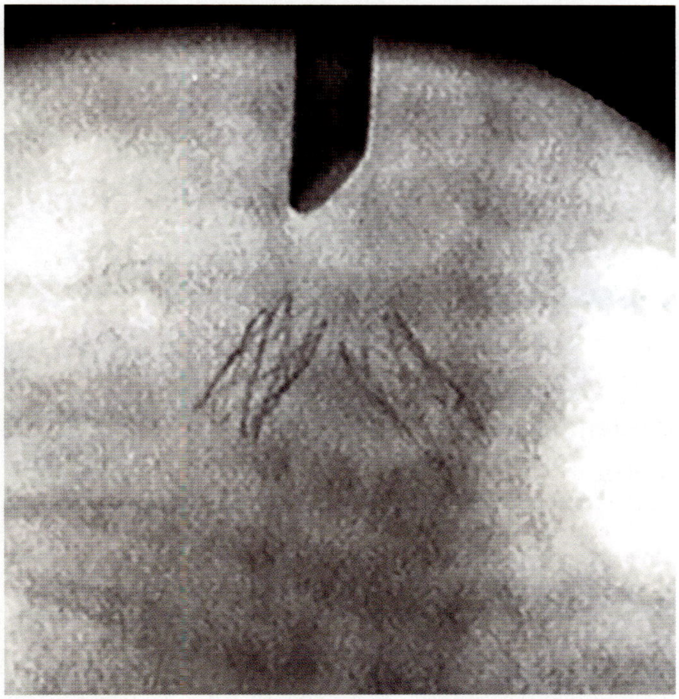

• **Fig. 14.10** Fluoroscopic image showing two metallic stents placed in both main bronchi.

**PEARL 14.6**

The proximal and distal ends of the stent can be flared with additional focused balloon dilation if necessary. This may reduce the potential for stent migration.

8. Checking and photodocumentation: Rod lens telescopes (0°) are used to examine the trachea and/or bronchi and confirm that the stent is in the right position and that no bleeding or damage to the airway is present. The procedure is documented with pictures or video recording (Video 14.2).
9. The rigid bronchoscope is removed from the airway and replaced by an endotracheal tube that should be fixed proximal to the upper rim of the stent if possible. The position of the tube should be checked with flexible bronchoscopy and a chest X-ray must be obtained when the procedure is completed (Pearl 14.7).

**PEARL 14.7**

When spontaneous ventilation is used, intubation at the end of the procedure is often not needed. However, the surgeon should have a clear idea of the size of tube and depth of placement that should be used if intubation is needed at any point while the stent is in situ. For proximal tracheal stents, this includes making sure the tube will pass through the stent easily if there is no space to place the tube between glottis and stent.

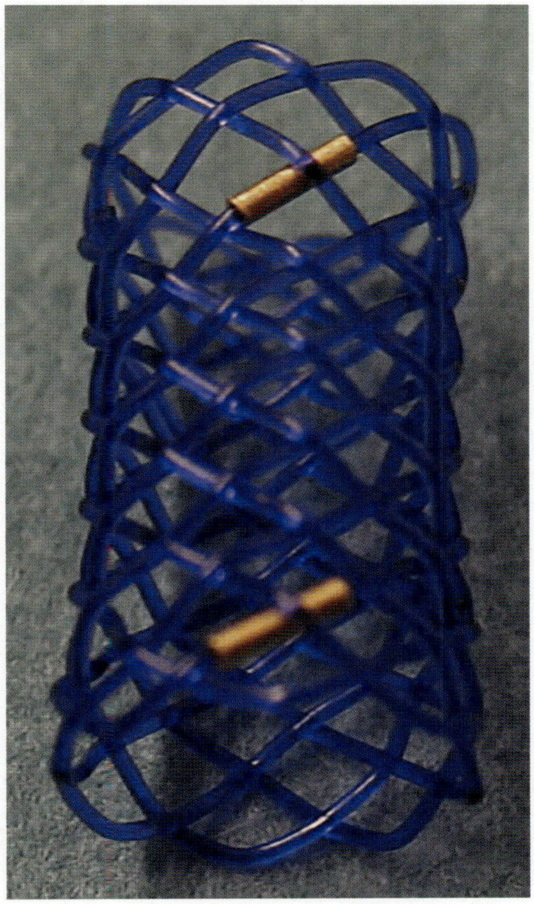

• **Fig. 14.11** Biodegradable stent made of a polydioxanone (PDO) monofilament.

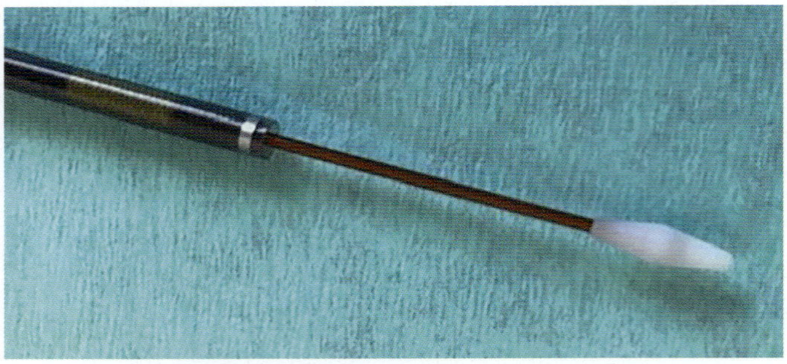

• **Fig. 14.12** Biodegradable stent insertion device.

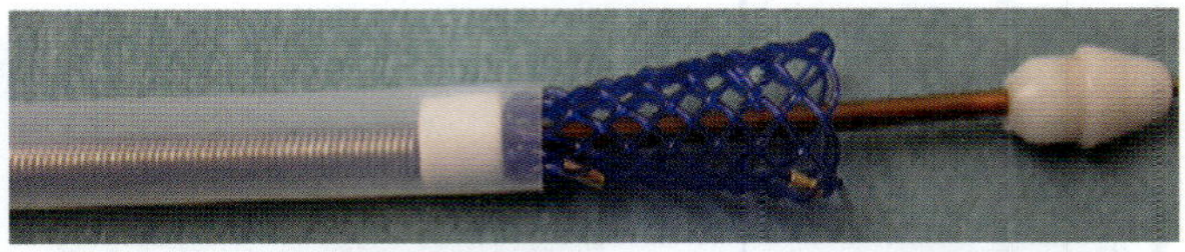

• **Fig. 14.13** Biodegradable stent being loaded in the insertion device.

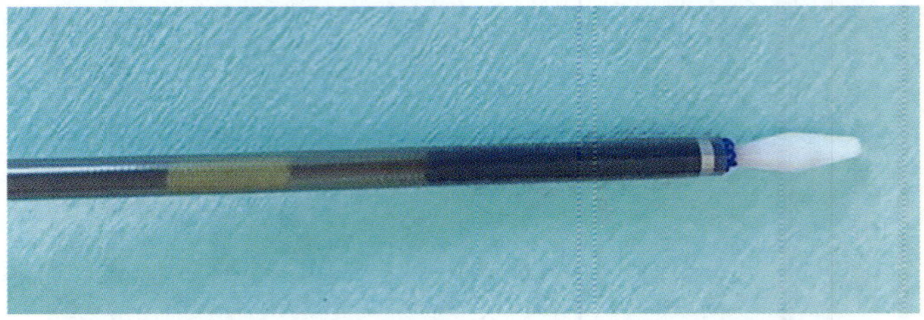

• **Fig. 14.14** Biodegradable stent completely loaded and ready to be placed in the airway.

## Biodegradable Stents

Biodegradable stents most frequently used in children consist of a polydioxanone (PDO) monofilament which is a semicrystalline polymer that degrades completely by hydrolysis at 14 to 15 weeks. They are custom made and a dedicated insertion device is necessary to deploy the stent in the airway (Figs. 14.11 and 14.12).

Steps 1, 2, 3, and 4 are similar to those described above for metallic stents.

5. Stent loading: The PDO stent is loaded in the distal part of the insertion device (Figs. 14.13 and 14.14). This type of stent is radiotransparent, so two gold marks are present at each end of the stent to detect it when performing fluoroscopy. The device is then inserted into the main port of the rigid bronchoscope and advanced until the two gold marks are visible on the x-ray screen (Fig. 14.15, Video 14.3).

6. Stent placement: This step is performed under continuous fluoroscopic imaging. If the distal part of the trachea needs to be stented, the delivering device is advanced until the distal gold mark of the stent matches the radiopaque needle placed on the chest to indicate the position of the carina. Next, the outer plastic sheath of the instrument is gently removed and the stent is delivered to the desired place. Care must be taken not to move the stent upward when withdrawing the plastic sheath of the device (Video 14.3). Ventilation through the working channel is restarted immediately after the whole instrument is completely removed from the rigid bronchoscope. If a main bronchus needs to be stented, the tip of the rigid bronchoscope is placed in its entrance and the PDO stent is delivered in the same way as above. In this setting, no needle mark is necessary because the distal end of the rigid bronchoscope marks the

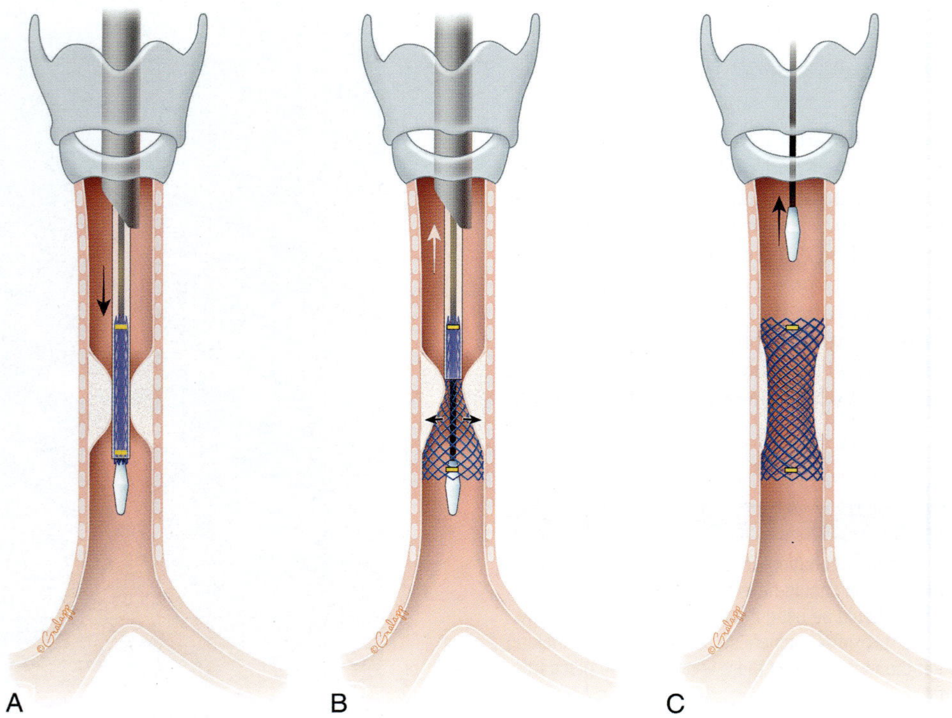


• **Fig. 14.15** Artist rendering demonstrating the placement of a biodegradable stent in the trachea. (© 2024 Chris Gralapp.)

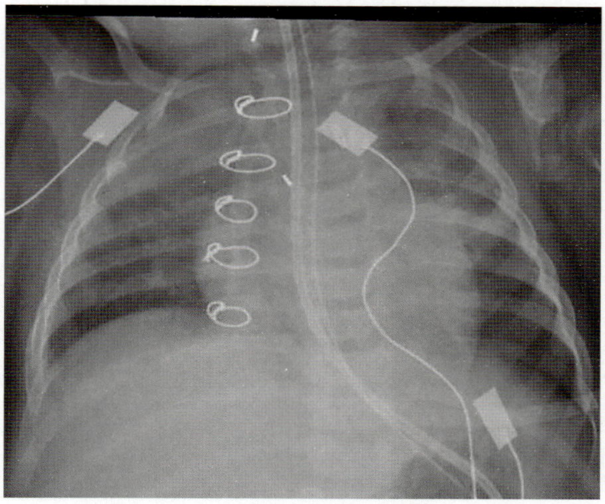

• **Fig. 14.16** Chest x-ray showing the two radiopaque marks delimiting the biodegradable stent in the trachea.

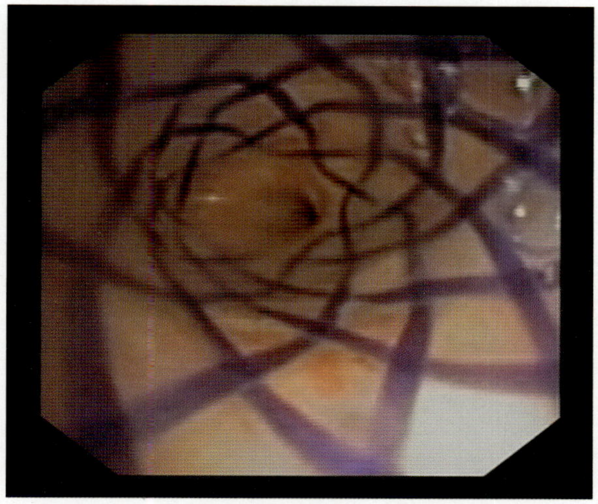

• **Fig. 14.17** Endoscopic view of a biodegradable stent immediately after placement in the trachea.

carina (Video 14.4). This step should be accomplished in less than 20 seconds.

Steps 7 and 8 are similar to those described for metallic stent placement (Figs. 14.16 and 14.17).

In patients with severe tracheal stenosis, balloon dilation may be necessary before placing the stent (Video 14.5). In cases of tracheo- or bronchomalacia, the stent diameter should be 10% to 15% larger than the estimated airway cross section determined in the CT scan (Video 14.6).

## Bibliography


1. Nicolai T. Airway stents in children. *Pediatr Pulmonol.* 2008;43:330–344.
2. Antón-Pacheco JL, Luna C, García E, et al. Initial experience with a new biodegradable airway stent in children: is this the stent we were waiting for? *Pediatr Pulmonol.* 2016;51:607–612.
3. Stramiello JA, Mohammadzadeh A, Ryan J, Brigger MT. The role of bioresorbable intraluminal airway stents in pediatric tracheobronchial obstruction: a systematic review. *Int J Pediatr Otorhinolaryngol.* 2020;139:110405.
4. Vondrys D, Elliott MJ, McLaren CA, Noctor C, Roebuck DJ. First experience with biodegradable airway stents in children. *Ann Thorac Surg.* 2011;92:1870–1874.
5. Minen F, Durward A, James P, et al. Single-center review on safety of biodegradable airway stenting in pediatric population. *Pediatr Pulmonol.* 2023;58(12):3437–3446.
6. Wallis C, McLaren CA. Tracheobronchial stenting for airway malacia. *Paediatr Respir Rev.* 2018;27:48–59.
7. Antón-Pacheco JL, Cabezali D, Tejedor R, et al. The role of airway stenting in pediatric tracheobronchial obstruction. *Eur J Cardiothorac Surg.* 2008;33:1069–1075.
8. Rocío Morante-Valverde, María López Díaz, Ma Carmen Luna-Paredes, et al. Further experience with polydioxanone airway stents in children. *Pediatr Pulmonol.* 2024;59(10):2517–2522.
9. Antón-Pacheco JL. Tracheobronchial stents in children. *Semin Pediatr Surg.* 2016;25(3):179–185.
10. Li L, Zhang X, Shi J, et al. Airway Stents from now to the future: a narrative review. *Respiration.* 2023;102(6):439–448.

# 15

# Endoscopic Suprastomal Stent Placement

ROMAINE F. JOHNSON

## Background

Pediatric laryngotracheal reconstruction (PLTR) is a surgical technique that aims to correct congenital or acquired airway obstruction in children, primarily caused by laryngotracheal stenosis.[1] The most frequent indications for PLTR include subglottic stenosis, tracheal stenosis, and laryngeal web or cleft. Suprastomal stenting is a widely used method in PLTR to maintain airway patency and prevent the collapse of the reconstructed airway.[2,3] The procedure is usually carried out under general anesthesia and typically placed during open double-staged PLTR. Double stage refers to leaving a tracheostomy in place to allow for the reconstructed area to heal. Suprastomal stents are contraindicated without a tracheostomy, as it would lead to severe airway obstruction.

Currently, the option of endoscopic suprastomal stent placement is available in select patients.[3,4] The procedure involves using an endoscope, a stent delivery system, and specialized instruments to insert the stent above the stoma and secure it in place. In pediatric patients, the size, shape, and flexibility of the stent must be carefully considered to ensure a proper fit and minimize the risk of complications.[5] The procedure's success is highly dependent on the surgeon's expertise, the healthcare institution's familiarity with postoperative care, as well as the patient's cooperation and adherence to postoperative care instructions. Endoscopic suprastomal stenting is considered a safe and effective technique in PLTR, but it is essential to closely monitor the patient's progress and adjust the stent as needed to ensure optimal results.

## Patient Selection

Patient selection is a critical aspect of performing an endoscopic suprastomal stent in pediatric patients. The procedure is typically recommended for pediatric patients with laryngotracheal stenosis who require stenting for more than 7 days post PLTR and whose stenosis and/or anatomy are suitable for endoscopic reconstruction. For example, an endoscopic posterior costochondral graft may be a good option for these patients. It is important to note that in cases where the stenosis or anatomy is not amenable to endoscopic reconstruction, open stent placement should be considered the preferred approach. Factors that should be considered when selecting patients for this procedure include the degree of stenosis, the size and shape of the airway, and the patient's overall health and tolerance for the procedure. A thorough preoperative evaluation, including a complete medical history, physical examination, and appropriate endoscopic evaluations, is essential to ensure that the patient is a suitable candidate for the procedure and to minimize the risk of complications.

## Key Aspects of the Consent Process

The consent process for endoscopic suprastomal stent placement in pediatric patients involves educating the patient and their family about the risks and benefits of the procedure. The following are some procedure-specific risks that should be discussed, in addition to the standard risks of any airway procedure:

- Risks associated with endoscopic stent placement, including but not limited to stent dislodgement, infection, bleeding, granulation tissue formation, and scarring. It is essential to discuss these risks with the patient and their family and to provide them with written information about the procedure. It is also important to emphasize that the procedure's goal is to improve the patient's airway and breathing. However, it is important to acknowledge that there is no guarantee of success, and the patient may need additional procedures in the future.

## Equipment

- Camera system and light cords: This includes brands such as Stryker, Storz, and Olympus, which are used to visualize the airway during the procedure.
- Basic Bronchoscopy Pediatric Set with Proximal Illumination: This instrument set is used to view the airway and deliver the stent. Instruments include but are not limited to:
  - Hopkins Straight Forward Telescope 0 degree, 2.9 mm diameter, 36 mm length
  - Pediatric Bronchoscopes, sizes 3.5 to 6
  - Prismatic light deflector with optic cables
  - Optical Forceps, 2 × 2 with teeth or alligators
- Operative microscope 400 mm lens: This is used to magnify the surgical field and provide better visibility during the procedure (Pearl 15.1).

**PEARL 15.1**

The editors typically perform the procedure with telescope magnification and do not use microscope.

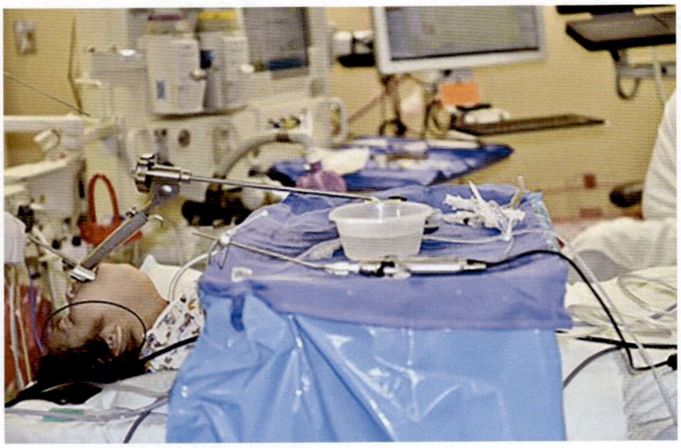

• **Fig. 15.1** Intraoperative image of patient positioning.

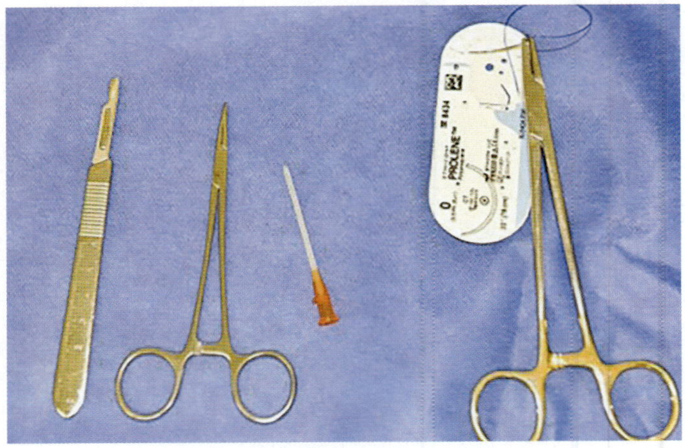

• **Fig. 15.2** Intraoperative image of instruments used to secure stent including 18 G angiocath

- Basic Pediatric Laryngoscopy Set
  - Lindholm Operating Laryngoscope for Children
  - Benjamin Operating Laryngoscope for Children
  - Benjamin-Lindholm Operating Laryngoscope for Newborns and Infants
- Frazier-tip suction tubes
- Grasping forceps
- Scissors, straight and curved
- Lindholm Distending Forceps (i.e., Vocal cord spreaders): These are used to spread the vocal cords and provide better access to the airway. These are optional.
- Laryngoscope Holder and Chest Support (Suspension apparatus): Used to suspend the larynx in view.
- Dental guards or gauze: These are used to protect the teeth during the procedure.
- Sterile rubber band: This stabilizes the vocal cord spreaders to keep them from moving if using the spreaders.
- Basic tracheostomy or neck dissection set: This includes the common instruments used in soft tissue surgery, such as scissors, forceps, and small retractors.

## Special equipment

Suprastomal stents are used to maintain airway patency and prevent collapse of the reconstructed airway in PLTR. They can be purchased separately and are made by various companies, including

- Rutter Suprastomal Stent (Boston Scientific)
- Mehta Laryngeal Stent (Hood Laboratories)
- Montgomery T-tubes (various suppliers)

It is important to note that the choice of stent will depend on the specific needs of the patient and the surgeon's preference. The Rutter and Mehta stents are premade and ready to use, while the Montgomery T-tube can be used to fashion a stent in the operating room. It is crucial to ensure that the stent is of the appropriate size and shape for the patient and is flexible enough to allow some give during insertion. The procedure may require multiple stents, as mistakes or errors in fashioning the stent can occur. The stent may need to be adjusted or replaced several times to ensure optimal placement and subsequent results.

It is important to note that the following steps presume that the surgeon is proficient with endoscopic approaches to repairing stenosis or obstruction using various techniques, including graft placement, scar excision, and dilations.

Steps in the procedure

1. Patient positioning: Standard suspension laryngoscopy setup and approach, including a surgical time-out to confirm patient identity and procedure details (Fig. 15.1).
2. Instruments used in making skin incision and securing the stent are shown in Fig. 15.2.
3. Laryngeal exposure: Confirm that the larynx can be seen with both a telescope and microscope. It is not uncommon to alternate between both imaging views to ensure proper visualization of the entire larynx, anterior commissure, postcricoid, and immediate subglottis.
4. Laryngeal spreaders (optional step): The spreaders are placed upside down, so the handles are facing up. The spreaders are placed so the graspers sit in the false vocal folds and ventricles, avoiding placement at the level of the true vocal folds. Once adequate displacement is obtained, a rubber band is used to suspend the spreaders to the suspension apparatus (Pearl 15.2).

**PEARL 15.2**

The rubber band should provide enough tension to prevent the spreaders' sagging into the surgeon's view of the larynx, while not being so tight that it drives the blades of the spreaders into the paraglottic space.

5. Visualization: Use the Hopkins rod telescope and microscope to visualize stent placement. The operative microscope allows for bimanual instrumentation, but the telescope is usually sufficient. The operating microscope is often used in the initial repair of the stenosis/obstruction.
6. Repair of stenosis: Various approaches according to surgeon preference.
7. Estimating size and length of stent needed: An uncuffed endotracheal tube can determine the appropriate size of the stent. Most often, the Cotton-Meyer grading system is used to determine the appropriate airway size. The length of the stent varies, but generally the stent should span the repair area and extend proximally to the mid-epiglottis level (Pearl 15.3).

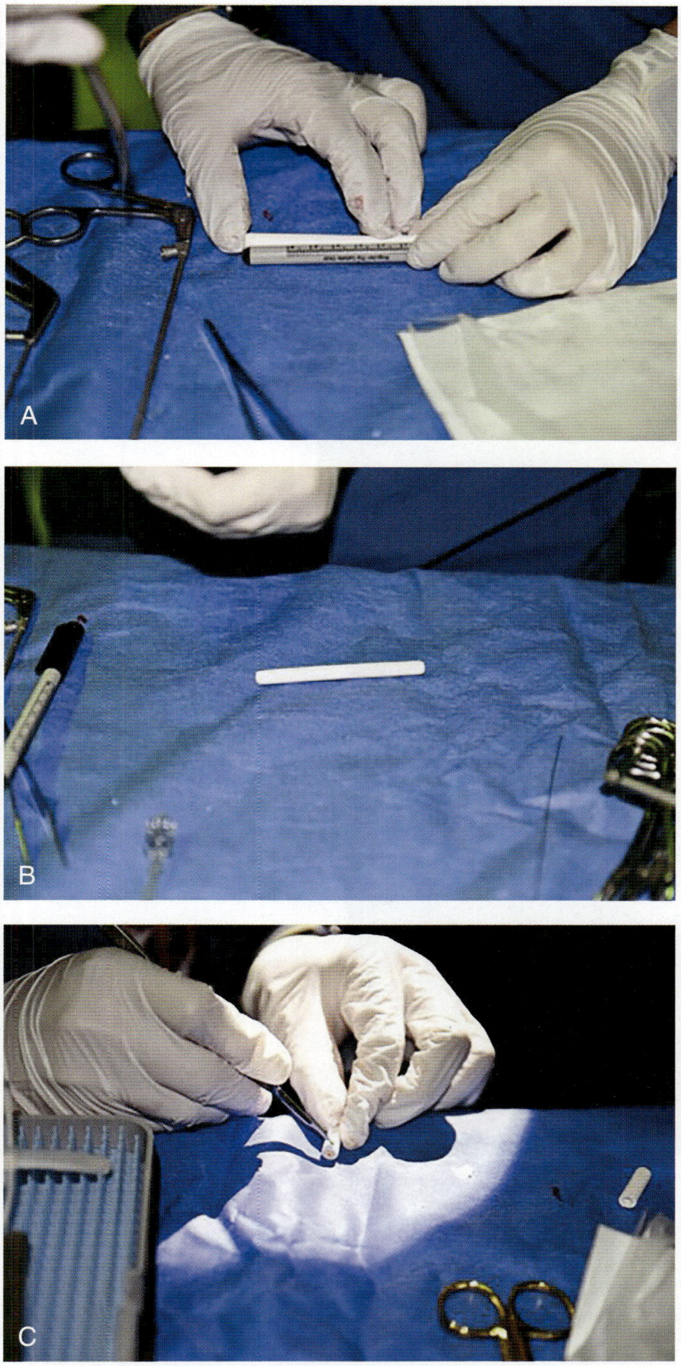


• **Fig. 15.3** Intraoperative image of stent measurement and cutting.

**PEARL 15.3**

Another similar approach is to trim the stent length such that the top of the stent sits just below the upper edge of the aryepiglottic folds when in position.

8. Placement of stent and ensuring proper placement: Using the telescope for visualization, the stent is carefully inserted into the airway using alligator forceps. The stent should sit just above the tracheostomy tube at the distal end, and the superior end should be adjusted according to the extent of the laryngeal component of the repair. The length of the stent can be estimated by measuring the distance from the tracheostomy stoma to the level of the aryepiglottic folds. Once the appropriate length is determined, the stent is trimmed and inserted into the airway (Figs. 15.3A-C–15.6).

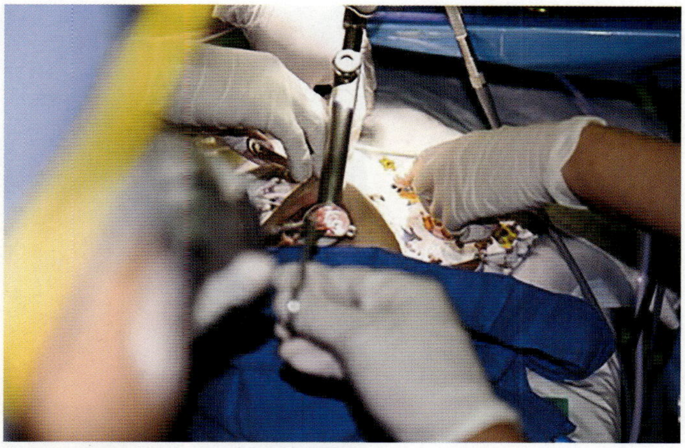

• **Fig. 15.4** Intraoperative image of endoscopic suprastomal stent placement, over-the-shoulder view of surgeon.

9. Securing the stent with an external transtracheal suture: A small external right neck skin incision (stab incision) is made slightly lateral to the airway, down to platysma. The surgical assistant passes the suture through the soft tissue and trachea (Pearl 15.4), making sure to avoid injury to the great vessels in the neck (Fig. 15.7) (Pearl 15.5). The needle passes through the stent and out of a small stab incision in the left neck. The stent is then removed transorally, and the cap is placed if desired. In addition, some surgeons will taper the distal end of the stent to reduce rubbing against the tracheostomy tube (Pearl 15.6).

**PEARL 15.4**

Some surgeons will place a slender rigid telescope inside the stent and visualize the needle's passage through the lumen of the stent.

**PEARL 15.5**

Suture and needle choice vary by surgeon preference. Usually, a 2-0 or 3-0 Prolene is a reasonable choice. A large curved or straight needle, such as a CT needle, is required. In some cases, using a free needle allows broader selection of needle sizes for a given suture.

**PEARL 15.6**

Use caution when making any tapering cuts on the stent itself. Any sharp edges have the potential to create granulation tissue where they interface with the airway mucosa. While cutting the stent is occasionally necessary, maintaining the factory "machined edge" of the stent is ideal when possible.

10. Securing the suture with a subcutaneous angiocath: The needle is passed as described through the right neck incision, through the trachea and stent, and directed toward the

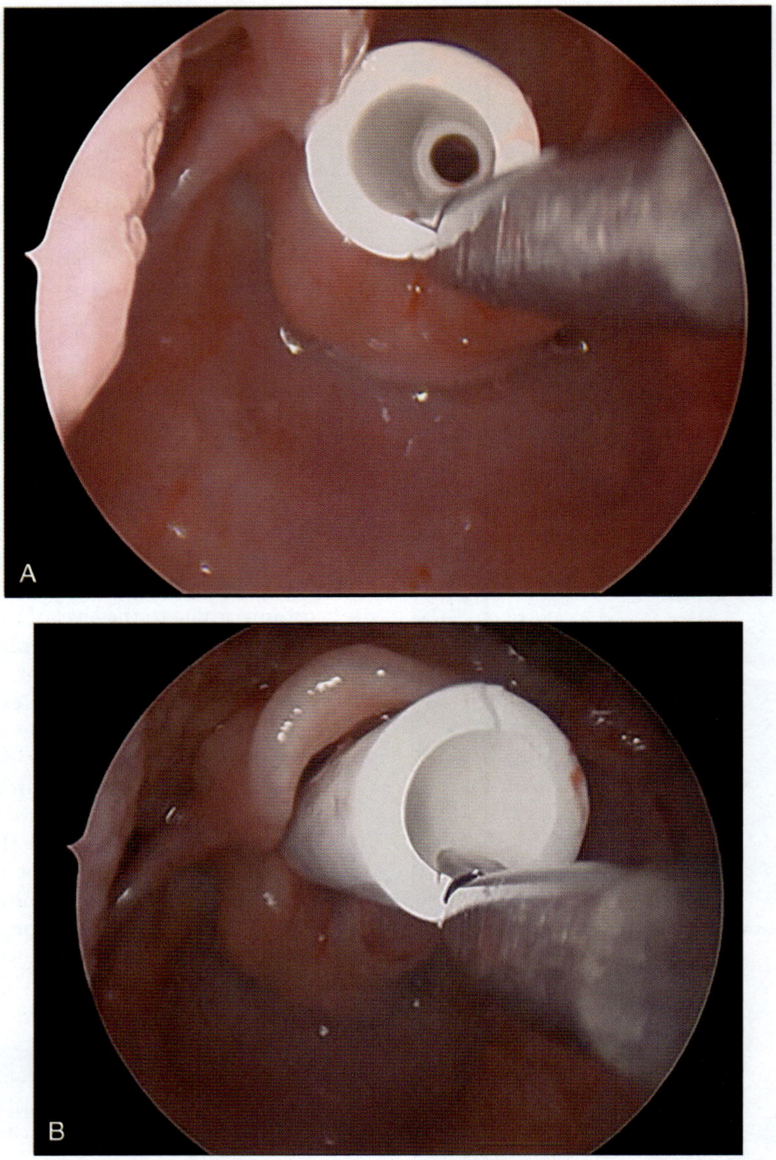

• **Fig. 15.5** (A) Intraoperative image of laryngeal view in suspension using the telescope. (B) Endoscopic views of suprastomal stent being placed using alligator forceps.

left neck skin. A tiny stab incision is made in the neck skin at the exit point of the needle in the left neck. The needle and suture are passed back through the opening, just deep to the platysma, and out the initial stab incision, such that both suture tails now protrude from the right neck incision (Figs. 15.8–15.11). After stent placement but before tying the suture, the stent can be evaluated with the suture tails on tension, and again after tying the stent in place, if desired (Fig. 15.12). A 14–18-gauge angiocath (IV catheter) is then used to secure the suture by threading it over one limb of the suture and tying at least 15 to 20 tight knots. This step helps prevent the suture from becoming deeply embedded in the tissue, prevents the suture from loosening over time, and minimizes the risk of complications of stent migration or during later stent removal. The neck incisions are closed. The angiocath should be palpable but not taut against the undersurface of the skin (Pearl 15.7).

**PEARL 15.7**

The angiocatheter, when placed on tension itself (slightly bowed when tying the suture), will straighten in the event that the suture loosens. As the angiocatheter straightens out, it maintains tension on the suture to reduce the risk of stent mobility within the airway. Additionally, the placement of several knots as described, improves the ability to identify the suture at the time of stent removal, which may be particularly helpful in patients who have undergone longer term (6-8 week) stent placement.

11. The angiocatheter, when placed on tension itself (slightly bowed when tying the suture), will straighten in the event that the suture loosens. As the angiocatheter straightens out, it maintains

(*Continued text on page 90*)

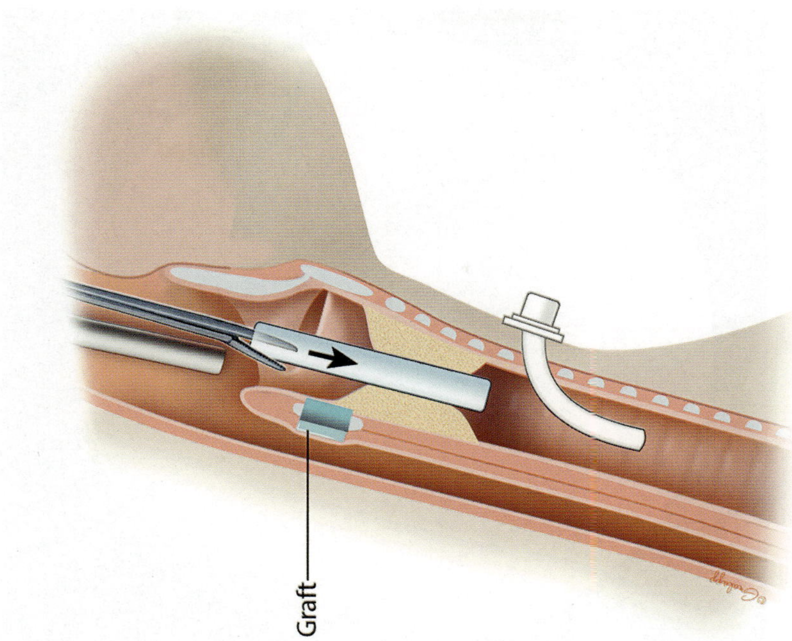


• **Fig. 15.6** Illustration of suprastomal stent being placed using alligator forceps and telescope for visualization. (© 2024 Chris Gralapp.)

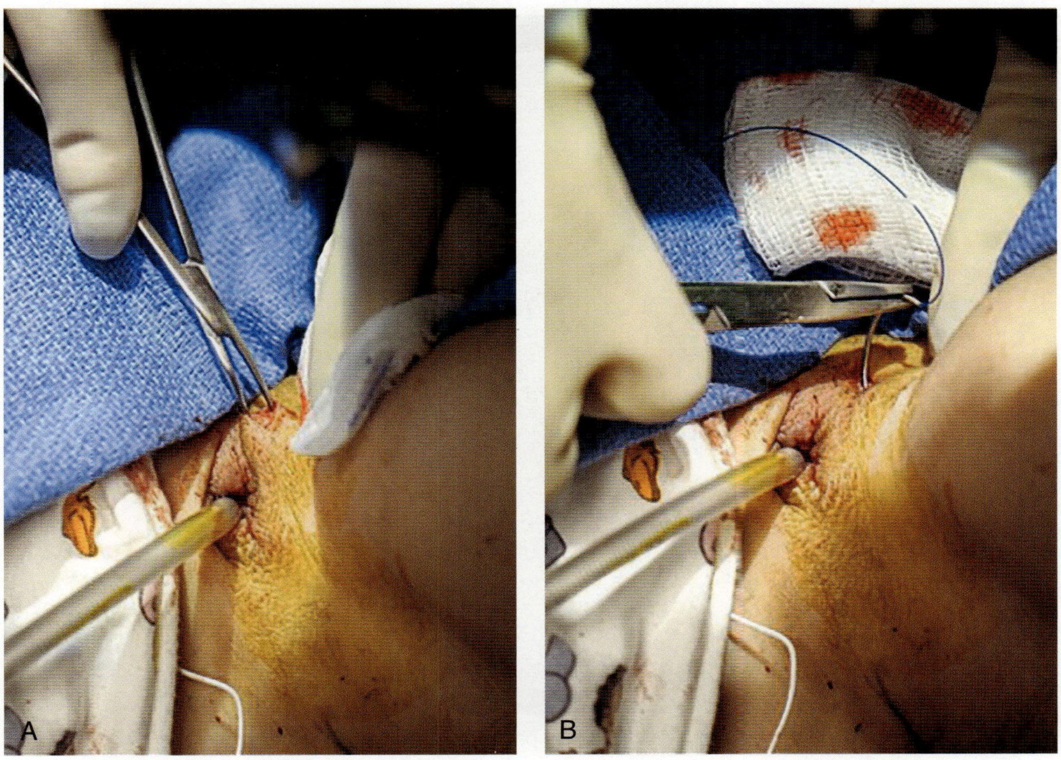


• **Fig. 15.7** (A) A small incision is made in the right neck. (B) A needle is passed through the right neck incision, toward the trachea and stent.

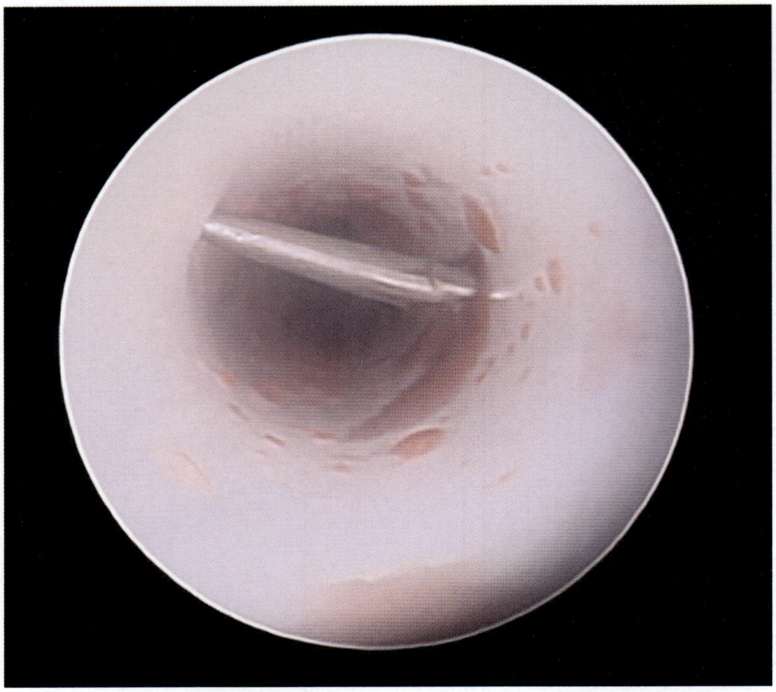

• **Fig. 15.8** Intraluminal view of needle passing through the suprastomal stent.

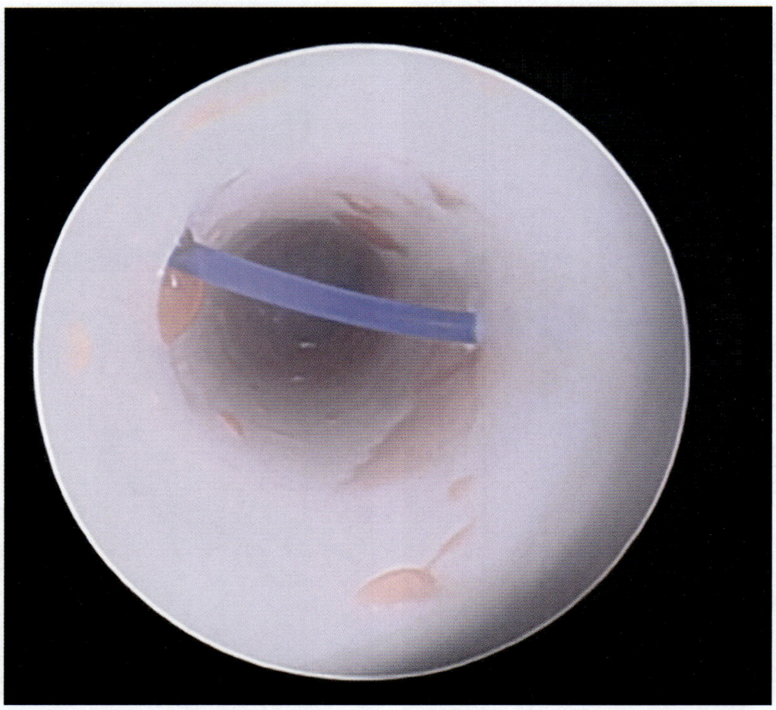

• **Fig. 15.9** Intraluminal view of suture passing through the suprastomal stent.

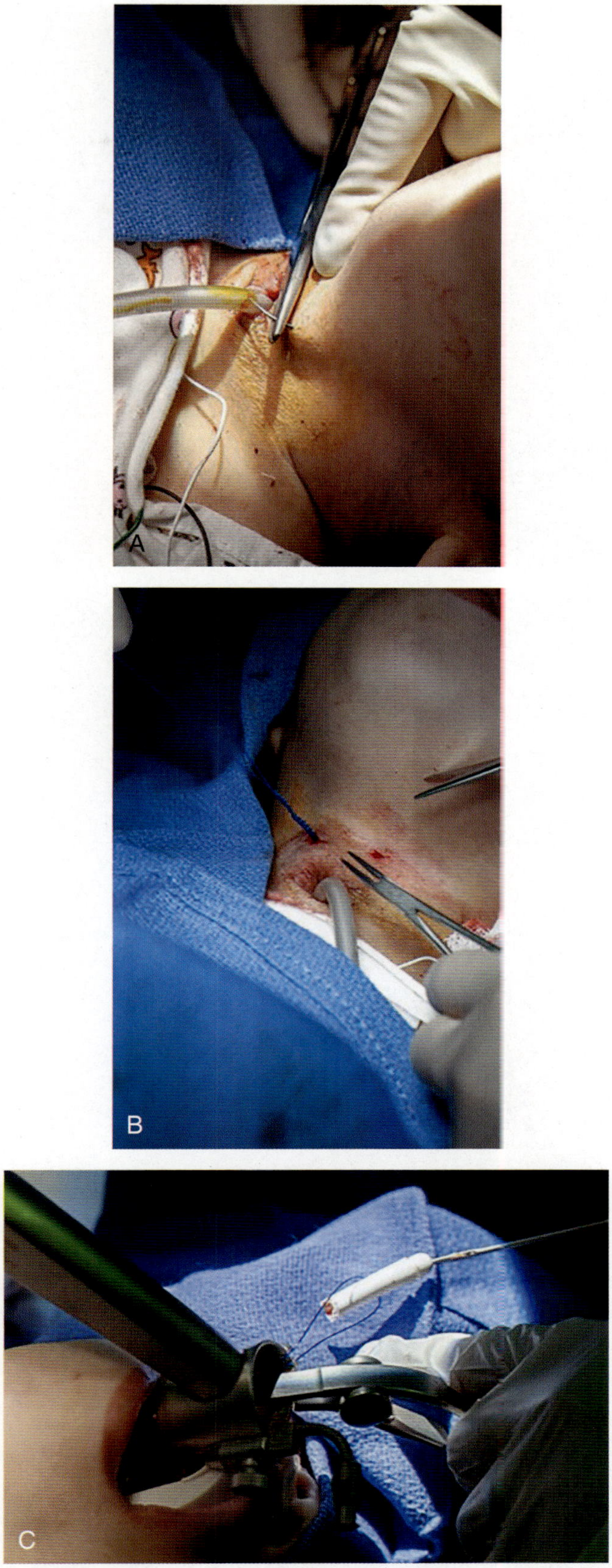

• **Fig. 15.10** Intraoperative views of suture being placed through skin and tracheal. (A) Suture is passed through the stab incision (right neck), and through the trachea to the contralateral neck where the needle in this image is being grasped through a small stab incision on the left. (B) The tail of the suture from the left neck is tunneled back to the right neck deep to platysma and pulled out through the right neck incision. (C) The stent is grasped with an alligator forcep before being inserted into the airway. The two suture tails from the right neck are pulled simultaneously while the stent is inserted into the airway under direct visualization, before being tied.

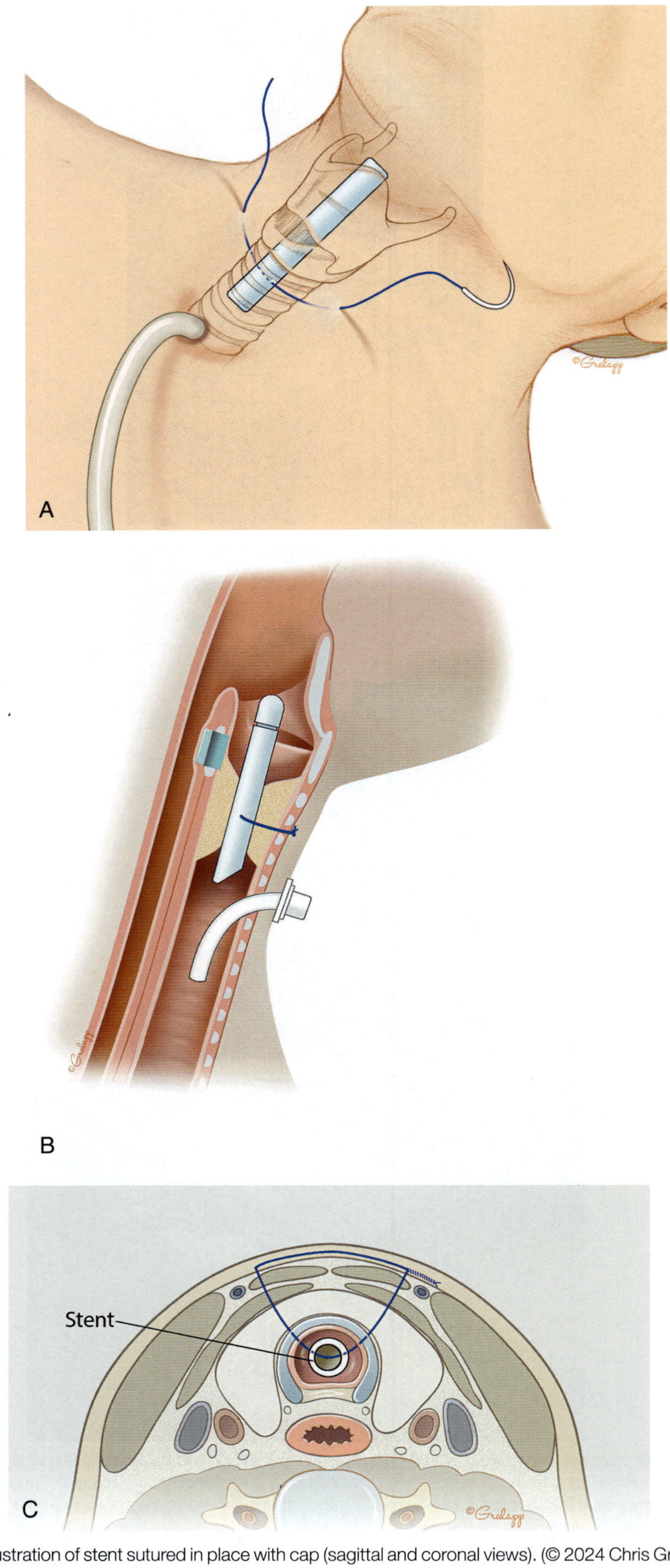


• **Fig. 15.11** Illustration of stent sutured in place with cap (sagittal and coronal views). (© 2024 Chris Gralapp.)

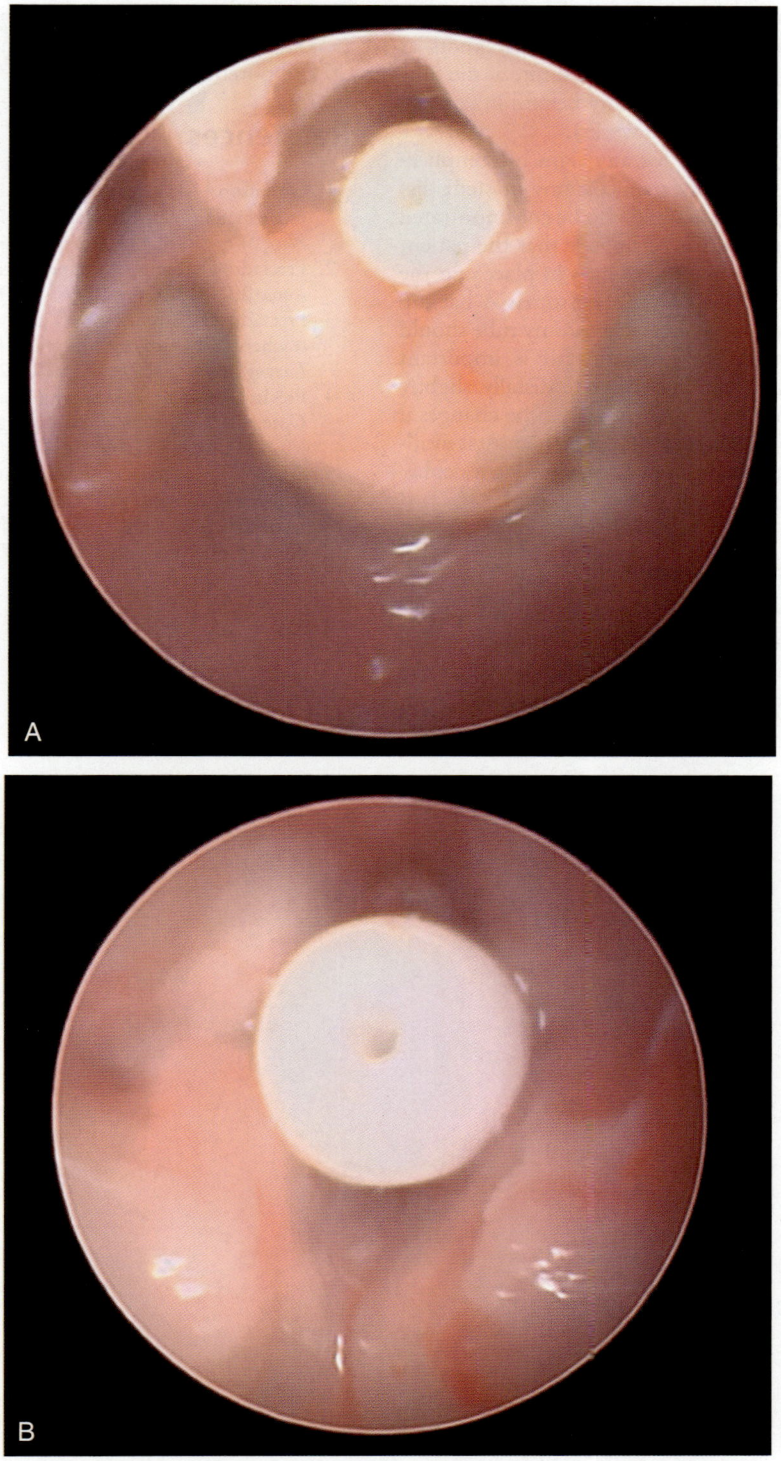

• **Fig. 15.12** Intraoperative view of stent with cap in place before and after final position.

tension on the suture to reduce the risk of stent mobility within the airway. Additionally, the placement of several knots as described, improves the ability to identify the suture at the time of stent removal, which may be particularly helpful in patients who have undergone longer term (6-8 weeks).

12. The patient should be monitored for any signs of complications, such as bleeding, infection, tracheostomy or stent dislodgement, and mucus plugs. It should also be communicated to all providers, including the use of signage that the patient cannot be intubated orally while the stent is in place and the airway must be established via the tracheostoma. A backup tracheostomy tube and a downsized tracheostomy tube should be confirmed to be immediately available. It is important to recognize that the stent can also migrate distally slightly enough to cause resistance with tracheostomy tube changes if it interferes with the stoma. As such, having a hemostat available at the bedside can aid in pushing a migrated stent cephalad in case of emergency.

## Additional Considerations

- Suprastomal stents are typically left in place for 2 to 8 weeks. Longer durations may lead to increased granulation tissue formation and difficulty locating the securing suture, which can require more extensive neck exploration during removal.
- During the stent placement period, the tracheostomy tube size may need to be increased to account for increased secretions and potential mucus plugs.

## References


1. Gustafson LM, Hartley BE, Liu JH, et al. Single-stage laryngotracheal reconstruction in children: a review of 200 cases. *Otolaryngol Head Neck Surg*. 2000;123(4):430–434. doi:10.1067/mhn.2000.109007.
2. Preciado D. Stenting in pediatric airway reconstruction. *Laryngoscope*. 2012;122(Suppl 4):S97–S98. doi:10.1002/lary.23808.
3. Preciado D. A randomized study of suprastomal stents in laryngotracheoplasty surgery for grade III subglottic stenosis in children. *Laryngoscope*. 2014;124(1):207–213. doi:10.1002/lary.24141.
4. Preciado D, Zalzal G. Laryngeal and tracheal stents in children. *Curr Opin Otolaryngol Head Neck Surg*. 2008;16(1):83–85. doi:10.1097/MOO.0b013e3282f433f4.
5. Smith DF, de Alarcon A, Jefferson ND, et al. Short- versus long-term stenting in children with subglottic stenosis undergoing laryngotracheal reconstruction. *Otolaryngol Head Neck Surg*. 2018;158(2):375–380. doi:10.1177/0194599817737757.

# 16

# Endoscopic Management of Collapse at the Tracheostomy Site

BRIAC THIERRY

## Introduction

Suprastomal collapse is one of the local complications induced by long-standing tracheostomies. It is an **obstruction of the airway** due to the loss of biomechanical properties of the tracheal cartilage rings above the tracheostomy site. Several etiologies have been suggested for the genesis of this process, including chronic chondritis. Both long-term tracheostomy and long-term ventilation may increase the risk of this complication. There are **two main types** of collapses: (1) an **anterior form**, which is typically static; and (2) an **antero-lateral one**, which is often dynamic. The degree of collapse ranges from mild to severe and may hinder decannulation efforts.[1]

The gold standard for the diagnosis of suprastomal collapse is laryngotracheal endoscopy under spontaneous ventilation, with the tracheostomy tube first left in place and then removed (Pearl 16.1).

**PEARL 16.1**

Gentle stomal occlusion with the tracheostomy tube removed and the patient breathing spontaneously may unveil otherwise elusive dynamic collapse. This is discussed in more detail in the description of procedure later.

Various surgical treatments have been reported in the literature, ranging from endoscopic excision to laryngotracheoplasty or tracheal wall stiffening with resorbable mini-plates.[1–3] The recommended first-line treatment is based on endoscopic approaches for anterior forms and open approaches for combined anterior and lateral forms.

In this chapter, we focus on endoscopic evaluation and treatment. *The main differential diagnosis of suprastomal collapse is suprastomal granuloma. It is linked with mucosal damage by the cannula. Its treatment is endoscopic. For these reasons, we have chosen to include it in this chapter.*

## Preoperative Evaluation

Most of the time, diagnosis of suprastomal collapse is made during the pre-decannulation endoscopic workup.[4] This workup is scheduled when the disease that motivated the tracheostomy has resolved. Its objective is to assess for the possibility of safe decannulation. The workup often includes a test of cannula capping, a sleep study with the cannula capped, and an endoscopy of the upper and lower airway looking for any obstruction between the nasal cavities and the main bronchi. Assessment of the laryngeal, tracheal, and bronchial airway relies on laryngotracheal endoscopy under general anesthesia with spontaneous breathing with the tracheostomy tube initially left in place and then removed. If a suprastomal collapse is observed, it can be classified as:

- anterior (Figs. 16.1 and 16.2) or anterior and lateral (Fig. 16.3 and Video 16.1)
- and as mild (0–50%), moderate (50–75%) or severe (more than 75%) as a function of the percentage of obstruction of the airway lumen

A suprastomal granuloma can also be present (Figs. 16.4 and 16.5) with any combination of the above classifications.

If the suprastomal lesion (collapse or granuloma) is treatable endoscopically, this treatment is often performed during the diagnostic endoscopy.

Suprastomal lesions are also suspected when there is a change in the dynamic airway parameters of the patient, such as new difficulty in tolerating a speaking valve that was previously accommodated. The evaluation and management of suprastomal and peristomal lesions in this scenario is essentially the same as when considering decannulation.

## Key Aspects of the Informed Consent

Consent involves a discussion of risks, benefits, and alternatives surrounding the predecannulation work up: capping trial, sleep study, airway endoscopy.

Description of the endoscopic procedure:

- Evaluation of airway patency
- Description of the primary lesions that might be observed, especially suprastomal collapse and/or peristomal granuloma
- Description of possible endoscopic treatments:
  - Excision of anterior suprastomal collapse with cold instruments or with powered instruments such as microdebrider, LASER, or coblation devices; specify information concerning the risks of airway fire if LASER is used
  - Excision of granuloma

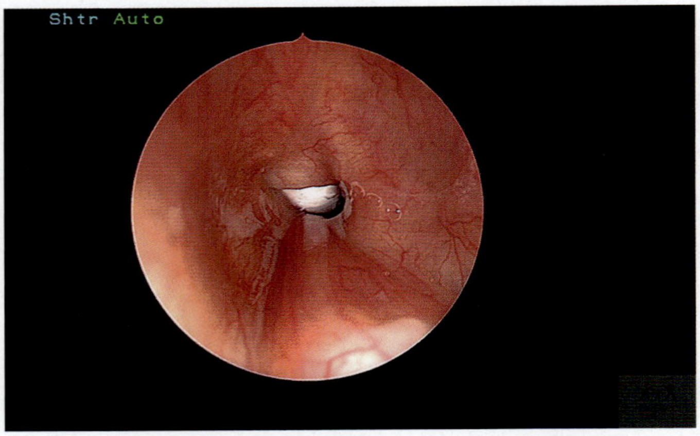


• **Fig. 16.1** Endoscopic view of the collapse of the anterior wall.

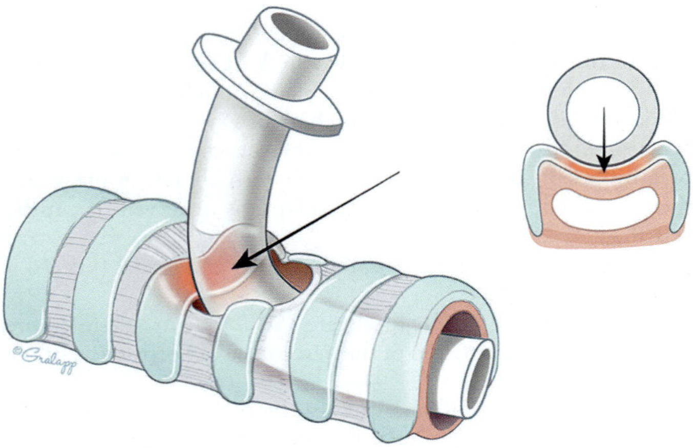

• **Fig. 16.2** Schematic *lateral* and *axial* views of the anterior collapse. The cannula is weighing on the cartilage above. (© 2024 Chris Gralapp.)

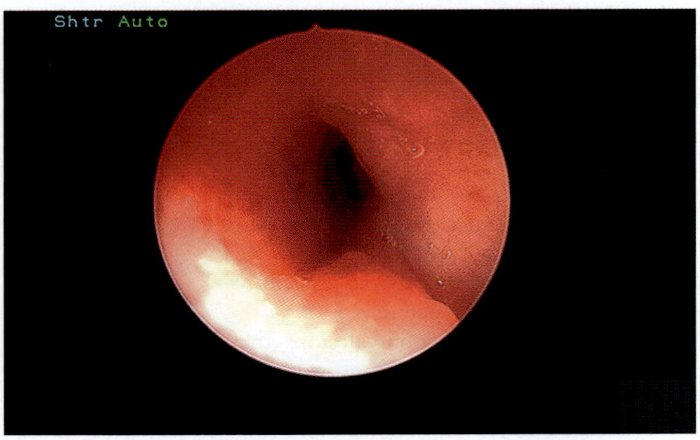


• **Fig. 16.3** Endoscopic view of an *anterior and lateral* severe collapse.

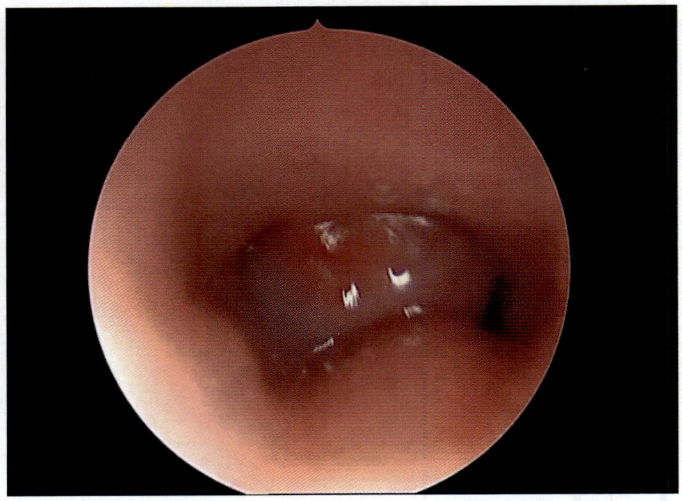

• **Fig. 16.4** Endoscopic view of a complete airway obstruction by a suprastomal granuloma (see also Video 16.2).

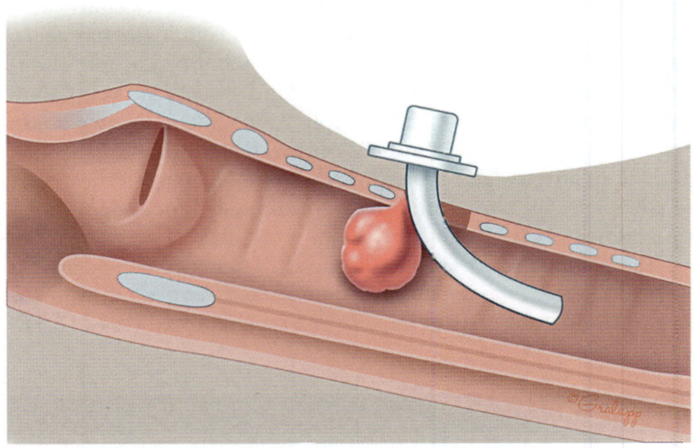

• **Fig. 16.5** Schematic lateral view of the cannula and the pedicle of the granuloma. (© 2024 Chris Gralapp.)

- Parental information regarding the necessity of open surgery in case of anterior and lateral collapse. If indicated, this procedure will be scheduled as a separate procedure following the diagnostic endoscopy.
- The need for a second look or additional procedures prior to continuing down the decannulation pathway should be discussed.

## Equipment

- Laryngoscope of appropriate size
- All necessary material for suspension laryngoscopy – see Chapter 2
- Hopkins rod telescope with 0 degree and 70 degree view angles

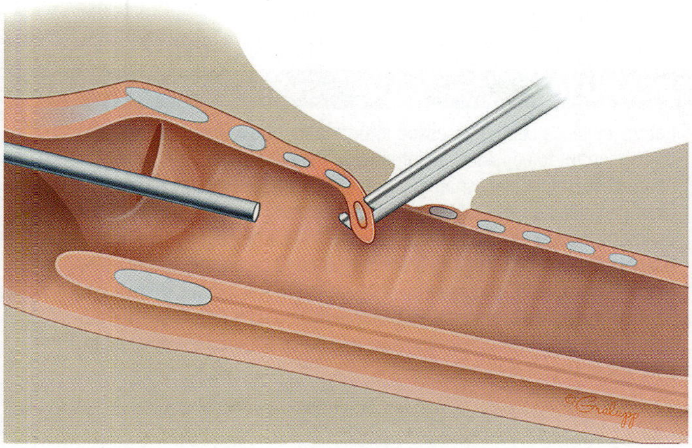

• **Fig. 16.6** Excision of collapsus of the anterior wall with through-cut endonasal forceps. (© 2024 Chris Gralapp.)

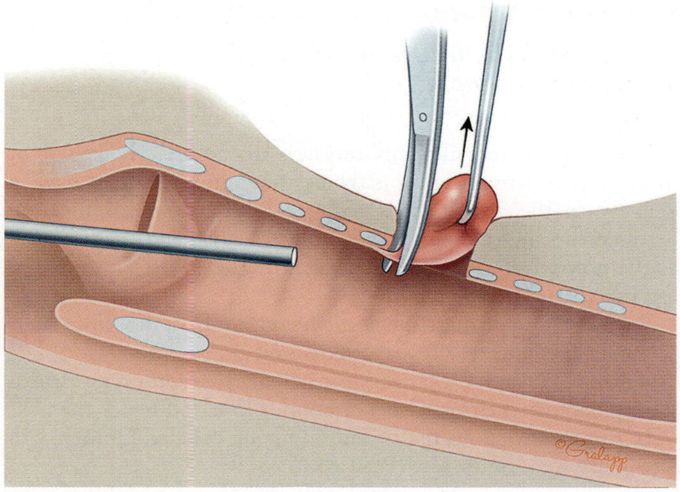

• **Fig. 16.7** Excision of suprastomal granuloma with Gillies hook and scissors. Same technique applies to large suprastomal anterior collapse. (© 2024 Chris Gralapp.)

- Laryngeal atomizer or means to anesthetize the larynx and trachea
- If LASER is used, appropriate LASER safety equipment, LASER generator, and micromanipulator that can be coupled with the operating microscope
- Laryngeal micro-instruments (forceps, scissors, etc.)
- Weil-Blakesley through-cutting forceps, Kerrison rongeur, or similar instruments for possible transcervical excision or debulking (see Fig. 16.6)
- Gillies hooks
- Scissors
- Bipolar forceps
- Cottonoid pledgets soaked in Epinephrine 1:50,000

## Patient Positioning

The patient is placed in a supine position with no shoulder roll and a gel donut around the head.

The tracheostomy site should remain accessible during the entire procedure in order to remove the cannula, to cap it, or to insert forceps through the stoma at any moment.

## General Anesthesia

Because the cannula will be removed during the procedure, it is helpful to provide:

- Intravenous general anesthesia maintaining spontaneous ventilation (avoid inhaled anesthesia if possible)
- Supplementary ventilation by Transnasal Humidified Rapid-Insufflation Ventilatory Exchange (THRIVE) or any device for oxygen diffusion

## Surgical Steps

### *Airway Assessment*

Airway assessment starts with nasal and pharyngeal flexible endoscopy in an awake patient. It continues with laryngotracheal endoscopy under spontaneous ventilation. Several tips can be used to increase the sensitivity of this exam:

1. Perform the endoscopy with the cannula initially left in place, and then removed
2. Switch off the THRIVE during the supra-stomal assessment in order to limit the ventilation artifacts that could mask a dynamic upper tracheal obstruction
3. After removing the cannula, occlude the stoma taking care not to apply additional pressure on local tissues and subsequently to the airway
4. Create a subglottic depression with a suction tube placed under the vocal folds

## Excision of Anterior Collapse With Cold Instruments by Combined Approach (see Video 16.3)

- Setup of the laryngeal suspension
- Visualization of the suprastomal anterior collapse with a 0-degree telescope
- Introduction of a Weil-Blakesley through-cutting forceps through the stoma
- Removal of the airway obstruction with the Weil-Blakesley through-cutting forceps under endoscopic visualization
- In case of bleeding, topical application of cottonoid pledgets soaked in epinephrine 1:50,000 or cauterization with bipolar forceps introduced through the stoma
- It is possible to improve the exposure of large collapses with a Gillies hook introduced through the stoma. The pedicle is then cut with thin sharp surgical scissors introduced through the stoma. In Fig. 16.7, we demonstrate the technique for granuloma excision, but the same technique applies to anterior collapse.
- At the end of the procedure, the endoscopist performs a final evaluation of airway patency and to ensure hemostasis.

## Excision of Anterior Collapse With LASER

### *Two Key Points in the Use of LASER to Treat Suprastomal Collapse*

- Safety

The major potential complication is airway fire. The key point to avoid such complication is the accurate monitoring of oxygen delivery to the airway. This requires excellent communication between the anesthesiology and surgical teams, and the lowering of the proportion of oxygen delivered by the THRIVE device to less than 30%

- In the setting of most subglottic lesions, only optical/fiber lasers can be used due to access/exposure limitations.

Fiber KTP or $CO_2$ lasers are particularly appropriate in this setting because their tissue penetration is low, and hence the risks of burning contiguous tissues and inducing collateral injury with secondary stenosis are low (Pearl 16.2).

**PEARL 16.2**

When using either $CO_2$ or KTP laser, it is important to understand the depth of penetration and potential for collateral thermal spread. The goal of incising tissue, rather than burning tissue superficially, is important to consider when using a laser in the airway.

### *Procedure*

- Laryngoscope suspension
- Patient protection: wet cloth on the face
- Caregivers' protection: protective glasses appropriate for the laser being used
- Patient's oxygenation must be set at safe levels by the anesthesiologist before the surgeon uses the laser
- Local anesthesia is applied to the stenotic area (lidocaine 1% up to 4 mg/kg)
- De-obstruction of the stenotic area (Pearl 16.3)
- Reduce local bleeding with 1:1000 epinephrine soaked cottonoid pledgets

**PEARL 16.3**

Lateral collapse can be assessed after treating the anterior collapse. It is important to consider the integrity of the peristomal framework. In obstructive, minimally dynamic (rigid) laterally based airway intrusion, the laser can also be used to address these lesions. The decision to perform unilateral wedge excision on the encroaching cartilage, or bilateral excision (staged or in a single setting) are highly dependent on the rigidity of the tracheal framework and severity of obstruction. This is thus patient and operator dependent. In addition, balloon dilation with or without steroid injection at the incision/excision site, can be considered as adjuncts to excision of lateral collapse.

## References


1. Doody J, Alkhateeb A, Balakrishnan K, et al. International Pediatric Otolaryngology Group (IPOG) consensus recommendations: management of suprastomal collapse in the pediatric population. *Int J Pediatr Otorhinolaryngol.* 2020;139:110427. doi:10.1016/j.ijporl.2020.110427.
2. Onder SS, Ishii A, Sandu K. Surgical options in suprastomal collapse-induced severe airway obstruction. *Eur Arch Otorhinolaryngol.* 2020;277(12):3415–3421. doi:10.1007/s00405-020-06339-3.
3. Tawfik A, Ebada HA, El-Fattah AMA, Kamal E. Surgical management of suprastomal tracheal collapse in children. *Int J Pediatr Otorhinolaryngol.* 2019;118:188–191. doi:10.1016/j.ijporl.2019.01.008.
4. Sharif-Askary B, Cheng TZ, Brown CS, Campbell JC, Yong Ji KS, Raynor EM. Airway findings in children with tracheostomies: when is diagnostic bronchoscopy and laryngoscopy indicated? *Int J Pediatr Otorhinolaryngol.* 2019;117:73–77. doi:10.1016/j.ijporl.2018.11.021.

17

# Endoscopic Management of Anterior Glottic Webs

DIEGO PRECIADO

## Background

Anterior glottic webs can be congenital or acquired. In truth, the term "congenital laryngeal web" is something of a misnomer, as these lesions are in fact a form of laryngeal atresia. A vast majority of congenital "webs" include thickening of the subglottic airway due to failure of programmed resorption of the laryngotracheal groove during the 10th week of embryogenesis.[1] These lesions therefore may result in some degree of airway obstruction and not simply vocal disturbance. The most common and widely accepted classification for congenital laryngeal atresia was first proposed by Seymour Cohen in 1985.[2] These lesions are graded from 1 to 4 depending on their severity (Table 17.1 and Fig. 17.1). The degree of luminal narrowing and subglottic involvement will dictate the symptomatology, but in general, most of the children will present in the first few months of life with airway obstruction symptoms or an abnormal cry.[3] While the subglottic narrowing can sometimes be appreciated on lateral plain film x-rays, the gold standard for the evaluation of these lesions is microdirect laryngoscopy and bronchoscopy under spontaneous ventilation anesthesia.

## Operative Procedure

### Patient Selection

In general, Cohen grades 1 and 2 are amenable to endoscopic intervention, while more severe lesions will require an open approach with laryngotracheoplasty cartilage graft expansion techniques or extended cricotracheal resection to achieve surgical success. However, as technology and surgical instrumentation evolve and improve, endoscopic procedures of the airway have become increasingly common, and indications for endoscopic airway surgery continue to grow, including procedures for more severe forms of congenital laryngeal atresia.

### Key Aspects of Informed Consent

In addition to the standard consent discussion for endoscopic airway operations, the surgeon should discuss risks of web recurrence, dysphonia or aphonia (either temporary due to keel placement or a longer-term problem if the vocal cords and superficial lamina propria are not well formed), dysphagia and/or coughing while a keel is in place, dislodgement of the keel into the airway requiring emergent removal, and need for additional procedures.

In children with congenital glottic webs, a discussion of possible underlying genetic causes is also worthwhile. Although there is no single gene mutation resulting in congenital laryngeal atresia, there is a strong association of this pathology in patients with 22q11.2 microdeletion,[4,5] with up to 20% of children with this chromosomal deletion noted to have some degree of congenital laryngeal atresia or anterior glottic web.[6] As such, patients with a congenital web should be offered further evaluation for possible 22q deletion.

It is important to consider that many children with 22q deletion syndromes will have congenital heart disease and may require a preoperative cardiac evaluation and cardiac anesthesia.

### Equipment

- Standard age-appropriate suspension laryngoscopy setup
- 0-, 30-, and 70-degree Hopkins rod telescopes with appropriate camera and image capture setup
- Operating microscope
- Laryngeal spreaders
- Blitzer knife (optional)
- Angled and straight endoscopic scissors
- Laser (optional) with micromanipulator attachment for microscope
- Thin silastic sheeting
- Soft-tissue instruments
- Lichtenberger endolaryngeal needle driver (optional)

### Patient Positioning

Per surgeon preference; standard endoscopic airway surgery positioning is generally appropriate.

### Steps of Procedure

Techniques for repair in general include establishing the anterior commissure with minimal cicatricial tissue at the vibrating surface of the glottis while achieving an open airway lumen. Endoscopic laser anterior commissurotomy simply divides the glottic web in the midline. Cutting the web on one side of the glottis and suturing it to the contralateral side to provide mucosal coverage has also been proposed (Fig. 17.2).[7,8]

**TABLE 17.1 COHEN Classification System From Descriptions in Cohen[2]**

| | Glottic Percentage | Subglottic stenosis | Thickness | Vocal Folds | Voice | Airway obstruction |
|---|---|---|---|---|---|---|
| **Type 1** | <35% | Little to none | Uniform | Identifiable | Hoarse | Minimal |
| **Type 2** | 35–50% | Minimal SGS at anterior portion of the web | Thin or Thick | Identifiable | Hoarse/Weak | With infection/trauma |
| **Type 3** | 50–75% | Anterior subglottic stenosis | Thick anterior and thinner posterior | Mostly visible, possibly obscured | Weak | Moderately severe, Frequent Tracheostomy |
| **Type 4** | 75–90% | Severely narrowed | Uniformly thick | Not identifiable | Aphonic | Severe, Tracheostomy shortly after birth |

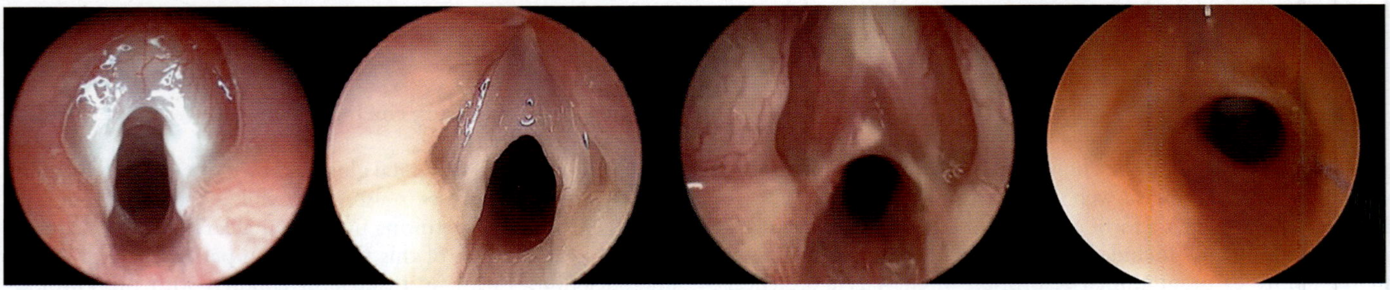

• **Fig. 17.1** Cohen scale from 1 to 4 (note the lack of discernable vocal folds in grade 4).

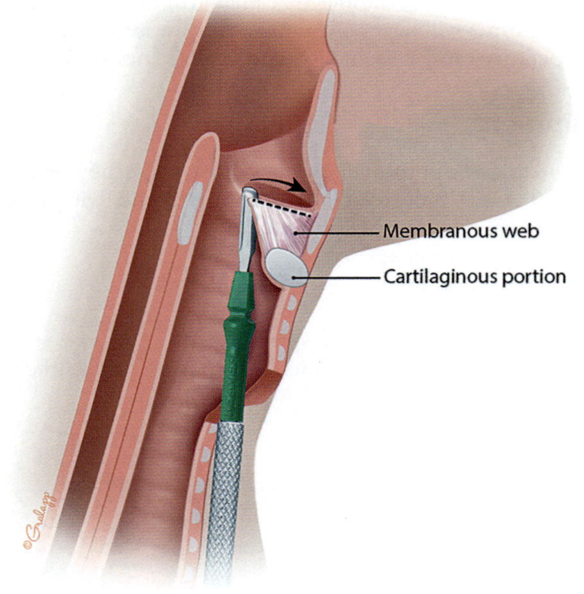


• **Fig. 17.2** Glottic web. (© 2024 Chris Gralapp.)

Perhaps the most popular technique involves division of the web with endoscopic guidance (Video 17.1) with the temporary placement of a silastic "keel" or sheet,[3,9–11] which may decrease the risk of web recurrence. Briefly, the technique is as follows:

1. Suspension laryngoscopy with microlaryngeal division of the web (laser or cold technique). This can most easily be done in the midline. Care should be taken to align the incision with the anterior commissure (Pearl 17.1).

**PEARL 17.1**

Also at this time, after division of the web, additional visualization and palpation of the subglottic component of the web, when present, should be performed. Sizing the airway again after web division using standard Myer-Cotton technique is appropriate. This allows for an objective assessment of the size of the airway and helps to eliminate any optical illusions, which may make the subglottic airway appear larger than it really is. If a firm subglottic cartilaginous component is present, this should also be addressed.

2. A small horizontal skin incision is made externally, over the thyroid cartilage.
3. A Prolene stitch (4-0 or 3-0) on a straight needle is then passed through the midline of the lower thyroid cartilage, aiming to be below the level of the glottis, and visualized telescopically in the airway. The needle is grasped and pulled out the mouth.
4. A hollow large-bore needle is then passed through the midline of the upper thyroid cartilage, aiming to be above the web, and visualized in the airway.
5. Next, a "keel" (typically a thin silastic sheet) is mattressed by the prolene stitch, which had been pulled out of the mouth and directed endoscopically to cover the raw surface of the web, with the keel secured by the Prolene. The free end of the Prolene suture is passed into the lumen of the large-bore hollow needle and withdrawn back through the neck incision externally.
6. After the keel is positioned, the suture is tied under the skin, typically over a small angiocath tube or sterile button, to maintain the material intact and easy to localize later upon removal of the sheet.

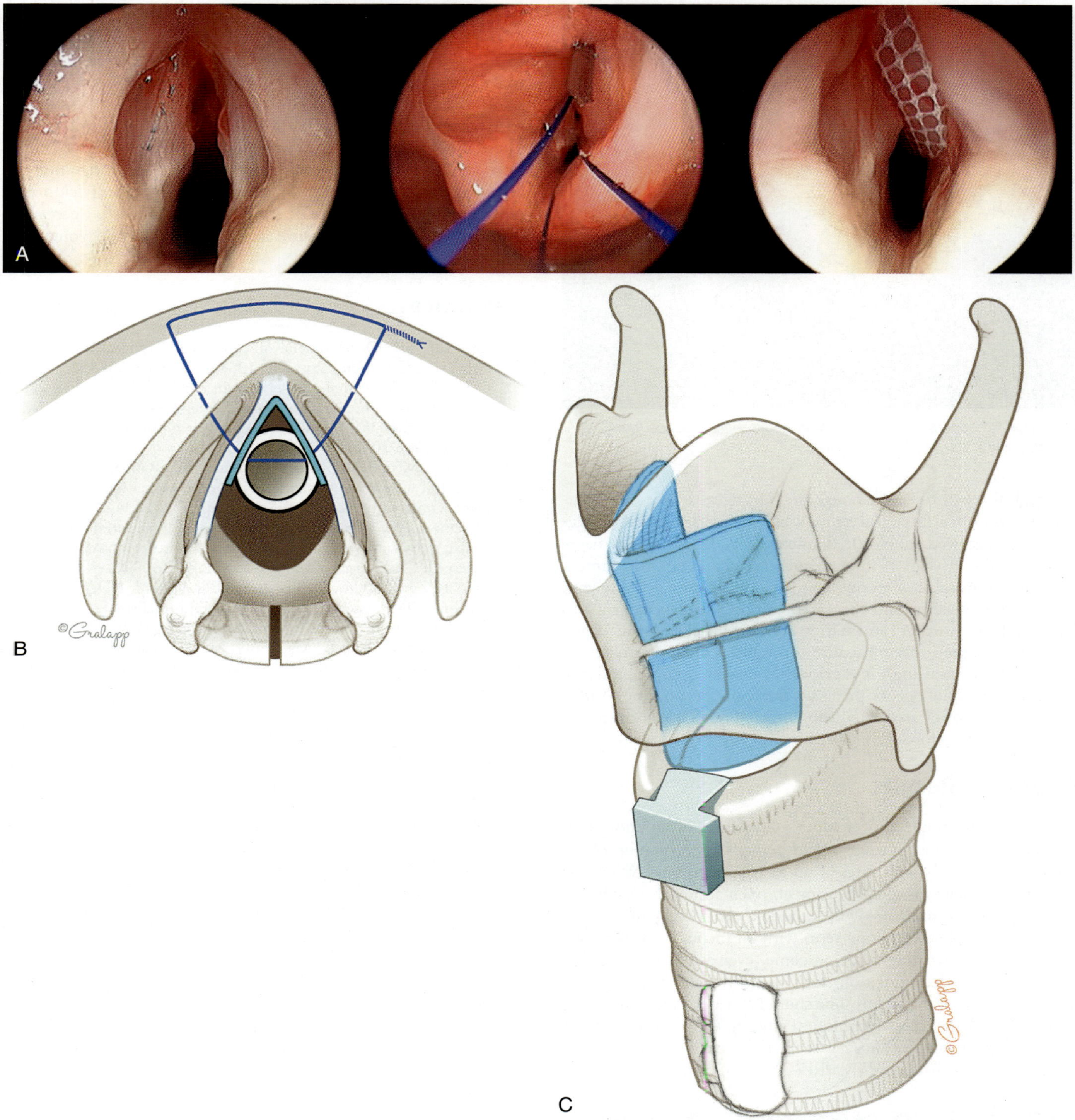


• **Fig. 17.3** Endoscopic silastic keel placement (A), which may be combined with laryngeal stent placement (B), with anterior cartilage graft to address subglottic component of the web (C). Note that the anterior graft portion of the operation must be done via a transcervical approach. (B and C © 2024 Chris Gralapp.)

7. The sheet is typically kept in place for 2 to 3 weeks. In patients without tracheostomy tubes, it is critical to monitor for any granulation tissue development, which could cause airway obstruction.
8. Other surgeons prefer to attempt web lysis with endoscopic lateralization and placement of a silastic sheet. An example of such technique is shown in Fig. 17.3.

Some variations of the described technique involve buccal mucosal or perichondrium grafts for interposition, or an epiglottic flap for large anterior commissural defects in lieu of the laryngeal keel (reviewed in Lahav et al.[12]); these are techniques usually best suited for older patients or adults with true acquired webs suffering from voice disturbances.

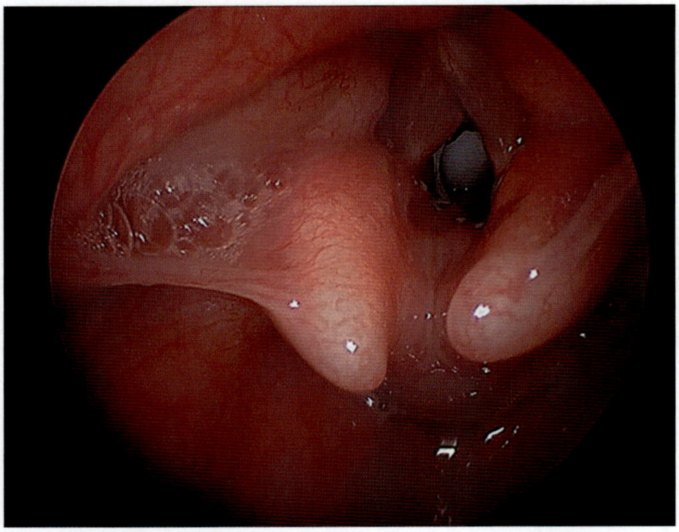

• **Fig. 17.4** Postoperative anterior commissure incongruence, years after laryngoplasty.

Surgical repair of severe congenital laryngeal atresia cases usually involves open laryngeal surgery using cartilage grafts to augment the narrowed subglottic diameter (Fig. 17.3C), with placement of stents[13] (Fig. 17.3B) to preserve the subglottic lumen, anterior commissure anatomy, and provide a luminal framework around which healing and contracture occur. Readers can refer to Chapter 15 for further information about stent placement. When splitting the anterior commissure through an open approach (in preparation for grafting), it is critical to use endoscopic guidance to ensure the split occurs precisely through the midline (Video 17.1). Treatment of associated subglottic stenosis is critical to the success of surgery for severe glottic webs.[13]

## Treatment Results

In general, one should expect some mild degree of anterior commissure blunting and to some extent perhaps a reformation of the anterior glottic web, with rates of up to 70% reported.[4] When the severity of the stenosis dictates using an open approach to split the anterior glottic commissure with secondary expansion grafting, it is very common to end up long term with an incongruent commissure and an unfavorable voice outcome, even when patients successfully achieve decannulation (Fig. 17.4). In terms of decannulation or avoiding tracheotomy, one should expect surgical success of greater than 80% across techniques, although some authors have reported higher re adhesion/recurrence rates in higher Cohen classification (3 or 4) patients[10] (Pearl 17.2).

**PEARL 17.2**

It is important to understand that the appearance of the surgical outcome does not always correspond with the voice outcome. Even in the absence of anterior commissure blunting or residual web, pediatric voice outcomes are highly variable.

## Conclusion

In summary, most congenital laryngeal webs are in fact not true webs, but a form of congenital subglottic stenosis/laryngeal atresia. In that sense, expansion of the lumen is frequently necessary, which may be a limiting factor for some endoscopic techniques. These lesions are more common in patients with 22q11.2 deletion syndrome. Lower-grade lesions, whether congenital or acquired, are most frequently managed with web division and temporary endoscopic silastic sheet (keel) placement. Recreation of a true anterior commissure is often difficult, and voice outcomes vary.

## References


1. Zaw-Tun HI. Development of congenital laryngeal atresias and clefts. *Ann Otol Rhinol Laryngol.* 1988;97(4 Pt 1):353–358.
2. Cohen SR. Congenital glottic webs in children. A retrospective review of 51 patients. *Ann Otol Rhinol Laryngol Suppl.* 1985;121:2–16.
3. Kuo IC, Rutter M. Surgical management of anterior glottic webs. *Front Pediatr.* 2020;8:555040.
4. Lawlor CM, Dombrowski ND, Nuss RC, Rahbar R, Choi SS. Laryngeal web in the pediatric population: evaluation and management. *Otolaryngol Head Neck Surg.* 2020;162(2):234–240.
5. Miyamoto RC, Cotton RT, Rope AF, et al. Association of anterior glottic webs with velocardiofacial syndrome (chromosome 22q11.2 deletion). *Otolaryngol Head Neck Surg.* 2004;130(4):415–417.
6. Sacca R, Zur KB, Crowley TB, Zackai EH, Valverde KD, McDonald-McGinn DM. Association of airway abnormalities with 22q11.2 deletion syndrome. *Int J Pediatr Otorhinolaryngol.* 2017;96:11–14.
7. Xiao Y, Wang J, Han D, Ma L, Ye J, Xu W. Vocal cord mucosal flap for the treatment of acquired anterior laryngeal web. *Chin Med J (Engl).* 2014;127(7):1294–1297.
8. Yilmaz T. Surgical treatment of glottic web using butterfly mucosal flap technique: experience on 12 patients. *Laryngoscope.* 2019;129(6):1423–1427.
9. Hsueh JY, Tsai CS, Hsu HT. Intralaryngeal approach to laryngeal web using lateralization with silastic. *Laryngoscope.* 2000;110(10 Pt 1):1780–1782.
10. Benmansour N, Remacle M, Matar N, Lawson G, Bachy V, Van Der Vorst V. Endoscopic treatment of anterior glottic webs according to Lichtenberger technique and results on 18 patients. *Eur Arch Otorhinolaryngol.* 2012;269(9):2075–2080.
11. Paniello RC, Desai SC, Allen CT, Khosla SM. Endoscopic keel placement to treat and prevent anterior glottic webs. *Ann Otol Rhinol Laryngol.* 2013;122(11):672–678.
12. Lahav Y, Shoffel-Havakuk H, Halperin D. Acquired glottic stenosis-the ongoing challenge: a review of etiology, pathogenesis, and surgical management. *J Voice.* 2015;29(5) 646 e1–646 e10.
13. Tunkel DE. A novel stent for treatment of combined anterior glottic web-subglottic stenosis. *Int J Pediatr Otorhinolaryngol.* 2005;69(7):893–896.

# SECTION IV

# Surgery for Voice

18

# True Vocal Fold Injection Medialization

KATE HEATHCOTE AND MICHELLE WYATT

## Background

The indication for true vocal fold injection medialization (IM) is glottic insufficiency. Symptoms of glottic insufficiency are dysphonia, aspiration, and ineffective cough. In children, glottic insufficiency is usually caused by unilateral vocal fold paralysis (VFP) secondary to recurrent laryngeal nerve trauma during cardiac surgery. A meta-analysis of over 5600 patients having had such intervention showed an incidence of VCP of nearly 10%.[1] However, studies involving routine laryngoscopy after cardiac surgery showed an incidence of VFP of closer to 30%, with rates particularly high for those who had patent ductus arteriosus repair.[2]

Repair of esophageal atresia with or without an associated trachea-esophageal fistula also has a high incidence of VFP, with rates up to 22% reported.[3] Idiopathic paralysis is less common but can occur; glottic insufficiency may also occur as a result of direct vocal fold trauma, typically from intubation.

It is important to note that there is a spontaneous recovery rate associated with unilateral vocal fold palsy. After PDA ligation, recovery rates up to 33% have been noted,[4] while with idiopathic causes, up to 40% can resolve.[5] This recovery can occur after several months or even up to 1 to 2 years later, and this possibility must be considered when proposing treatment options.

## Operative Assessment

In children, the relative indication for injection medialization (IM) of the vocal folds varies, often depending on the age of the child as well as the symptomatology. Modification of feeds is often the first-line management of patients with VFP when aspiration is a concern. Regarding the length of time before consideration of injection, the average duration obtained from a survey of the American Society of Pediatric Otolaryngology (ASPO) members was 3.5 months after diagnosis. However, earlier intervention was proposed by respondents of the ASPO survey if patients were poor candidates for medical therapy or their pulmonary status was tenuous enough to warrant aggressive management of aspiration.[6] In a separate study, an increased incidence of diet advancement was noted in children who were injected within six months of the onset of the VFP.[7]

## Patient Selection

Under 2 years of age: Vocal fold medialization can be considered when there is aspiration and ineffective cough in the context of unilateral vocal fold paralysis (UVFP). Unilateral vocal fold paralysis is diagnosed by awake flexible nasendoscopy and/or ultrasound of the larynx. On evaluation of swallow, these children may be considered at risk of aspiration and nasogastric feeding instigated. As stated earlier, a significant proportion of children can recover vocal fold movement, but persistence of these issues, such that longer-term enteral feeding is being considered, should trigger more active intervention to facilitate continuation of oral feeding.

Vocal fold medialization may prevent aspiration and provide an effective cough such that oral feeds may be continued and oral aversion and other feeding issues avoided. Many infants with UVFP have other medical issues associated with prematurity or congenital conditions, and avoiding further lung damage from aspiration should be prioritized.

However, there are concerns that medialization could lead to respiratory compromise in the very young due to narrowing of the glottic inlet. There is much debate in specialist Pediatric Otolaryngology Units as to the "safe" age for injection. Some would consider waiting until a child is over 2 years, but others will intervene in those under 1 year of age.[6] Careful postoperative monitoring and supportive airway management are vital if this intervention is to be considered.

We advocate for assessment of the larynx under general anesthetic to allow simultaneous assessment of cricoarytenoid joint mobility, possible injection augmentation of the vocal folds, and possible laryngeal electromyography. We see this as a step in the pathway to nonselective laryngeal reinnervation (NSR).

**In children aged 2 to 5 years** with UVFP from an early age, the problem of aspiration has often resolved with either recovery of the paralysis or adaptation of the swallow. Injection medialization may be considered if this is not the case or if it is a new onset. Again, IM is a useful tool in cases where a temporary

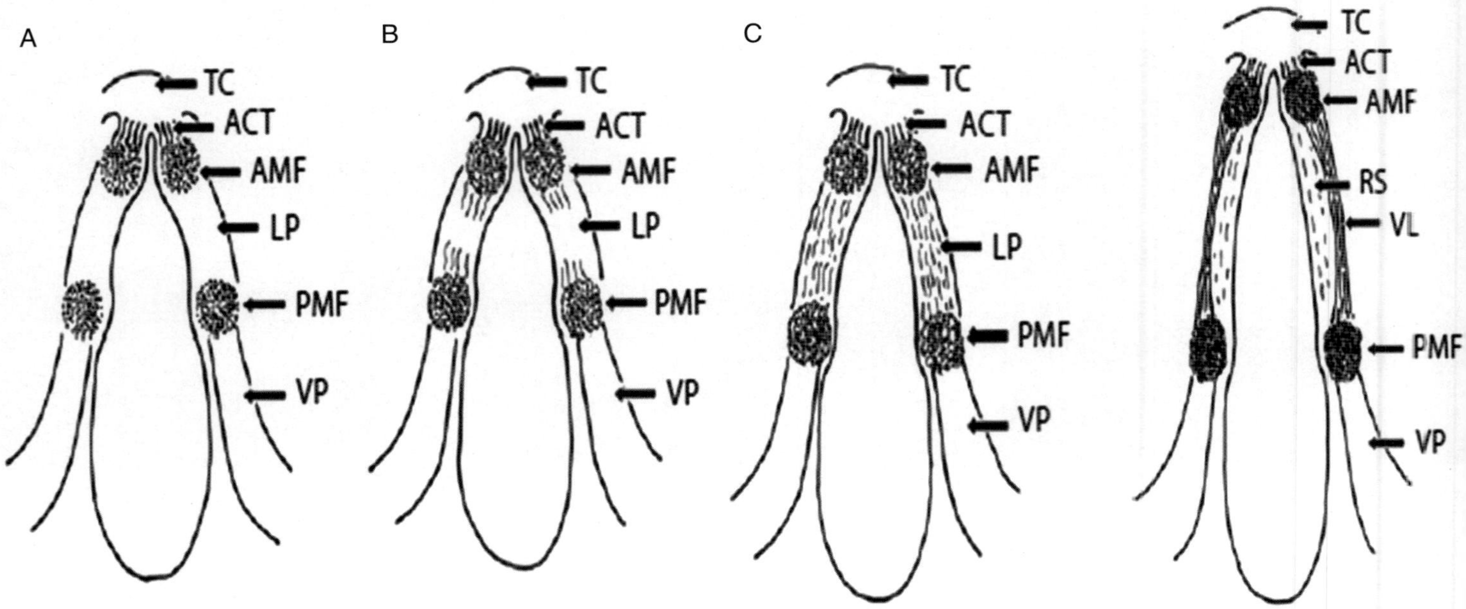


• **Fig. 18.1** From left to right: human newborn, infant, child, and adult maculae flavae and vocal fold mucosa. *ACT*, Anterior commissure tendon; *AMF*, anterior macula flava; *LP*, lamina propria; *PMF*, posterior macula flava; *RS*, Reinke's space; *TC*, thyroid cartilage; *VL*, vocal ligament; *VP*, vocal process of arytenoid cartilage. (From Sato K, Umeno H, Nakashima T. Functional histology of the macula flava in the human vocal fold—Part 2: Its role in the growth and development of the vocal fold. *Folia Phoniatr Logop* 2010;62(6):263–270.)

improvement is required to avoid enteral feeding and improve cough, or while awaiting recovery of vocal fold mobility or the effects of NSR.

**In children over 5 years old,** normalization of voice is essential for social and educational development. In new cases, or those where recovery may still occur, an IM is useful; however, in well-established UVFP, repeated IM is less desirable and the option of a definitive intervention (NSR) should be considered.

**In teenagers** with new-onset UVFP, aspiration is less commonly an issue, but IM can be performed to re-establish voice. This supports their social and educational needs while awaiting possible recovery of vocal fold function. In properly selected teenagers, it may be possible to perform this as an in-office procedure under local anesthetic. Injection medialization can be a useful trial for improving glottic competence prior to pursuing NSR in teenagers.

In cases of vocal fold trauma where the vocal folds need augmenting to achieve glottic closure, the procedure is best performed under general anesthetic. This allows the clinician to palpate and target the injection to the deficient region of the vocal fold. Injection augmentation is a useful trial prior to open thyroplasty, as it allows understanding of whether normal voicing can be achieved despite the compensatory mechanisms that may have developed, such as supraglottic phonation. It may also help elevate vocal fold scar prior to thyroplasty.

## Key Aspects of Informed Consent

With the exception of carefully selected older children, general anesthesia (GA) is required for IM in the pediatric population. The standard implications of this must be considered and discussed with the patient and their family.

Under GA, the larynx is approached with the child in suspension laryngoscopy and so has the associated risks of injury to the lips, teeth, and tongue. Care must be taken if there is an underlying coagulopathy, which is not uncommon in children with cardiac conditions. There is also the risk of airway obstruction by overinjection and reaction to the specific compound used. This is discussed further below.

A particular concern with injecting a child is related to the fact that it may affect development of the vocal fold structure. Children are not born with the classic three-layered structure of the lamina propria (LP) that exists in the adult.

### *Development of the Vocal Fold*

The newborn LP is a loose monolayered structure with no vocal ligament. It has cellular regions called macula flavae at the anterior and posterior ends from which the fibrous components of the vocal fold developed. Two layers start to appear at around 2 months of age, and by 11 months, three layers can be determined, but it takes until the age of 7 for this process to be complete. The adult structure, where the layers are defined by differing elastin and collagen components, does not develop until around 13 years. The superficial layer remains hypocellular while the middle is predominantly elastin and the deeper layer collagen.[8] This evolution in structure is reflected by the membranous portion of the vocal fold being much shorter before adolescence (Fig. 18.1).

The low risk of injection negatively influencing the developing vocal fold is thought to be outweighed by the potential benefits. This must be discussed with the child and family beforehand and informed consent obtained. From a practical perspective, great care is taken to keep the needle placement as lateral as possible to ensure the injectable is delivered into the paraglottic space rather than more superficial tissues (Figs. 18.2 and 18.3).

## Operative Approach

### Equipment

#### *Types of Injectables*

**Autologous Fat**

Using the body's own tissue has advantages in avoiding a foreign body reaction and avoiding the cost associated with a commercial material. However, extraction and preparation prolong the procedure, and there is a risk of morbidity at the donor site. The most common location for fat harvest is the abdomen, but children may not necessarily have the reserves that adults do. Fat lasts for a variable time as it is redistributed by the body, and as such, it is not possible to predict the duration of the effect. As such, overinjection is often proposed in adults, but this could cause airway limitation or compromise in a younger child (Pearl 18.1).

> **PEARL 18.1**
>
> Fat is a good option for patients with vocal fold volume deficiency, for example in the setting of atrophy. A percentage of the fat frequently remains for many years and can be thought of as permanent augmentation material. Unfortunately, the percentage of fat that will remain is difficult to predict, and subsequent injections may be needed.

**Calcium Hydroxylapatite (CaHA)**

This injectable is composed of microspheres of CaHA in a carboxymethylcellulose carrier, and studies have shown it to be effective for up to 18 months. It is available off the shelf and ready to inject. Side effects that have been reported include inflammation, migration of the microspheres, and the fact that, if injected too superficially, it may interfere with the pliability of the vocal fold (Pearl 18.2). Also, this product comes with a recommendation for slight overinjection to counteract the anticipated reduction of volume that occurs in the first few days after administration. These features have resulted in the fact that use of the carrier agent (carboxymethylcellulose) alone is preferred in children.

> **PEARL 18.2**
>
> A misplaced injection may be difficult to correct, and injection material has been discovered in the larynx many years after injection.

**Carboxymethylcellulose Gel**

Sodium carboxymethylcellulose in combination with glycerin in a gel carrier of sterile water is available as an injectable. It has an excellent safety profile, but its duration of action is 3 months at best. This also requires no preparation and is sold directly ready to administer.

**Hyaluronic Acid Gels**

These substances are animal- or bacterial-derived variations of the naturally occurring extracellular matrix glycosaminoglycan found in various human tissues, including the vocal fold LP. They have a relatively good safety profile for vocal fold medialization and last for around 4 to 6 months. They are available pre-prepared and have the advantage that overinjection is not recommended.

With this substance, inflammatory side effects have been reported, with airway compromise occurring as a result.[9] Hyaluronidase is the enzyme that breaks down these gels and can therefore be used to help reverse unwanted side effects if an unfavorable reaction occurs (Pearl 18.3).

> **PEARL 18.3**
>
> Although reactions are very rare, having hyaluronidase available and accessible at your institution is worthwhile prior to using this injectable material. Some of these preparations include local anesthetic, which may reduce postoperative discomfort.

Of note, licensing of injectables for use in the pediatric larynx is very limited and varies between jurisdictions and must be discussed as part of the preoperative consent process. There is consensus that certain materials should never be considered in children, and these include Bioplastique, silicone, and Teflon (Pearl 18.4).

> **PEARL 18.4**
>
> Although excellent outcomes may occur in experienced hands, similar to Teflon and silicone injections in the past, many would advise against using CaHA in young children as well.

#### *Operative Setup*

**Under GA**

We recommend IM, when performed under GA, to be done with the larynx suspended using an appropriately sized Lindholm laryngoscope. The child is breathing spontaneously with total intravenous anesthesia with oxygenation via a nasopharyngeal airway. Atomized local anesthetic is delivered prior to instrumentation to reduce the risk of laryngospasm.

There are various options for the needle used to deliver the injectable. We prefer the Butterfly Winged Infusion set with a 27-gauge × ¾-inch needle. The flanges are trimmed to facilitate access. The piece of residual flange is held with crocodile forceps and the needle is bent upward at the base as required to optimize visualization of the tip as it is inserted.

Alternatively, a long rigid needle is available, with a 24-gauge tip and a 16-gauge, 25-cm long malleable shaft, which may be required for some injectables. Also, a 22-gauge spinal needle may be appropriate, depending on the size of the child and type of injectable used.

**Under Local Anesthetic**

If the procedure is performed with the patient awake, the child is sat in a dental chair. Of note, fat is not suitable for this route due to the pressure required for its delivery. Both nostrils are anesthetized and decongested (we use cophenylcaine and xylometazoline). The most patent nostril is cannulated with a

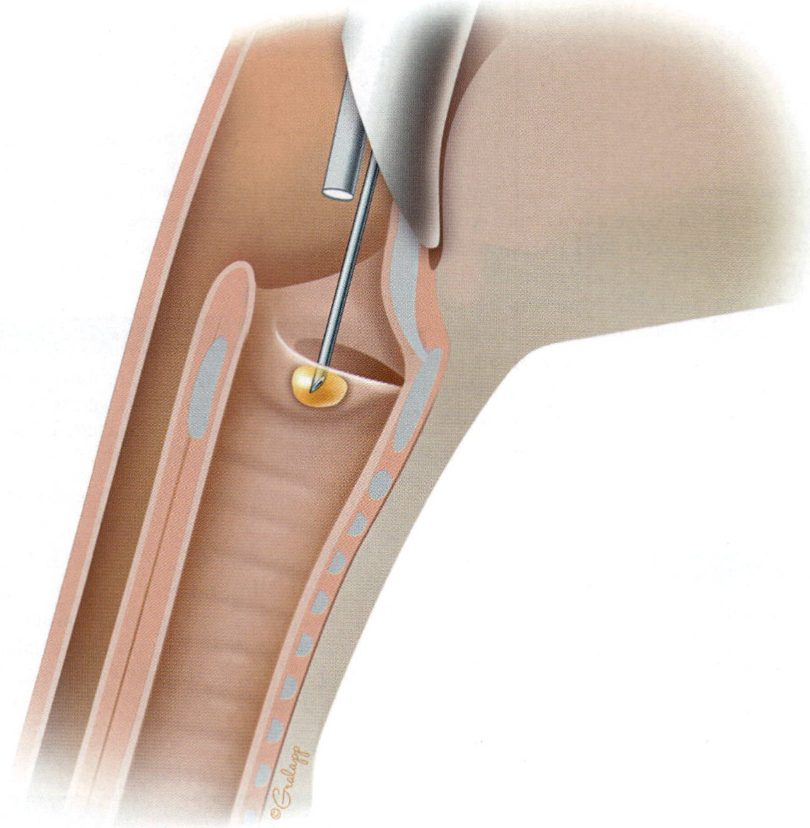


• **Fig. 18.2** Endoscopic injection medialization of the vocal fold—sagittal view. (© 2024 Chris Gralapp.)

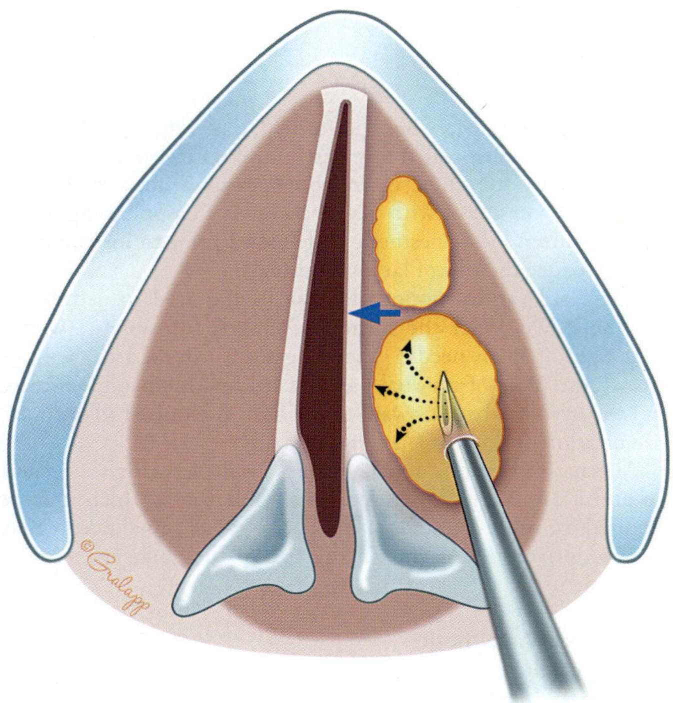


• **Fig. 18.3** Endoscopic injection medialization of the vocal fold—axial view. Note the placement of the injectable in the paraglottic space rather than the substance of the true vocal cord itself. (© 2024 Chris Gralapp.)

lubricated appropriately sized flexible nasendoscope to enable visualization of the larynx. To anesthetize the larynx, we use a dental syringe and needle containing 2% lidocaine with 1 in 80,000 epinephrine introduced superiorly via a transcervical approach through the thyrohyoid membrane. The needle is positioned above the vocal folds, and the anesthetic is dripped slowly over them as the child phonates. The injectable is then placed via the same route with a commercial product of choice attached to a suitable needle. We use a 23-gauge, 6-cm needle, which we bend to achieve the appropriate angle.

The local anesthetic technique is advantageous in determining the amount of filler required to achieve closure, as the patient is able to phonate and demonstrate the degree of closure achieved.

### Additional Operative Tips

**Priming of the Injectable.** In all cases the needle of choice must be primed with the injectable prior to introducing it into the patient. It is recommended to prime the cannula and the needle just prior to injection and to flush the apparatus just after injection so that the material does not harden in the cannula.

**Delivery of the Injectable.** Ensure the syringe is held in a manner that adequate pressure can be applied without having to alter the hand position once the needle is in the tissues. We recommend that the piston of the syringe should rest on the thenar eminence rather than the thumb.

**How Much to Inject.** The volume placed is limited by the space available, which reflects the child's age. There is a balance to achieve between adequate treatment of glottic insufficiency and avoiding any airway compromise. Families should be warned about possible additional noise of breathing post intervention, including stridor, but airway compromise must be avoided.

**Post Operative Management.** One dose of intravenous dexamethasone (0.25–0.5 mg/kg) is given as standard perioperatively and can be repeated at a lower or similar dose if required afterward. We recommend admission overnight with regular airway observations including oxygen saturations. Routine antibiotics are not required. Speech and language therapy input is recommended to determine the timing of appropriate swallow assessment and management. Our patients are reviewed clinically the next day to form a discharge feeding plan.

## Conclusion

We would like to propose that symptomatic UVFP is treated in early childhood to minimize the psychosocial, developmental, and potentially educational impact. Late injections, performed years after the development of vocal fold immobility, may result in a sub-optimal outcome, as vocal limitations and compensatory maneuvers have often become embedded in the patient's persona.

## References

1. Strychowsky JE, Rukholm G, Gupta MK, Reid D. Unilateral vocal fold paralysis after congenital cardiothoracic surgery: a meta-analysis. *Pediatrics*. 2014;133:e1708–e1723.
2. Smith ME, King JD, Elsherif A, Muntz HR, Park AH, Kouretas PC. Should all newborns who undergo patent ductus arteriosus ligation be examined for vocal fold mobility? *Laryngoscope*. 2009;119:1606–1609.
3. Kovesi T, Porcaro F, Petreschi F, Trozzi M, Bottero S, Cutrera R. Vocal cord paralysis appears to be an acquired lesion in children with repaired esophageal atresia/tracheoesophageal fistula. *Int J Pediatr Otorhinolaryngol*. 2018;112:45–47.
4. Engeseth MS, Olsen NR, Maeland S, Halvorsen T, Goode A, Røksund OD. Left vocal cord paralysis after patent ductus arteriosus ligation: a systematic review. *Paediatr Respir Rev*. 2018;27:74–85.
5. Jabbour J, Martin T, Beste D, Robey T. Pediatric vocal fold immobility: natural history and the need for long-term follow-up. *JAMA Otolaryngol Head Neck Surg*. 2014;140:428–433.
6. Jang M, Gregory S, Jabbour J, Robey TC, Sulman C, Chun R. Injection laryngoplasty in infants with unilateral vocal cord paralysis: a survey of ASPO members. *Int J Pediatr Otorhinolaryngol*. 2020; 128:109671.
7. Meister KD, Johnson A, Sidell DR. Injection laryngoplasty for children with unilateral vocal fold paralysis: procedural limitations and swallow outcomes. *Otolaryngol Head Neck Surg*. 2019;160(3):540–545.
8. Hartnick CJ, Rehbar R, Prasad V. Development and maturation of the pediatric human vocal fold lamina propria. *Laryngoscope*. 2005;115(1):4–15.
9. Hamdan AL, Khalifee E. Adverse reaction to restylane: a review of 63 cases of injection laryngoplasty. *Ear Nose Throat J*. 2019;98(4): 212–216.

# 19

# Posterior Cricoid Reduction Laryngoplasty

ALESSANDRO DE ALARCON

## Background

Posterior cricoid reduction (PCR) is a procedure designed to address deficiencies of the posterior glottis, specifically posterior glottic diastasis. Posterior glottic diastasis is a condition where the posterior glottis is always open during phonation. The posterior diastasis may be a result of intubation (short or long term) leading to a loss of tissue and a "carved-out" or a hollowed-out appearance to the posterior glottis. Patients with a history of prior airway reconstruction with a posterior graft may have a large posterior diastasis due to the graft's causing a larger-than-normal space in the posterior glottis. Patients may present with a breathy dysphonia, short phonation times, aspiration, or supraglottic phonation. This chapter focuses on the endoscopic PCR for posterior glottic diastasis. For additional management options for posterior glottic diastasis, please refer to Chapter 20.

## Operative Endoscopic Assessment

### Patient Selection

Patients with a clinical suspicion of posterior glottic diastasis and a prior voice assessment, including stroboscopy, acoustic, aerodynamic, perceptual evaluation of voice, and voice-related quality of life, will benefit from a formal operative endoscopic assessment prior to proceeding to surgical repair.

### Key Aspects of Informed Consent

Standard risks of operative airway endoscopy should be discussed, including:

- Risks of general anesthesia
- Risks of injury to oral, pharyngeal, and airway structures

### Equipment

- Appropriately sized laryngoscope
- Hopkins rod telescope (0 degree)
- Equipment to spray medications on the larynx
- Small alligator forceps

## Steps to This Assessment

1. Patient positioning: The patient is positioned supine with head at the top of the table. The table is turned 90 degrees with the patient's left side toward the anesthesiology provider. A 5.0 to 6.0 endotracheal (ET) tube is positioned to insufflate and attached to the anesthetic circuit. No shoulder roll is used. If the patient's head tends to roll to one side or the other, a rolled towel or gel donut can be placed around the head. Particular care should be taken not to overextend the neck. When properly exposed, the glottis should be readily visible and accessible surgically.
2. Under telescopic or microscopic visualization and after application of topical laryngeal anesthetic, the airway is assessed from the supraglottis to the distal airway. This is particularly important in patients with a history of prior airway reconstruction to assess for other causes of the dysphonia as well as any potential areas that may cause problems for surgical correction of the posterior diastasis.
3. The posterior glottis should be closely inspected to visualize and confirm the diastasis. A small alligator is then used to palpate the arytenoid joints bilaterally to evaluate for fixation (Pearl 19.1).
4. The airway is then formally sized using appropriately sized ET tubes to gauge the airway size.
5. Airway assessment also ensures the feasibility of an endoscopic approach to the posterior diastasis.

Suspension laryngoscopy may be beneficial in cases where the exposure is difficult or to better assess arytenoid/vocal fold fixation.

**PEARL 19.1**

Palpation of the midline posterior cricoid to assess cartilage integrity is also useful.

## Operative Approach

### Patient Selection and Informed Consent

Patients should have undergone full assessment with an initial endoscopic assessment as well as a full voice evaluation (Pearl 19.2). CT imaging is a useful adjunct, specifically dynamic

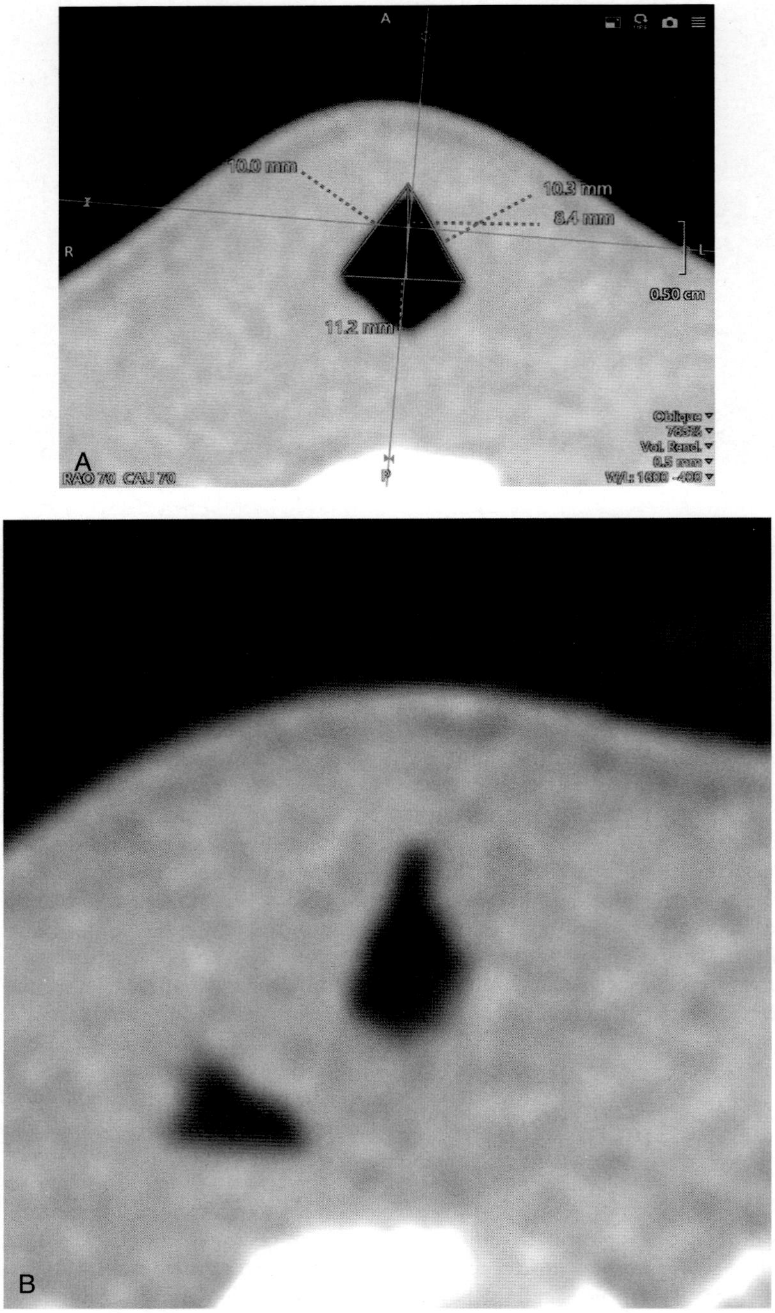


• **Fig. 19.1** (A) Dynamic CT image at the level of the glottis in the relaxed position. Examples of the measurements that can be taken including the length of the vocal fold and the maximum width at the vocal process, which in this case is 11.2 mm. (B) Dynamic CT image at the level of the glottis during phonation demonstrating the posterior gap.

**PEARL 19.2**

It has been objectively established that patients who participate in both voice therapy and surgical intervention have better outcomes than those who adhere to only one treatment regimen.

CT imaging allowing for direct measurement and visualization of the posterior gap. Images are taken statically and during sustained phonation (Fig. 19.1A and 19.1B). Three-dimensional (3D) reconstructions can aid in assessment; visualization from the subglottis toward the inferior surface of the glottis are key images of the gaps (Fig. 19.2A and 19.2B). Measurement of the posterior glottis can be made at the vocal process level to assess the static glottis and the residual posterior diastasis to aid in planning the exact amount of posterior cricoid to remove (Pearl 19.3). Ideal candidates have undergone their pubertal growth spurt. If a decision is made to proceed prior to the growth spurt, there

**PEARL 19.3**

At institutions where this advanced airway imaging is not available, the surgeon may consider comparing the current airway size (obtained with ET tube sizing as noted earlier) to the "ideal" airway size, as determined by calculating age-appropriate normal airway sizing. The difference in outer circumference between the current and ideal ET tube sizes indicates roughly the amount of PCR that might be appropriate.

is a possibility that the procedure may need to be repeated if the voice worsens again post completion of puberty (Pearl 19.4). Patients with a prior history of cricotracheal resection and an A-frame deformity are at high risk for destabilizing the cricoid and a resulting severely symptomatic A-frame. The airway should ideally size with at least a 6.0 ET tube before proceeding with reduction. Glottic fixation and arytenoid fixation are relative contraindications; in these patients, care should be taken to remove a smaller portion of the posterior cricoid to maintain an adequate airway.

**PEARL 19.4**

In younger patients or those with smaller airways, careful sizing is warranted, as PCR will naturally reduce the airway caliber. In patients with inadequate airway patency, despite the presence of pathologic diastasis, cricoid reduction could lead to airway obstruction. Allowing for adequate airway growth prior to intervention is usually the safer approach.

## Key Aspects of Informed Consent

Same as endoscopic assessment, with the following additional risks

- Airway fire during the use of the laser
- Posterior glottic stenosis if there is excessive scarring in the surgical bed
- Subglottic stenosis if the airway is significantly narrowed
- Postoperative stridor or airway obstruction due to swelling; typically, may last 12 to 24 hours and resolves with time and or administration of oral/IV steroids
- Granulation tissue formation on the incision site

## Equipment

- Laryngeal Suspension Laryngoscope
  - Large Lindholm
  - Zeitels modular glottiscope
- Microscope
- Hopkins rod telescope(s)
- Microlaryngeal Instruments
  - D-knife
  - Blitzer knife
  - Sickle Knife
  - Peak Woo Microfrance Laryngeal Scissors
  - Vocal fold spreaders
- Vocal Fold Spreaders
- Needle Driver
  - Preferred laparoscopic needle driver
- Knot Pusher
  - Preferred laparoscopic knot pusher

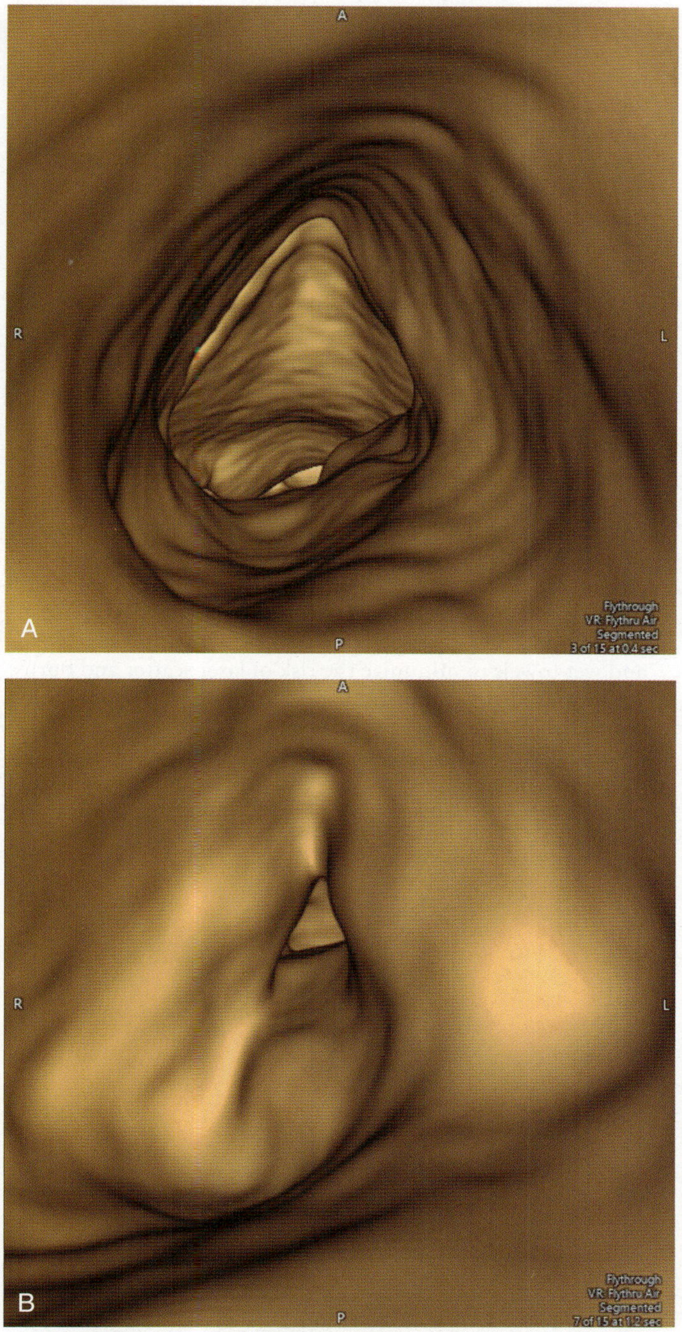


• **Fig. 19.2** (A) Dynamic CT 3D reconstruction visualizing the glottis from the subglottis in the relaxed position. (B) Dynamic CT 3D reconstruction visualizing the glottis from the subglottis during phonation demonstrating the persistent posterior gap.

- $CO_2$ Laser
  - Preferred Lumenis with Digital AcuBlade Scanning Micromanipulator and Software package
  - Settings
    - 10 to 16 watts
    - Continuous
    - Spot (circle) size 1.0 to 2.5 mm
    - Depth 2 to 3 mm
    - May switch to a 2.0 to 2.5 mm line to remove excess
- 4.0 to 5.0 PDS suture on an RB-1 or RB2 (noncutting needle)

## Steps of the Procedure

1. Patient positioning: As discussed earlier. The patient is then placed in suspension using a Lindholm or a Zeitels laryngoscope.
2. Laryngeal exposure: As discussed earlier. The surgeon must obtain an adequate view of the posterior glottis to adequately remove a sliver of the posterior glottis. Depending on the patient, a Lindholm may provide adequate exposure. In other cases, the Zeitels may provide better exposure. The Zeitels may be positioned to place the posterior glottis and posterior cricoid in direct view.
3. Laryngeal spreaders: May be placed to aid in exposure. These are placed with the handles aimed superiorly to leave the posterior glottis unobstructed by the instrument.
4. Visualization: The operating microscope provides handsfree visualization with binocular vision and depth perception. Focal length set to 400 mm.
5. $CO_2$ Laser: The appropriate generator and micromanipulator should be attached to the microscope and correct function confirmed. A laser with scanning software is preferred to aid in the speed and precision of the surgery. Laser safety precautions should include protecting the patient with wet eye pads and wet towels to minimize the risk of laser scatter and burns. Any exposed tissue can be damaged by the laser, including the teeth. Inspired oxygen fraction should be confirmed 30% or less. The laser should be tested to confirm correct function and good alignment with the visible aiming beam. All personnel in the operating room should wear appropriate eye protection.

**PEARL 19.5**

Particularly in patients with posterior glottic def ciency, scarring between the mucosa and underlying cricoid cartilage may make submucosal injection difficult.

6. Resection of the posterior cricoid: Lidocaine/epinephrine may be injected into the posterior cricoid and the interarytenoid space but is not essential if using the $CO_2$ laser (Pearl 19.5). If cold instruments are being used to resect a strip of cartilage, then injection is highly recommended. The $CO_2$ programmable laser greatly enhances speed and precision in resecting a sliver of the posterior cricoid. A spot size is chosen based on the desired width of the resection. The spot size should be slightly undersized relative to the exact width desired if the spot is in between sizes (i.e., the exact width is either too small or too large relative to the desired resection width.) Ideally, the width is based on the CT obtained beforehand; however, on average, 2 mm is a safe size in most teenagers and adults and will not result in airway compromise or excessive narrowing of the airway. Additional settings include 10 to 16 watts of power with a depth of 2 to 3 mm set in continuous mode or with a very minimal delay. Inspired oxygen fraction must be kept below 30% while the laser is used, to minimize risk of airway fire. A strip of the cricoid is then removed in its entirety from superior to inferior (Fig. 19.3A–19.3D). Care is taken to stay directly in the midline of the posterior cricoid. During the resection, a suction can be placed to deliver the cricoid on end to more effectively resect the strip. Oxymetazoline or

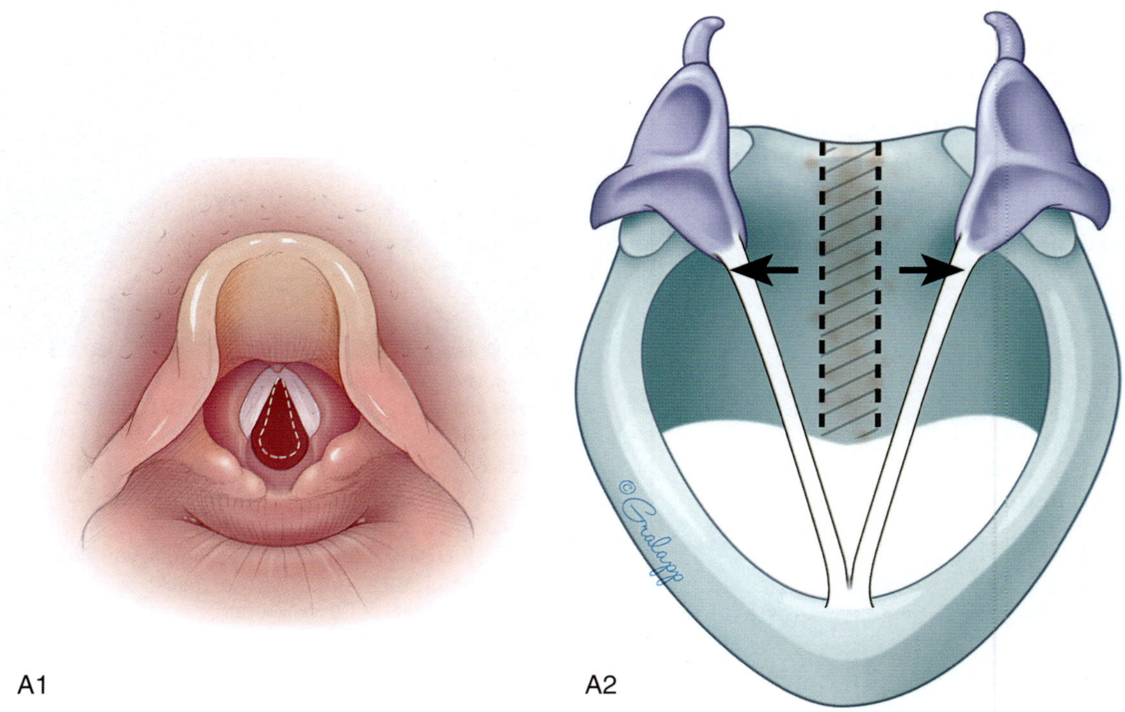


A1 A2

• **Fig. 19.3** (A) Illustration of the posterior diastasis and the planned resection of the cricoid. (© 2024 Chris Gralapp.)

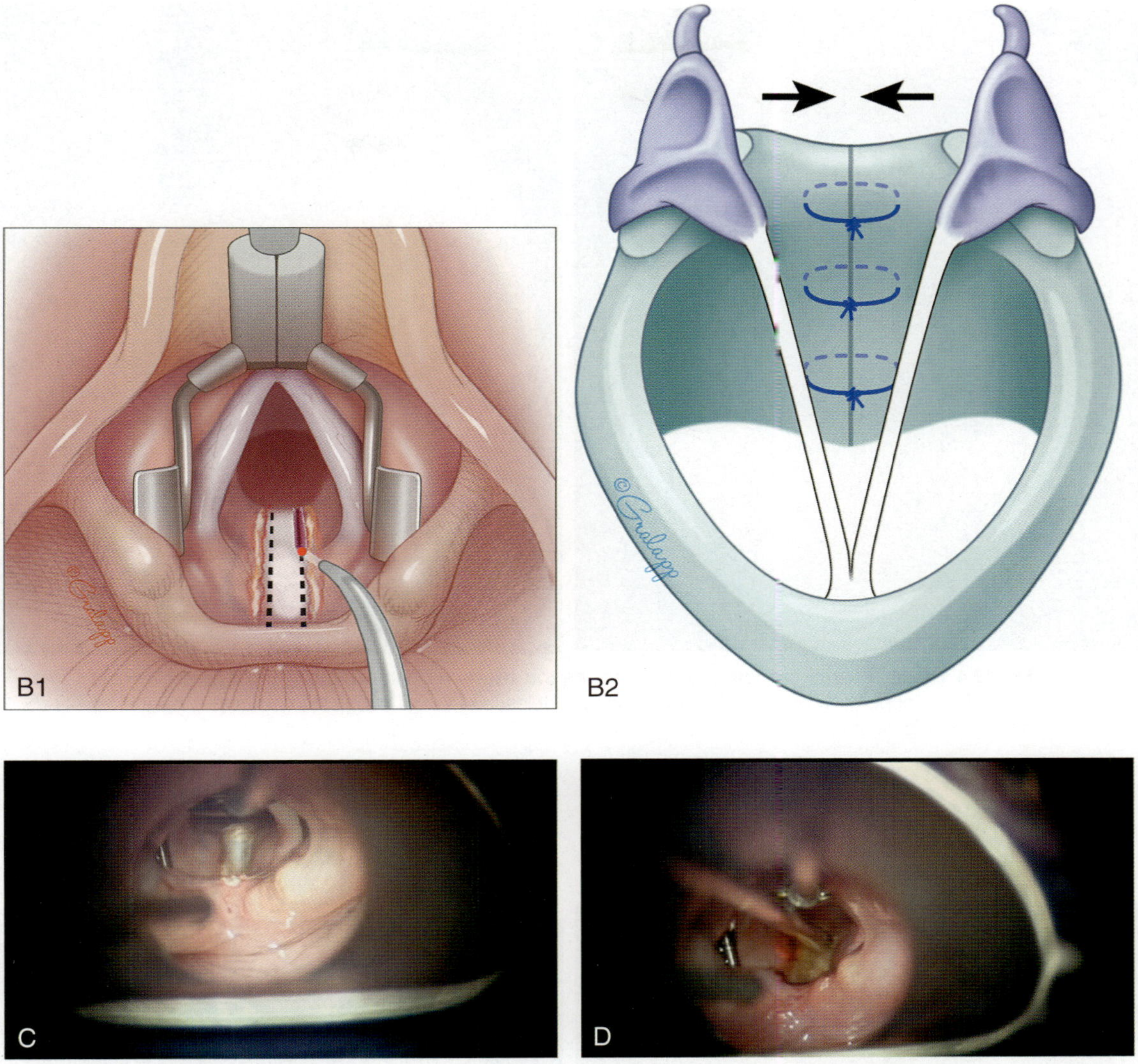


• **Fig. 19.3 cont'd** (B) Illustration of the resection of a strip of the posterior glottis and the resulting closure and narrowing/closure of the posterior diastasis. (C) Intraoperative photo demonstrating the initial resection of the cricoid with a trough of resected cricoid. (D) Intraoperative photo demonstrating the partial resection of the cricoid and removal of char with a rigid suction. (A and B © 2024 Chris Gralapp.)

epinephrine-soaked pledgets can be used to clean the surgical bed if there is excessive char. Hopkins rod telescopes can also be used intermittently to visualize the resection site. (Fig. 19.4A and 19.4B) The posterior perichondrium should be left intact. A straight-line laser setting may then be used of a length of 1.0 to 2.0 mm to remove any valleys or troughs in the resection site to ensure the edges of the cricoid come together evenly.

7. Suturing: The surgical bed is then closed to narrow the prior gap and close the resection site. 4-0 or 5-0 PDS on RB-1 or RB-2 taper needle is used. Two stitches are typically used and may be placed using the microscope or a Hopkins rod for visualization. The stitch is left with the knots in the airway lumen. Stitches are placed through mucosa and cricoid cartilage back through cricoid cartilage and mucosa to close the surgical defect. Care should be taken to keep the depth and level in the same planes. The most distal stitch is placed first followed by the most proximal. Sutures should be tied down once both are placed to allow ease of suture placement. (Fig. 19.5A and 19.5B). Readers should also refer to Chapter 4, Endoscopic Laryngeal Cleft Repair for additional details.

Photodocumentation: 0-degree telescopes or the microscope are used to document the repair and examine the trachea to ensure that suctioning of any blood or secretions is not required. The airway is sized at the end of the procedure to ensure that the airway has not been overly narrowed. Additionally, this serves as the documented airway size should the patient need to be intubated postoperatively.

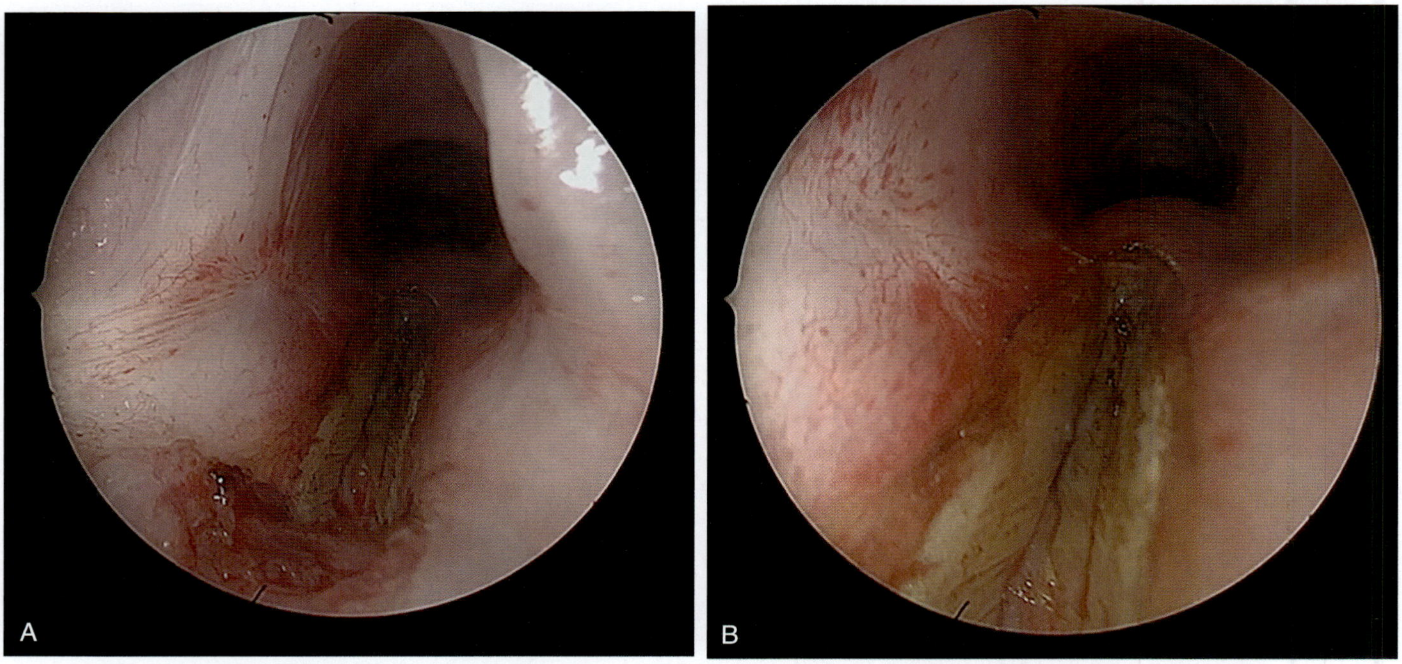

• **Fig. 19.4** (A) Intraoperative photo using a Hopkins rod telescope demonstrating the resected cricoid trough. (B) Intraoperative photo using a Hopkins rod telescope in the subglottis demonstrating the full resected cricoid section.

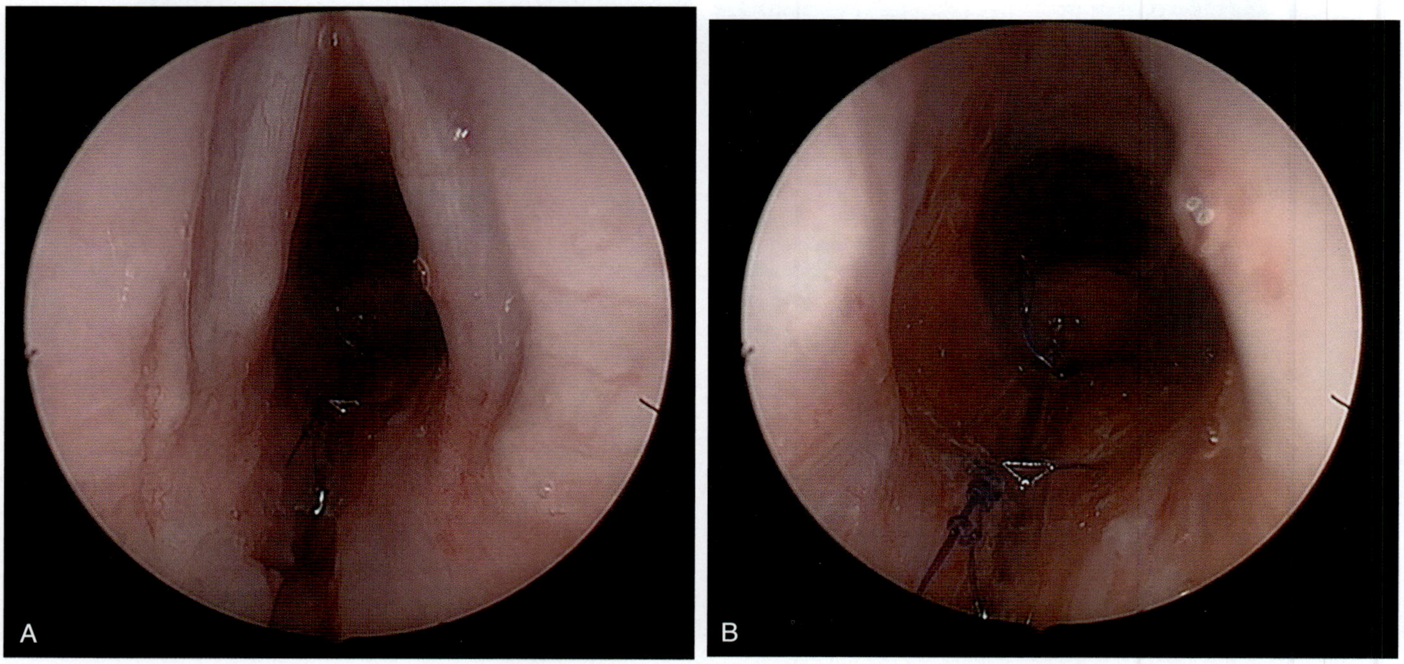

• **Fig. 19.5** (A) Intraoperative photo at closure with the completed two sutures. (B) Intraoperative photo at the closure in the posterior glottis visualizing the two sutures and the reduced posterior glottis.

## Bibliography

1. Zeitels SM, de Alarcon A, Burns JA, Lopez-Guerra G, Hillman RE. Posterior glottic diastasis: mechanically deceptive and often overlooked. *Ann Otol Rhinol Laryngol.* 2011;120:71–80.
2. Padia R, Smith ME. Posterior glottic insufficiency in children. *Ann Otol Rhinol Laryngol.* 2017;126:268–273.
3. de Alarcón A. Voice outcomes after pediatric airway reconstruction. *Laryngoscope.* 2012;122(Suppl 4):S84–S86.
4. Bliss M, Houtz D, Smith ME. Cricoid reduction laryngoplasty for treatment of dysphonia after pediatric laryngotracheal reconstruction. *Int J Pediatr Otorhinolaryngol.* 2015;79:80–82.
5. Sidell DR, Zacharias S, Balakrishnan K, Rutter MJ, de Alarcon A. Surgical management of posterior glottic diastasis in children. *Ann Otol Rhinol Laryngol.* 2015;124:72–78.
6. de Alarcon A, Zacharias S, Oren L, et al. Endoscopic posterior cricoid reduction: a surgical method to improve posterior glottic diastasis. *Laryngoscope.* 2019;129:S1–S9.
7. Bergeron M, Fleck RJ, Middlebrook C, et al. Preliminary assessment of dynamic voice CT in post-airway reconstruction patients. *Otolaryngol Head Neck Surg.* 2018;159:516–521.

# 20

# Endoscopic Posterior Glottic Rotation Flap for Posterior Glottic Insufficiency

JULINA ONGKASUWAN

## Background

While some individuals may develop posterior glottic stenosis (PGS) as a result of prolonged intubation, others may develop the inverse: posterior glottic insufficiency (PGI). Posteriorly directed pressure exerted by an endotracheal tube can result in erosion of the vocal processes and the posterior cricoid plate.[1] Posterior glottic insufficiency is also in contradistinction to posterior glottic diastasis (PGD) wherein the cricoarytenoid joints are moved further apart due, for example, secondary to the presence of a cartilage graft (Fig. 20.1). While both PGI and PGD can result in air escape through the posterior glottis, the underlying etiology of the incomplete glottic closure has implications for potential treatment modalities. In the case of PGD, posterior cricoid reduction (open vs. endoscopic) can be considered to move the cricoarytenoid joints closer together and obviate some of the air escape (Pearl 20.1).[2]

**PEARL 20.1**

Readers should also review Chapter 19 for another operative approach to this problem.

To complicate matters, PGI can cooccur with PGD, vocal fold immobility, and/or vocal fold atrophy. The constellation of findings can be more broadly grouped as post-intubation phonatory insufficiency (PIPI). It is the same patient population who were premature and had a prolonged intubation who may develop PGI, as well as subglottic stenosis requiring laryngotracheal reconstruction with placement of a posterior rib graft and resultant PGD. In addition, these premature infants may also have undergone patent ductus arteriosus (PDA) ligation with resultant recurrent laryngeal nerve (RLN) injury and vocal paralysis.[3,4]

## Clinical Assessment

Posterior glottic insufficiency may be difficult to diagnose via in-office laryngoscopy (Pearl 20.2). Patients will often present with a weak and breathy voice; in fact, clinicians may suspect vocal fold immobility based on their perceptual evaluation of voice. However, in isolated PGI, the vocal folds will appear mobile, and anterior glottic closure may be intact. The posterior glottis may be difficult to visualize due to hooding of the arytenoids (Fig. 20.2). To complicate matters, patients may also have associated membranous vocal fold atrophy, again related to prolonged intubation (Fig. 20.3).[5,6]

**PEARL 20.2**

Despite this limitation, in office laryngoscopy is important to assess vocal fold mobility and may also play a role in endoscopic swallow evaluation. Understanding baseline airway, voice, and swallow status is important before embarking on any glottic procedure.

A high index of suspicion is needed to make the diagnosis of PGI. The diagnosis is best made in the operating room with a microsuspension direct laryngoscopy with close inspection of the posterior glottis (Fig. 20.4). The presence of an endotracheal tube at the time of evaluation may make visualization of the posterior glottis challenging. Thus a tubeless spontaneous ventilation technique is preferred in children, and jet ventilation or high-flow nasal cannula (THRIVE) can be used in adults.

## Patient Selection and Consent

We have found that often it is older children (approximately age 10 years and up) who most commonly request the evaluation and management of postintubation voice disorders. Thus the patient should be included in the discussions regarding management. We typically do recommend a course of voice therapy prior to any surgical intervention (Pearl 20.3). If the patient does not think that their voice is adequate for their needs after voice therapy, then we discuss surgery. It is important to emphasize that improving glottic closure after prolonged intubation may require several staged surgeries, especially if there are multiple areas to be addressed.

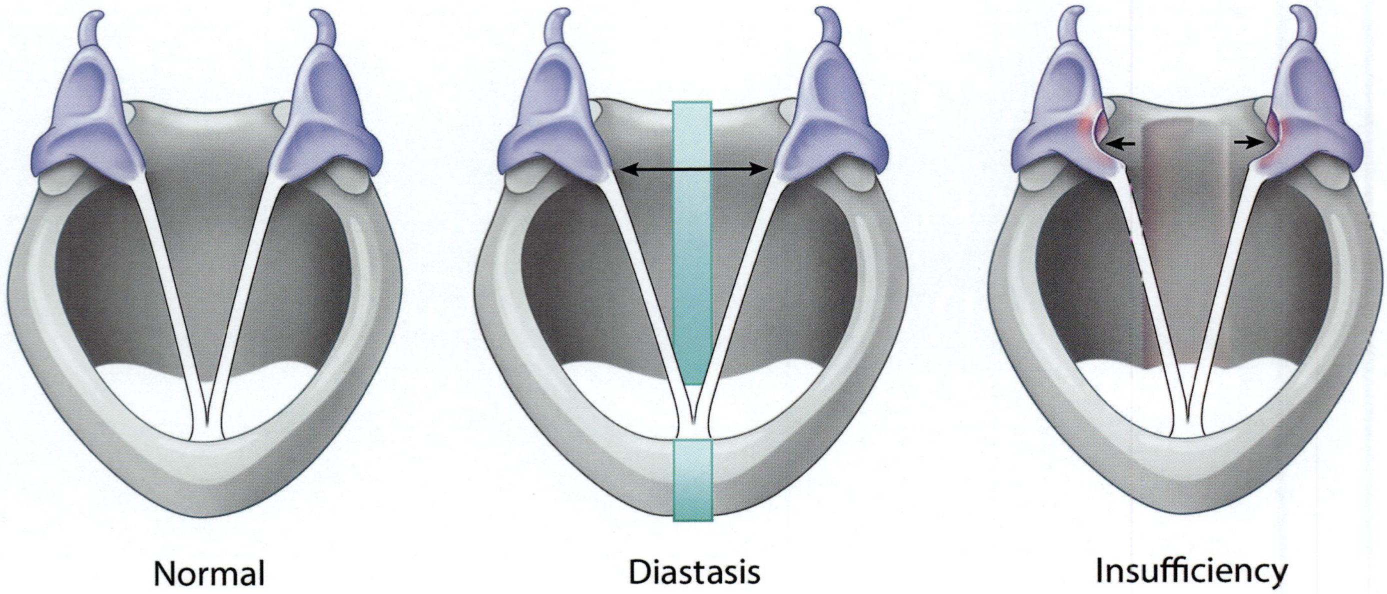


• **Fig. 20.1** Posterior glottic diastasis versus insufficiency. (© 2024 Chris Gralapp.)

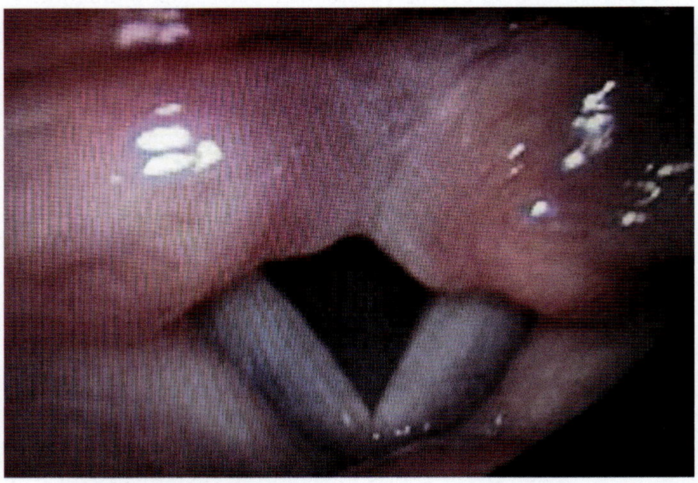

• **Fig. 20.2** Arytenoid hooding obscuring posterior glottis in office.

**PEARL 20.3**

Objective voice measures and a recording of the presurgical voice may be helpful in assessing improvement postoperatively.

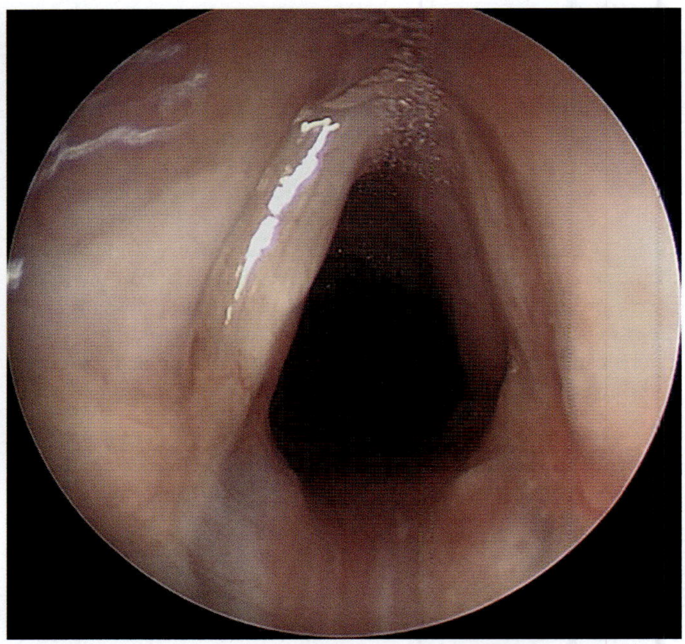

• **Fig. 20.3** Concurrent vocal fold atrophy and posterior glottic insufficiency.

For example, a patient may also require augmentation of the membranous vocal folds if there is significant coexistent atrophy (Fig. 20.5). When both vocal fold atrophy and PGI are present in PIPI, a trial membranous vocal fold augmentation with a short-acting filler material may help determine which area, membranous or cartilaginous vocal fold, to address first. It may not be possible to restore normal vocal fold pliability and vibration or glottic configuration. The goal of surgical intervention is to improve voice loudness and intelligibility and decrease the effort to phonate (Pearl 20.4).[7]

**PEARL 20.4**

The benefit of waiting until the child is of adolescent or pre-adolescent age is that the child can express for themselves what limitations, if any, their voice is causing in their life.

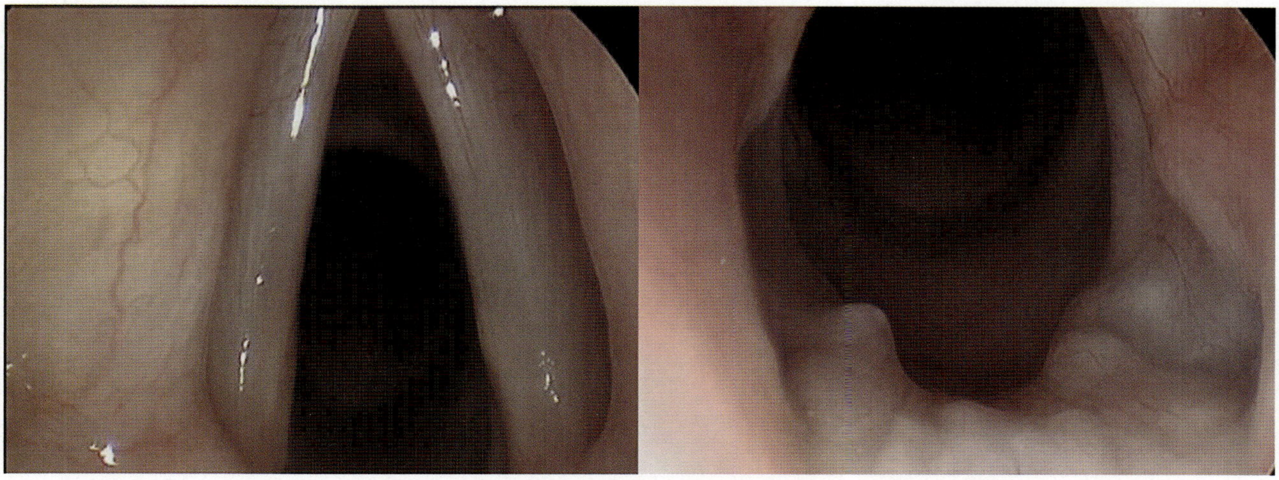

• **Fig. 20.4** Inspection of posterior glottis under anesthesia.

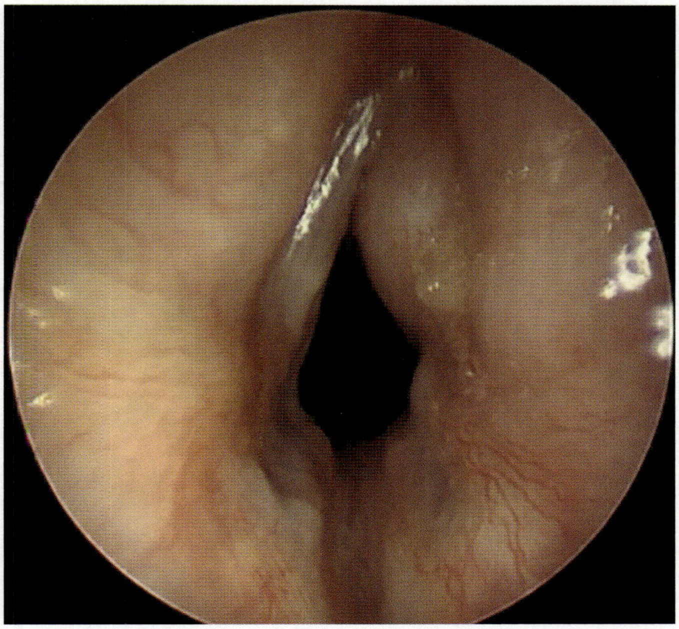

• **Fig. 20.5** Augmentation of vocal fold atrophy revealing posterior glottic insufficiency.

The endoscopic posterior rotation flap is best done in older children (approximately 6 years and up) when the larynx is larger and there is a little more room in which to maneuver. Consent should also include risks of dental injury as well as tongue numbness or dysgeusia.

## Operative Technique[8]

### Anesthetic and Ventilation Technique

The presence of an endotracheal tube in the posterior glottis can make it very difficult, or impossible, to maneuver endoscopically. Our preferred technique is total intravenous anesthesia (TIVA) with tubeless spontaneous ventilation; however, jet ventilation or THRIVE can be used as well. Collaboration with the anesthesia team preparing for a longer tubeless microsuspension case is essential to achieve the appropriate plane of anesthesia to allow oxygenation and ventilation in the setting of laser use and low entrained fraction of inspired oxygen ($FiO_2$). There is no need for perioperative antibiotics, though a dose of dexamethasone is usually given at the start of the case. Topical lidocaine is also applied to the larynx at the start of the case to help prevent laryngospasm.

### Positioning and Equipment

Microsuspension direct laryngoscopy is performed, ideally with a Lindholm laryngoscope, bed-mounted Mayo stand, and suspension arm.

Other equipment includes:

- Binocular microscope (400 mm lens or focal length)
- Laser ($CO_2$ with micromanipulator) with appropriate laser safety precautions
  - Low $FiO_2$
  - Wet towels to protect the patient's eyes and face
  - Eye protection for OR staff
  - Laser signage on doors
- Surgical stool with adjustable arm supports
- Bouchayer forceps, laryngeal flap elevator, 5-0 vicryl on an S14 needle (Pearl 20.5).

**PEARL 20.5**

An endoscopic needle driver and knot pusher are very useful for this procedure.

### Steps of the Procedure (Fig. 20.6)

The laser is used to outline a medially based U-shaped flap up the middle medial surface of the arytenoid (Fig. 20.6A). The incision is taken through the submucosal fat. The flap is grasped with a Bouchayer forcep and elevated using the laser. While elevating the flap medially, care must be taken not to buttonhole through the flap. At the most medial portion of the flap, where the PGI trough is located, the mucosa is often tightly adherent

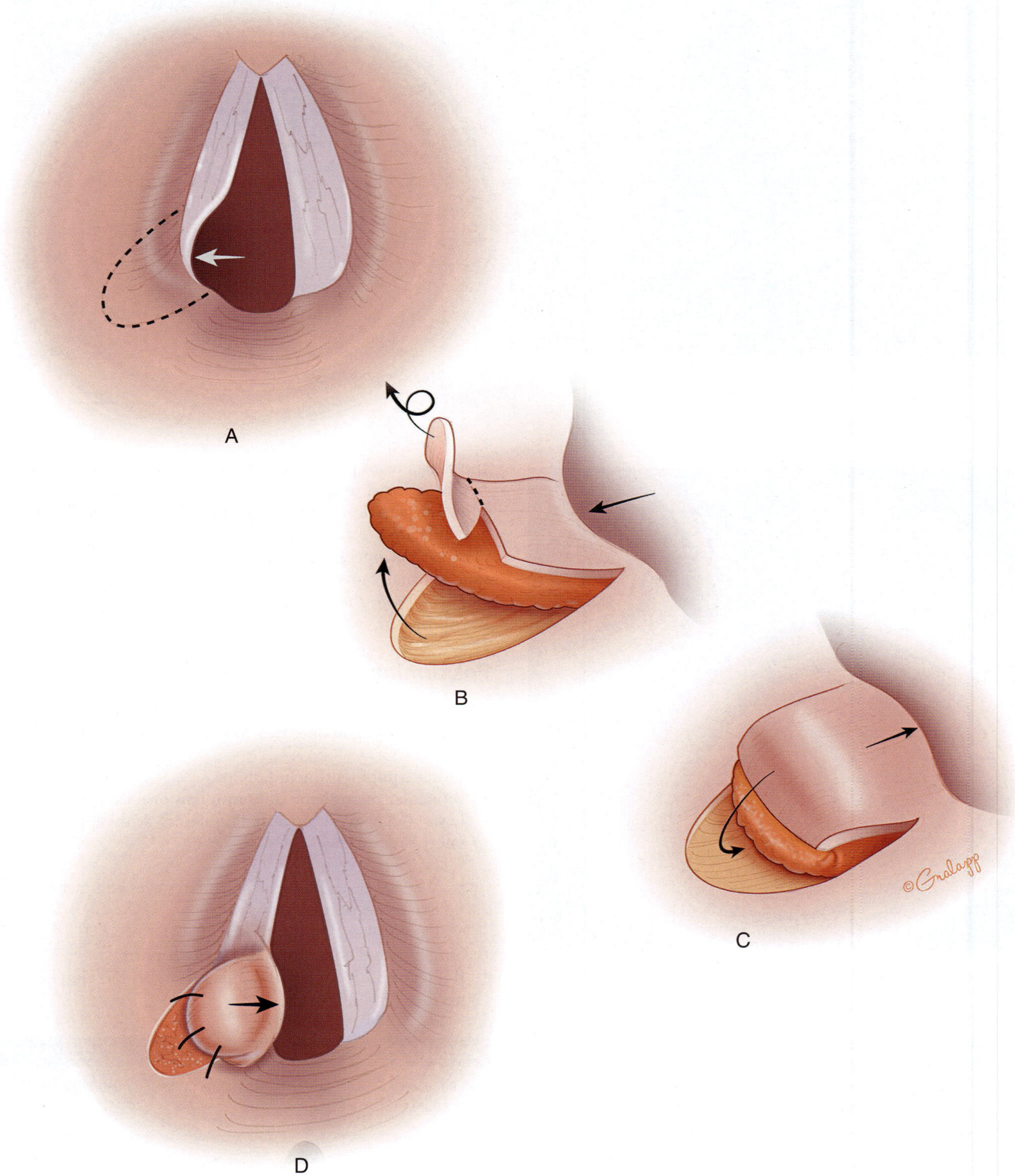


• **Fig. 20.6** Surgical procedure. (© 2024 Chris Gralapp.)

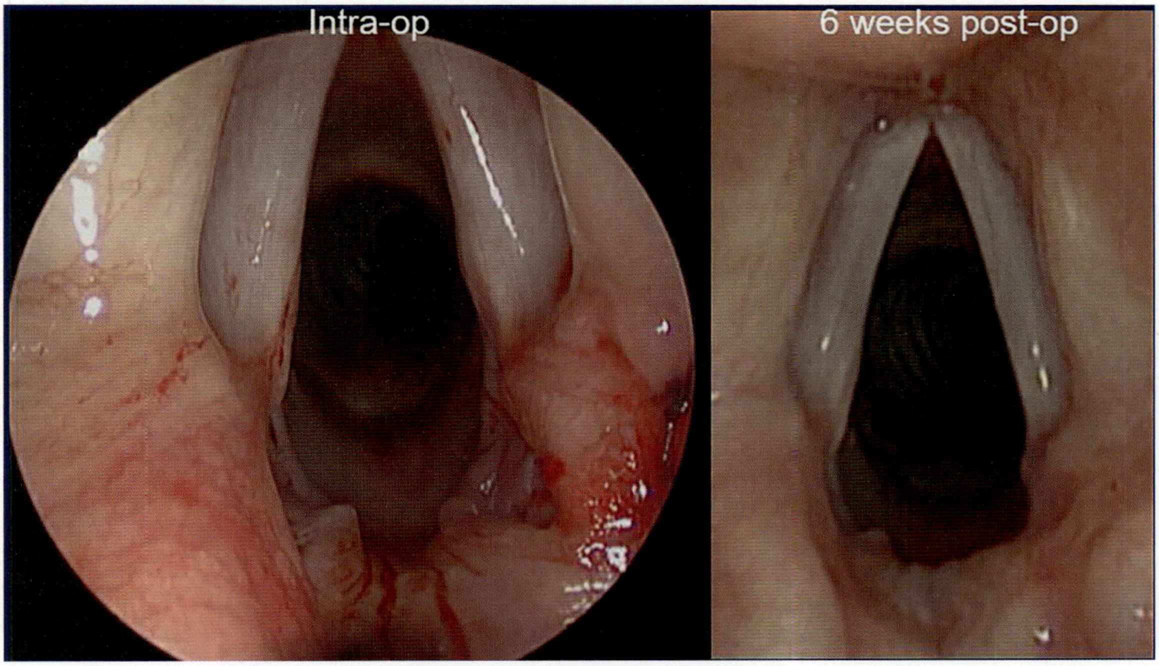


• **Fig. 20.7** Postoperative view of the larynx.

to the remnant vocal process cartilage. Typically, a slice of cartilage must be elevated with the flap. Similar to popping out a dent on a car, the trough is elevated and a pocket created just lateral to it using a laryngeal flap elevator. The lateral portion of the flap is demucosalized using the laser (Fig. 20.6B). The flap is then folded on itself and the lateral portion is tucked into the pocket just lateral to the trough (Fig. 20.6C). A 5-0 vicryl on an S14 needle is used to suture the flap into place (Fig. 20.6D). Laterally, the suture can be placed through vocal process cartilage, and medially, the suture is placed through the edge of mucosa on the flap. One or two sutures may be needed (Fig. 20.7).

## Postoperative Care

If PGI exists bilaterally, the sides can be staged if desired. Patients are typically kept overnight for observation. If there is concern for laryngeal edema, postoperative steroids can be given. Pain typically can be managed with acetaminophen and ibuprofen. There are no dietary or voice or activity restrictions postoperatively (Pearl 20.6).

**PEARL 20.6**

Repeat assessment of objective voice measures and review of presurgical and postsurgical voice recordings may help both the surgeon and patient better understand the impact of the procedure.

## References

1. Padia R, Smith ME. Posterior glottic insufficiency in children. *Ann Otol Rhinol Laryngol.* 2017;126(4):268–273.
2. de Alarcón A, Zacharias S, Oren L, et al. Endoscopic posterior cricoid reduction: a surgical method to improve posterior glottic diastasis. *Laryngoscope.* 2019;129(S2):S1–S9.
3. Ongkasuwan J, Espinosa MCL, Hollas S, et al. Predictors of voice outcome in pediatric non-selective laryngeal reinnervation. *Laryngoscope.* 2020;130:1525–1531.
4. Zur KB, Douglas J, Carroll LM. Intubation-related laryngeal deficiency and vocal fold immobility in pediatric premature patients. *Laryngoscope.* 2021;131(11):2550–2557.
5. Ramos PH, Lagos AE, Napolitano CA, Badía PI. Postintubation phonatory insufficiency: a challenging diagnosis. *J Voice.* 2020;S0892–1997:30261–30267.
6. Zeitels SM, de Alarcon A, Burns JA, Lopez-Guerra G, Hillman RE. Posterior glottic diastasis: mechanically deceptive and often overlooked. *Ann Otol Rhinol Laryngol.* 2011;120:71–80.
7. Sidell DR, Zacharias S, Balakrishnan K, Rutter MJ, de Alarcón A. Surgical management of posterior glottic diastasis in children. *Ann Otol Rhinol Laryngol.* 2015;124(1):72–78.
8. Kobayashi KR, You P, Devore D, Hollas S, Geraghty JR, Ongkasuwan J. Endoscopic posterior rotation flap for posterior glottic insufficiency. *Laryngoscope.* 2022;132(7):1452–1454.

# SECTION V

# Endoscopic Airway Resection Procedures

# 21 Endoscopic Tumor Resection

MARILENA TROZZI AND SERGIO BOTTERO

Tumors of the larynx, trachea, and bronchi are rare in children. By virtue of their location, these lesions can lead to significant morbidity and mortality by mechanical obstruction of the airway. Symptoms include stridor, cough, dysphonia, wheezing, or dyspnea. Airway tumors may be classified by tissue of origin and as benign or malignant; within this classification, the range of specific diagnoses is broad (Table 21.1).

There are numerous options available to treat malignant airway obstruction, including chemotherapy, radiation, airway stent placement, and bronchoscopic ablative techniques. The selection of a specific ablative technique depends primarily on the clinical urgency to restore airway patency and available technologies. If the patient is presenting with mild or subacute symptoms, then multiple modalities can be utilized, including those that have a delayed treatment response. If the patient is presenting with more severe symptoms or life-threatening malignant airway obstruction, the patient should be stabilized and then treated with an ablative therapy that will result in a more immediate effect. In addition to computed tomography, an initial bronchoscopy is performed to determine what the most appropriate modality may be. Techniques such as laser, electrocautery, argon plasma coagulation (APC), cryoprobe debulking, and airway stenting all result in immediate improvement in airway patency.

## Mechanical Debulking and Resection

Mechanical debulking remains the cornerstone on which most other endoscopic ablation modalities depend.

- Flexible mechanical debulking

Utilization of biopsy or debulking forceps through a flexible bronchoscope allows for precise removal of target endobronchial tissue. Mechanical flexible forceps exist in many forms and variations exist depending upon the manufacturer (Pearl 21.1). Salient features of these instruments include the size of the forceps (generally range from 1.2 to 2.8 mm or larger), the cup shapes (smooth vs. serrated), as well as the configurational design (rat tooth, alligator, needle fenestrated) (Fig. 21.1).

> **PEARL 21.1**
>
> Because a wide variety of flexible scope sizes exist, understanding the scope dimensions (e.g., outer diameter and working channel of the bronchoscope) is important. Decisions will be further influenced by the operation at hand and the instruments available that fit in the channel of your bronchoscope.

- Rigid forceps and related instruments

The rigid bronchoscope itself is a very effective debulking instrument and allows for other rigid instruments to be introduced through it, into the airway. Rigid coring of an endobronchial tumor is an effective means of rapidly removing an endobronchial tumor obstruction; however, extreme caution and expertise are required to ensure appropriate application without damage to adjacent or surrounding structures (Pearl 21.2). While severe bleeding is not common, some degree of hemorrhage is expected, and operators must have a plan and tools available to achieve hemostasis (e.g., electrocauterization, cold saline, laser, adrenaline).

> **PEARL 21.2**
>
> In addition, distalizing tumor fragments may pose a risk of airway obstruction if not recognized intraoperatively.

Principal rigid accessories (Fig. 21.2) are available for mechanical debulking and are delivered through the rigid bronchoscope. Rigid forceps of varying sizes and designs exist for the effective removal of endobronchial tissue. The basic features include length of the instrument, shaft diameter (generally 1.5–2.8 mm), and forceps design (cup, cutting, crocodile jaw, angulated, reverse grasping). Rigid accessory instruments are used either for direct debulking, or for removal of adjunctively ablated tissue.

## Microdebrider

The microdebrider (Fig. 21.3) is an instrument comprising three components: a long disposable rotating blade coupled to suction, a handpiece to control directionality, and a console that adjusts the revolution speed. During dissection, tissue is drawn up and into the blade while debris and blood are rapidly removed from the operating field through suction. As such, any specimens for

**TABLE 21.1** Types of airway tumors.

| Type of Tumor | Benign | Malignant |
|---|---|---|
| **Epithelial** | Squamous papilloma<br>Adenoma<br>Oncocytoma<br>Pleomorphic adenoma | Squamous cell carcinoma<br>Verrucous carcinoma<br>Spindle cell carcinoma<br>Squamous cell carcinoma<br>Adenosquamous carcinoma<br>Basal cell carcinoma<br>Malignant melanoma<br>Adenoid cystic carcinoma<br>Adenocarcinoma<br>Malignant mixed tumor<br>Mucoepidermoid carcinoma |
| **Mesenchymal** | Fibroma<br>Chondroma<br>Chondroblastoma<br>Hemangioma<br>Leiomyoma<br>Lipoma<br>Rhabdomyoma<br>Lymphangioma<br>Fibrous histiocytoma | Fibrosarcoma<br>Rhabdomyosarcoma<br>Chondrosarcoma<br>Liposarcoma<br>Angiosarcoma<br>Spindle cell sarcoma<br>Leiomyosarcoma<br>Malignant fibrous histiocytoma |
| **Neuroendocrine** | Neurofibroma<br>Schwannoma<br>Paraganglioma<br>Granular cell tumor | Malignant granular cell tumor<br>Carcinoid tumor |
| **Hematopoietic** | Plasmacytoma<br>Reticulocytoma<br>Hemangioendothelioma | Lymphoma<br>Leukemia<br>Malignant hemangioendothelioma |
| **Miscellaneous** | Hamartoma<br>Adenolipoma<br>Teratoma<br>Amyloidosis | Malignant teratoma<br>Metastatic carcinoma |

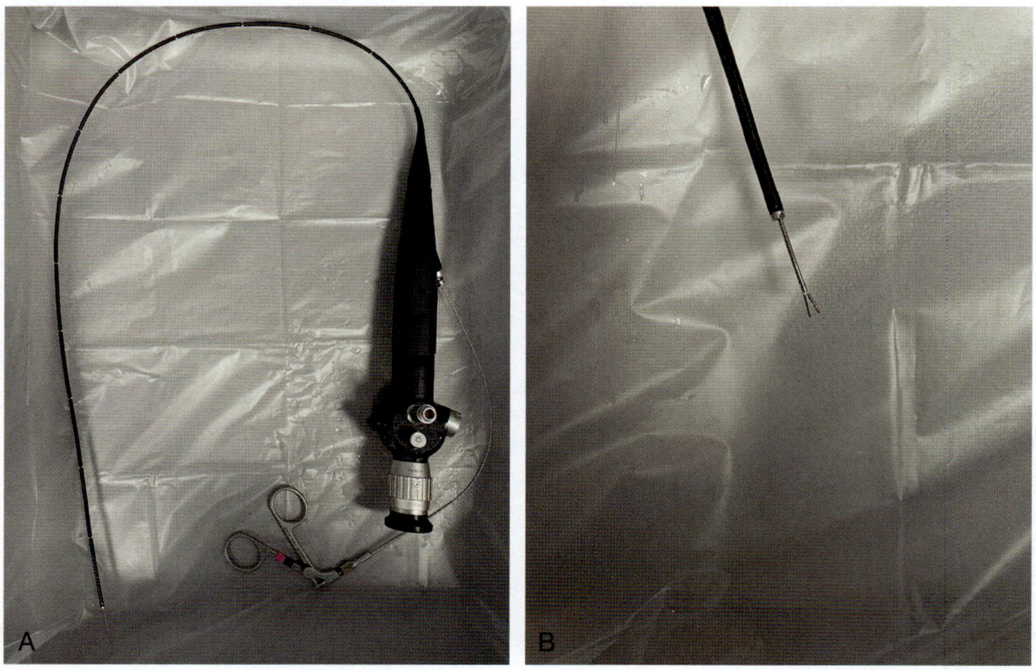

• **Fig. 21.1** A flexible 2.8 endoscope with crocodile forcep.

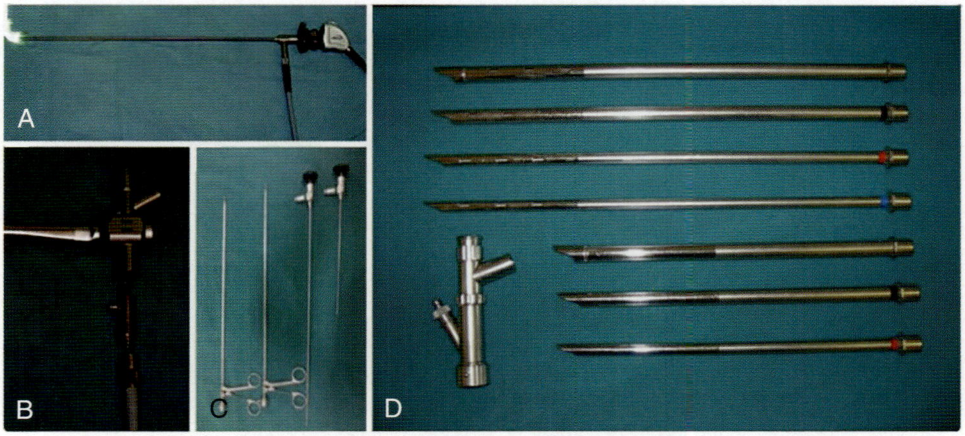


• **Fig. 21.2** Rigid bronchoscopy equipment.

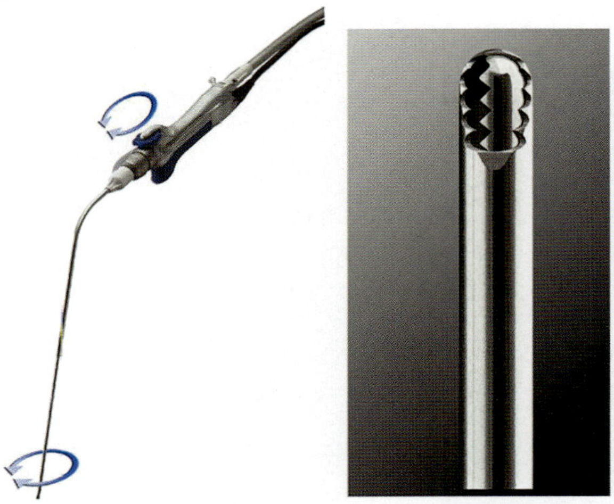

• **Fig. 21.3** The rotating tip tracheal microdebrider.

pathology or microbiology should ideally be taken prior to use of the microdebrider. The features of this debulking instrument allow for prompt debridement of endobronchial tumors; however, operators must be attentive as unintentional damage to normal tissue can occur (Pearl 21.3).

**PEARL 21.3**

For less aggressive cutting, it is recommended to use the blade at a higher revolutions per minute (RPM) because of the shorter opening time of the suction channel. For more efficient cutting, it is helpful to set the RPM between 500 and 800.

## Thermal Ablation

Thermal ablation techniques are used in cases of endobronchial disease or in patients with mixed endobronchial/extrinsic lesions. Heat thermal ablation modalities must be used with caution, especially in patients with high-flow oxygen (those on fraction of inspired oxygen greater than 0.4 secondary to risk of airway fire) and patients with airway stents or other artificial airway devices in place (endotracheal or tracheostomy tube), as there is a risk of

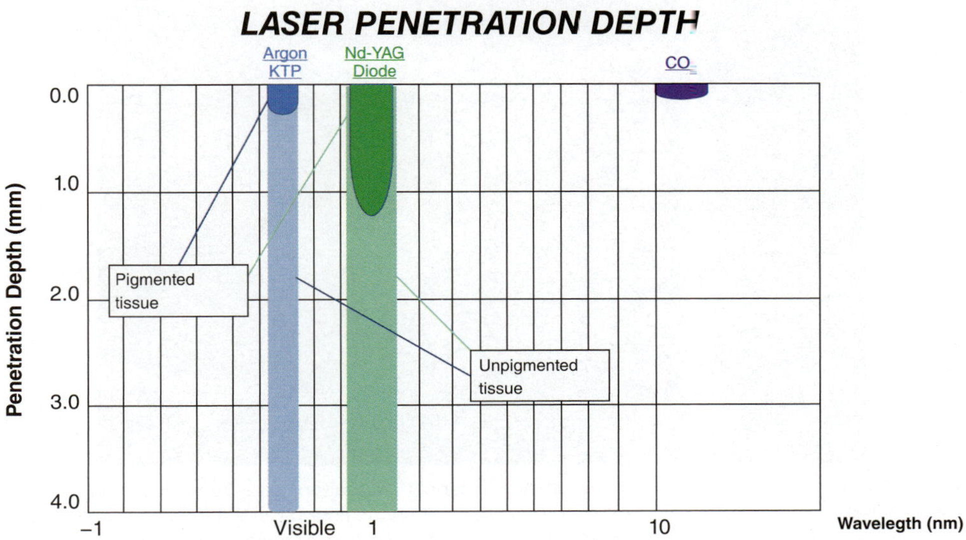


• **Fig. 21.4** Laser types and tissue penetration depth.

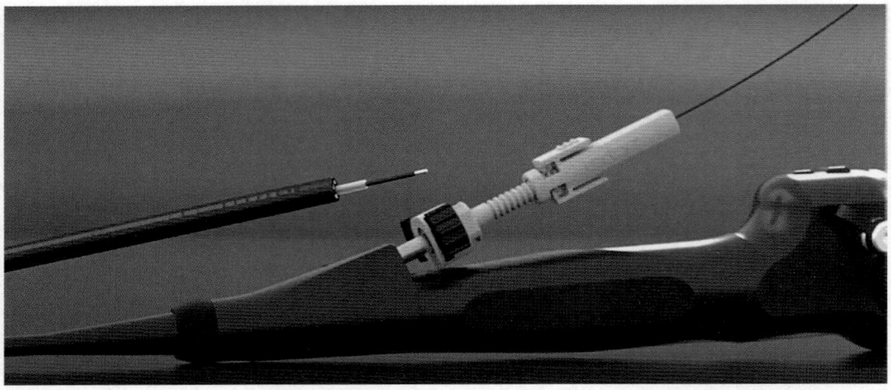

• **Fig. 21.5** The cryoprobe is inserted through the bronchoscope. Postop MRI T2-weighted scans 6 and 12 months later, showing the results of surgery, no evidence of residual disease.

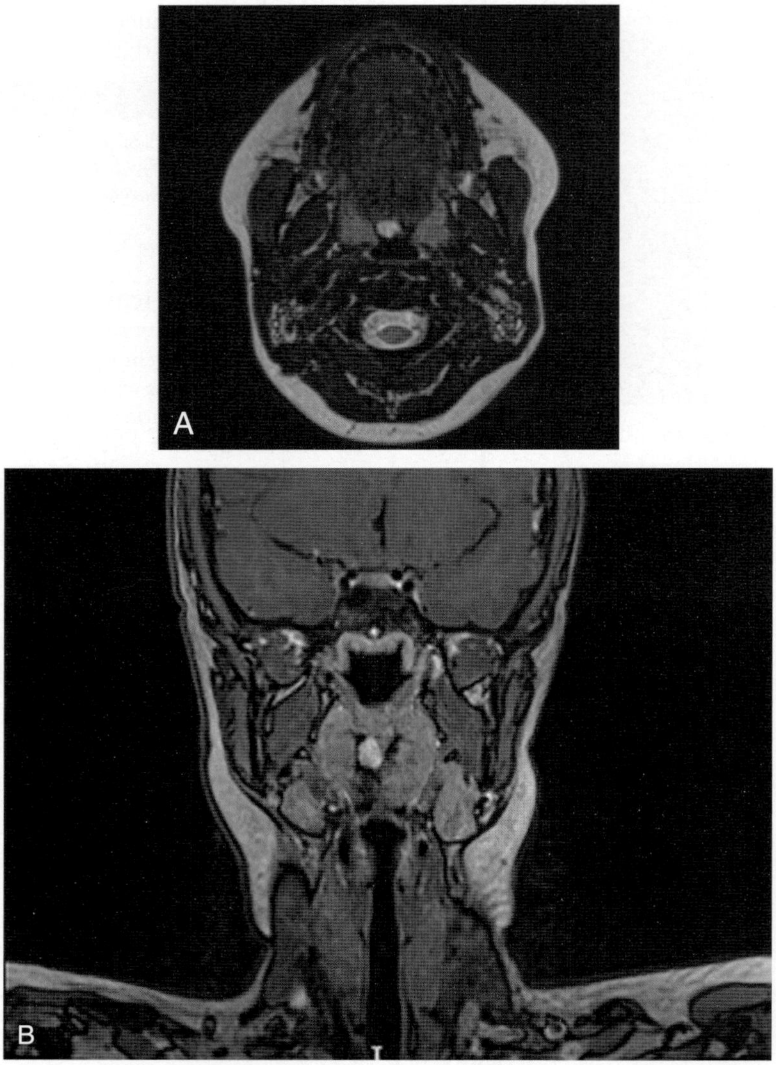

• **Fig. 21.6** Base of tongue schwannoma in a 15-year-old girl. Preop axial (A) and coronal (B) MRI T2-weighted scans showing a 1.2-cm round mass located on the right base of the tongue, with modest expansive features that appear hyperintense in T2 and which after administration of MDC becomes homogeneously impregnated. *MDC*, Methylated deoxycytidine.

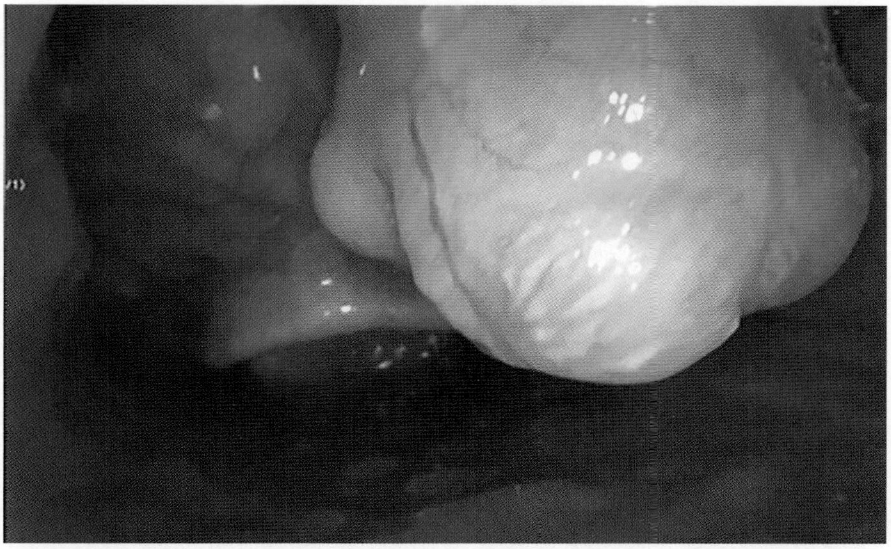

• **Fig. 21.7** Flexible endoscopy using a 3.5 endoscope, evidence of a sessile neoformation of the tongue base, right paramedian about 1 cm in diameter, hard-elastic, nonulcerated, pinkish in color, with intact mucosa lining it. In direct suspension microlaryngoscopy, excisional biopsy of the formation is performed.

melting or fire. Furthermore, thermal ablation in distal airways may have a higher risk of airway perforation.

### *Argon Plasma*

Argon plasma coagulation (APC) is an electrosurgical technique similar to laser or electrocautery. Argon plasma coagulation is used during bronchoscopic procedures to ablate malignant airway tumors, control hemoptysis, remove granulation tissue from stents or anastomoses, and treat a variety of benign disorders. A grounding pad is placed on the patient's back or thigh. Typical settings include a power of 30 Watts and an argon flow rate of less than 1 L/min. The argon flow rate determines the length of the flame. The probe tip is positioned several cm beyond the bronchoscope's tip to ensure that the bronchoscope will not be burned. The probe tip is placed within 1 cm of the target lesion; the electric current will not be conducted if the probe is farther than 1 cm from the target lesion. Caution must be used to ensure that the catheter does not come into direct contact with the target tissue.

As argon gas is expelled, a high-voltage electric current passing along the probe contacts the gas, ionizing it and conducting a monopolar current to the target lesion. The current is applied to the surface in 1- to 3-second bursts. The tissue effect is similar to that seen with electrocautery. In the process of debulking an endobronchial lesion, eschar is first formed with the application of APC and then removed using a forceps or a cryotherapy probe. Argon plasma coagulation is then applied to the underlying fresh tissue. This process is repeated until the tumor is removed. Upon completion of the ablation, APC may be applied to the tumor base to mitigate risk of postprocedure bleeding from the site.

### *Electrocautery*

Electrocautery is the use of an electrical probe, knife, biopsy forceps, or snare to conduct monopolar electrical current for heating tissue in contact with or in close proximity to the instrument. Electrical current is conducted by the insulated metal wire probe toward the target tissue. Due to the voltage difference between the probe and tissue, electron current density generates heat at the point of contact. Tissue resistance for electrons is high, resulting in vaporization, coagulation, or fulguration.

Thermal destruction of tissue can be used to induce coagulation or resection. Applying the energized instrument directly destroys the target tissue, such that activation creates an immediately visible effect of burning, desiccation, and vaporization. Resection can also be accomplished with more polypoid lesions by using a wire snare apparatus looped around the base of the lesion and energized. Applying traction to the snare while delivering energy excises the lesion at the base, after which the tissue is retrieved by assistance with bronchoscopic suction or graspers. Rigid electrocautery probes are available and used with rigid bronchoscopy while flexible electrodes can be used through the working channel of a flexible bronchoscope. Thus endobronchial electrocautery can be used as a primary modality or often in conjunction with mechanical debulking.

Endobronchial electrocautery is most commonly indicated for the treatment of symptomatic malignant airway obstructions that are not operative candidates, or as adjuncts to other treatment modalities.

Endobronchial electrocautery is usually well tolerated, but the application of electrocautery near the airway wall has a risk of perforation, potentially leading to pneumothorax and pneumomediastinum. Bleeding can result from tissue destruction, however, it generally stops as a result of thermocoagulation, but the risk can be greater depending on the location of the tumor in relation to adjacent vascular structures, as well as tumor type.

Coblator is a related bipolar device that conducts current through an ionized fluid (e.g., saline), creating a plasma that cuts or ablates tissue (Video 21.1); it can also provide a coagulating function. While coblation can be highly effective, it often leaves a layer of eschar or fibrinous debris that may require endoscopic debridement a few days later.

### *Laser therapy*

This treatment modality is appropriate for slow-growing tumors.

Bronchoscopic laser therapy (Videos 21.2 and 21.3) is a thermal ablative technique, which may have cutting and coagulant properties depending on the type of laser, thus making it a useful instrument for treating malignant airway disease. Laser therapy is an immediate-acting, palliative, or adjunctive therapy used to

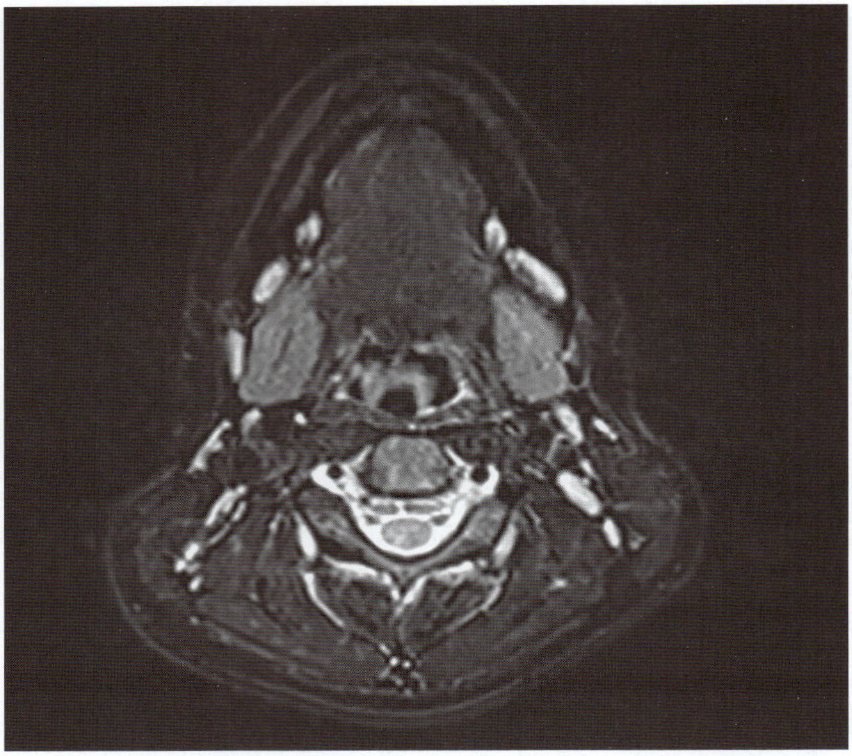

• **Fig. 21.8** Synovial biphasic sarcoma in 5-year-old female. The endoscopic view showing a sessile neoformation of the left piriform sinus and the ipsilateral hemilarynx.

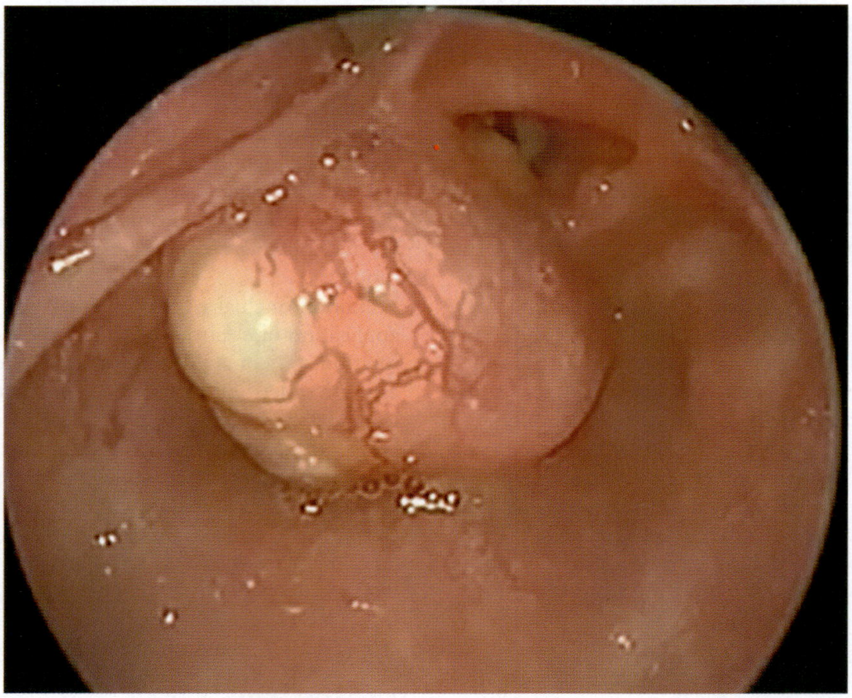

• **Fig. 21.9** After the induction chemotherapy, an endoscopic left hemilaryngectomy was performed in suspension direct laryngoscopy. After the patient was placed in the Boyce-Jackson position, direct suspension laryngoscopy revealed a voluminous neoformation starting from the left cricoarytenoid region, involving the pharyngo-epiglottic, aryepiglottic plica, the posterior portion of the ventricular fold and Morgagni's ventricle.

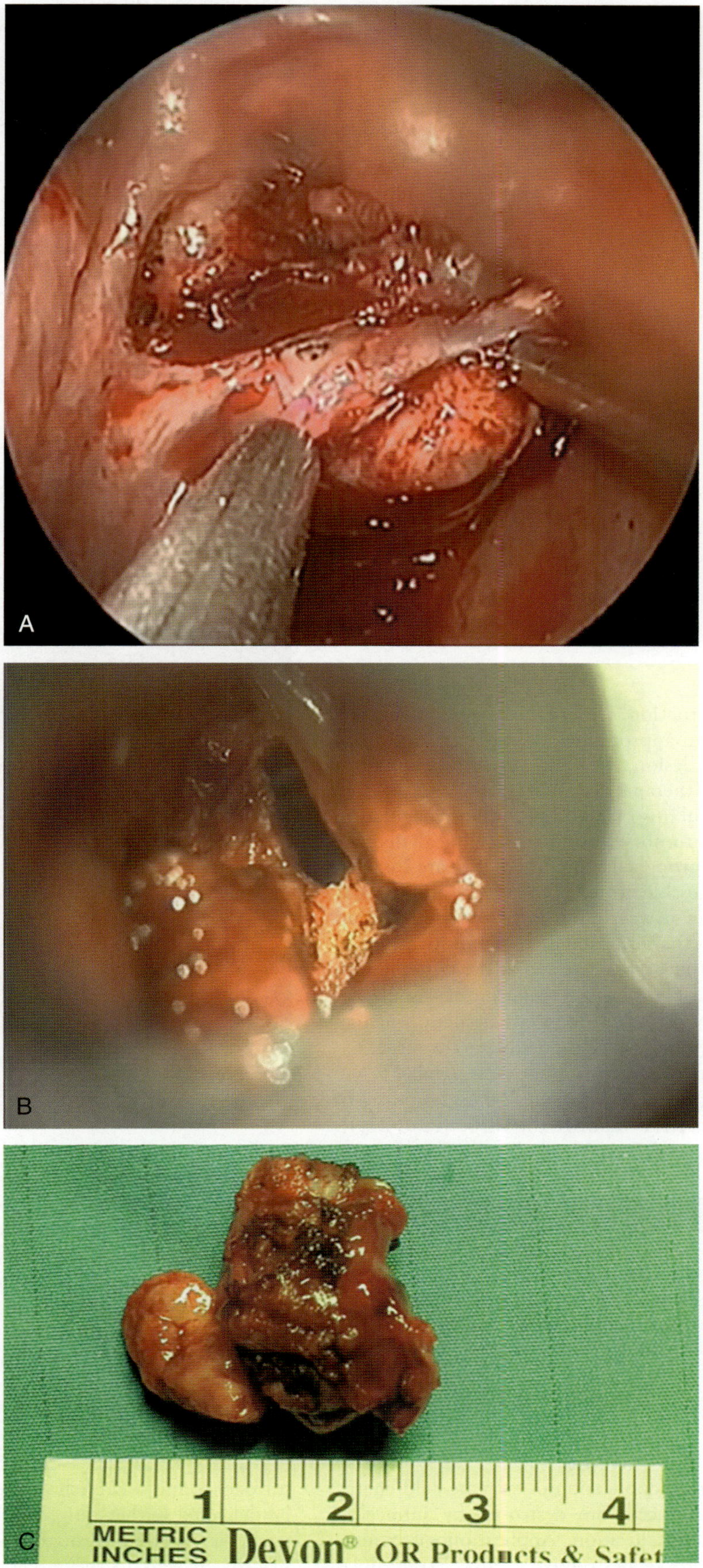


• **Fig. 21.10** (A and B) Progressive excision is performed microscopically and endoscopically with a $CO_2$ laser. (C) The hemilaryngectomy specimen.

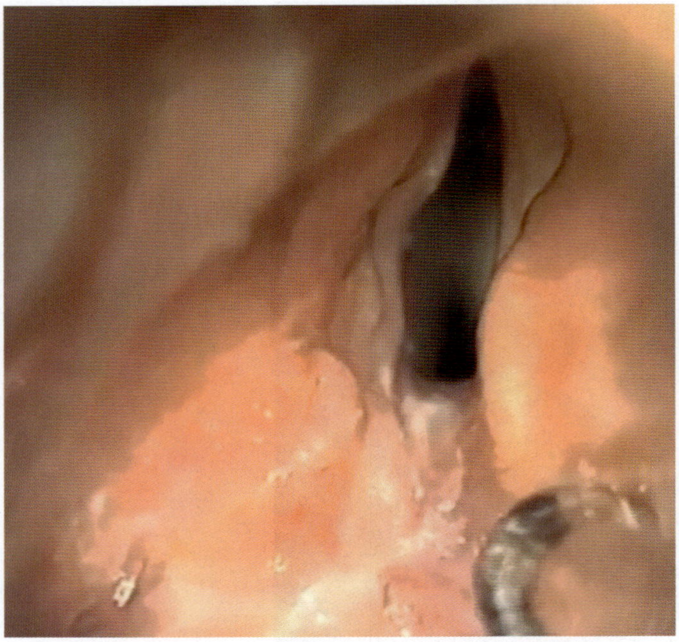

• **Fig. 21.11** The endoscopic follow-up showing no evidence of recurrent disease.

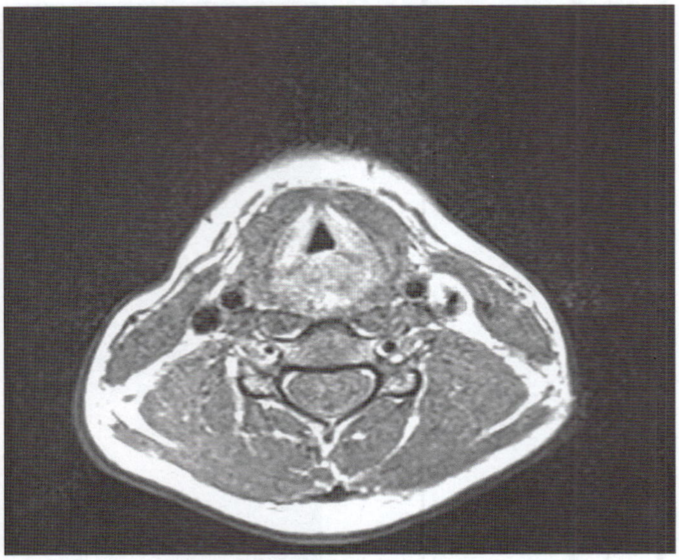

• **Fig. 21.12** Granular cell tumor in a 10-year-old female. Preop MRI T2-weighted scans showing a 2-cm mass located in the interarytenoid region.

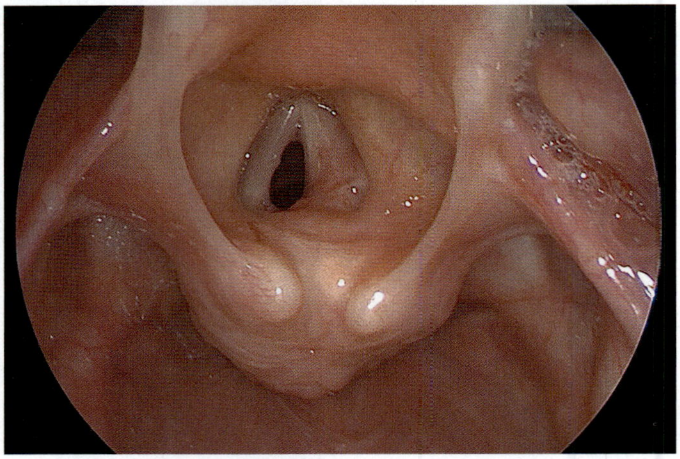

• **Fig. 21.13** Flexible endoscopy using a 3.5 endoscope, evidence of an exophytic tumor of the interarytenoid region.

relieve central airway obstruction. Different strategies to employ laser techniques depend on appropriate patient selection, properties of the obstructing lesion, and the concomitant use of adjunctive endobronchial therapies.

Lasers are used for debulking, as well as for photocoagulation and devascularization of tumors prior to mechanical debulking. Energy is delivered through flexible fibers that are inserted through either a rigid or flexible bronchoscope (Fig. 21.4). Lasers can remove an obstructing airway lesion in two ways: resection in combination with a mechanical modality, or vaporization. In using laser for resection, the laser is directed at the target lesion, devitalizing the lesion through photocoagulation of vascularity. The devitalized tissue is removed through either suction or forceps extraction. Vaporization of tissue is possible as the target tissue contains water. This involves aligning the laser parallel to the bronchial wall and aiming precisely at the lesion. Laser pulses of a few seconds or less are used to vaporize the tissue (Pearl 21.4). See Figs. 21.8–Figs. 21.11 and Figs. 21.14–21.16.

**PEARL 21.4**

The $CO_2$ laser should be used in the continuous wave (CW)/chopped mode, at an output power of 3 W, with a slightly defocused beam at 400 mm focal distance, along with a 70 to 100 ms duration of the laser strikes. With these conditions, the tumor can blanch and then vaporize without significantly carbonating, which results in minimal heat diffusion into the tissues around it.

## *Cryotherapy*

Cryotherapy is the controlled application of extreme cold energy to diseased tissue in which cells are destroyed by intracellular and extracellular cryocrystallization. Application of extreme cold energy causes a cascade of destructive events. Extracellular ice crystal formation causes an efflux of intracellular fluid, which results in cellular dehydration and increased toxicity. Intracellular ice crystal formation causes damage to intracellular organelles such as mitochondria and endoplasmic reticulum. Furthermore, cryotherapy has profound effects on the microcirculation: vasoconstriction, endothelial injury, and platelet aggregation. These effects lead to microthrombi formation and subsequent cellular death. Although application of cryotherapy may affect normal tissue, malignant tissue is particularly susceptible given its hypervascularity. The inherent cryosensitivity of a tissue depends mainly on its water content.

Application of cryotherapy requires a cryosurgery device (rigid or flexible cryoprobe, spray cryotherapy catheter), a cooling source known as a cryogen (either nitrous oxide or liquid nitrogen), and a bronchoscope through which the therapy can be delivered (either a rigid or flexible bronchoscope). The cryoprobe is inserted through the bronchoscope (Fig. 21.5) and placed adjacent to the target tissue such that direct contact is made. Repeated freeze-thaw cycles are applied, with a freeze time

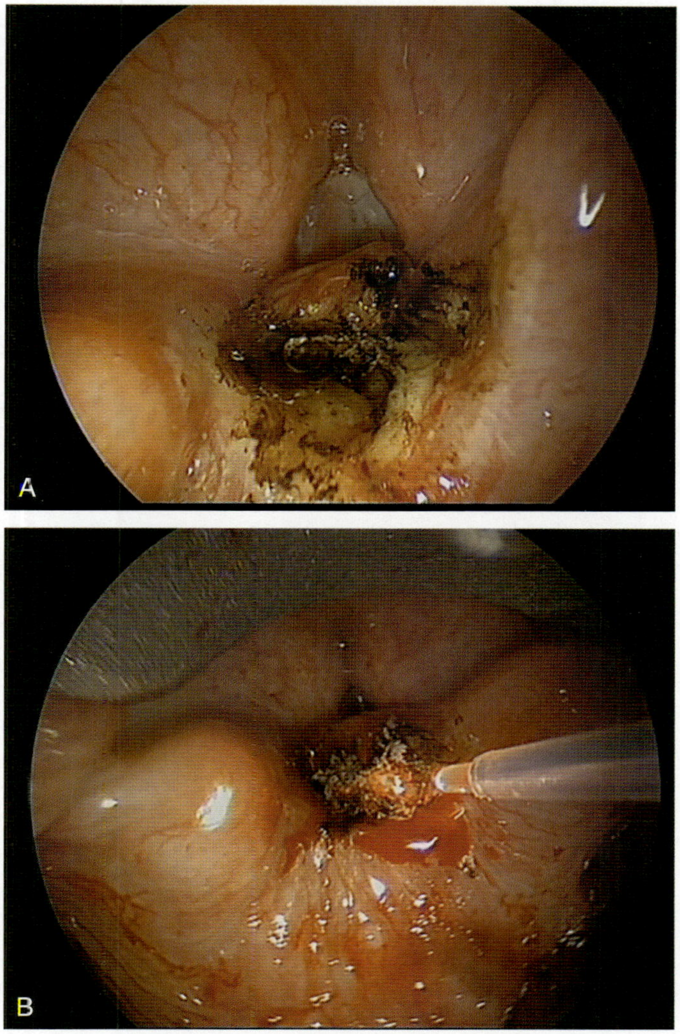

• **Fig. 21.14** In jet ventilation and in suspension direct laryngoscopy, a progressive excision is performed endoscopically with plasma ablation and $CO_2$ laser.

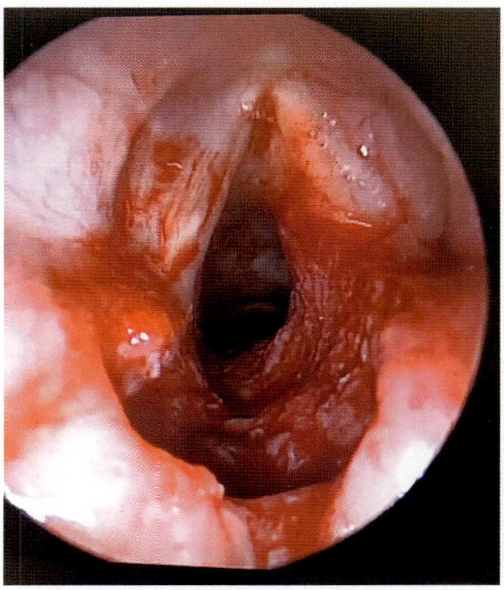

• **Fig. 21.15** The final endoscopic view.

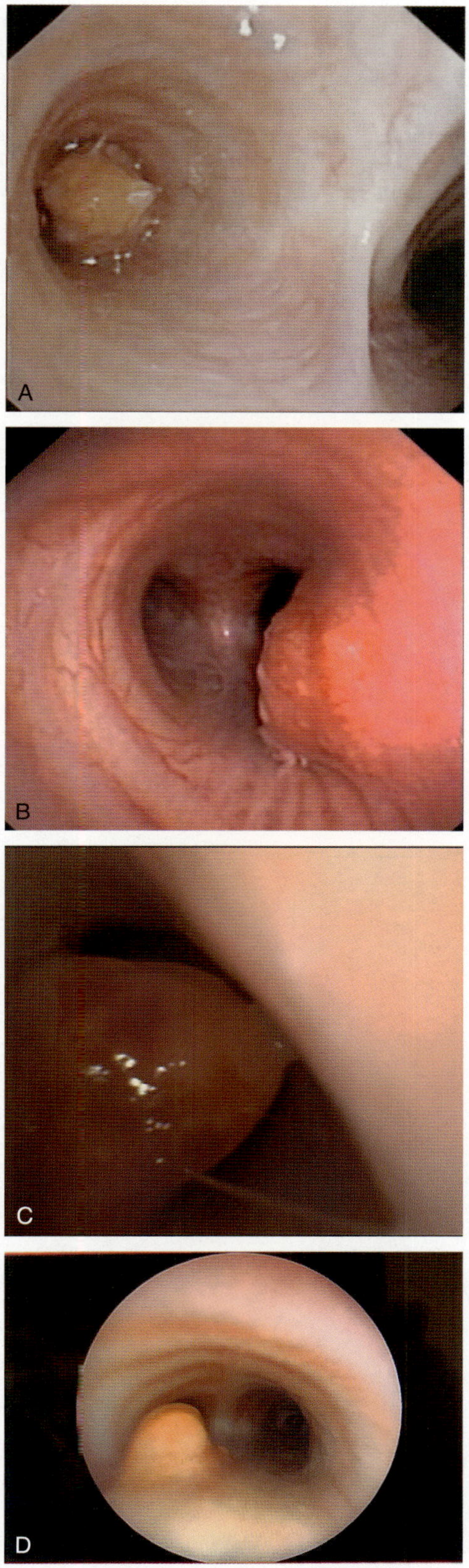

• **Fig. 21.16** Bronchoscopy endoscopic view: three different tracheal tumors aspects. (A) Pedunculated mass lesion almost entirely blocking the left main bronchus, suggesting bronchial carcinoid tumor. (B) Mucoepidermoid carcinoma with an irregular soft tissue thickening in the region of the right intrathoracic trachea. (C and D) Myofibroblastic tumor, which involved the left intrathoracic trachea.

varying depending on the cryogen used. The probe is moved to an untreated area, and repeated freeze-thaw cycles are applied until the entirety of the lesion has been treated. Over the ensuing days to weeks, tissue necrosis occurs followed by sloughing, which may be expectorated or may necessitate bronchoscopic removal.

Cryodebridement or cryorecanalization (Video 21.4) is a modality of tumor debulking in which a cryoprobe is inserted and placed in direct contact with the desired lesion. When the cryoprobe is activated, the contacted tissue is frozen and becomes adhered to the end of the probe. The probe is retracted along with large fragments of tissue. This technique is helpful for debulking endobronchial tumors in patients unable to tolerate lower fraction of inspired oxygen.

See Video 21.4.

# 22

# Recurrent Respiratory Papillomatosis

SHAZIA PEER

## Background

Recurrent respiratory papillomatosis (RRP) is a benign disease of the airway characterized by the presence of wart-like lesions, or papillomata, that may occur anywhere along the respiratory tract from the nasal vestibule to the terminal bronchi. It is caused by human papillomavirus (HPV). Types 6 and 11 are the causal strains in juvenile-onset RRP.

No cure currently exists, and management is aimed at alleviating symptoms that accompany recurrent disease. Surgical clearance of recurrent obstructive lesions while preserving voice is the mainstay of treatment. This recurrent and relapsing pattern of therapy can take a significant toll on patients, caregivers, and otolaryngologists.

More recently, primary prevention through comprehensive HPV vaccination programs that include RRP-linked strains has shown a significant reduction in the incidence of RRP in many developed nations. This is not reflected in developing nations, where HPV vaccination programs largely target oncogenic strains linked to cervical cancer.

## Initial Assessment and Diagnosis

Patients typically present with a triad of symptoms, of varying degrees, that include persistent hoarseness, stridor, and respiratory distress. Persistent hoarseness is the commonest feature. Altered voice quality or aphonia may also be present. Stridor, when present, is variable according to the degree of airway obstruction. It may be inspiratory or biphasic, present at baseline or only with exertion.

Patients may present in acute respiratory distress, making an urgent evaluation necessary. Recurrent respiratory papillomatosis should be high in the differential diagnosis on initial review of an unknown patient in the emergency room who presents in acute respiratory distress with a history of nonresolving dysphonia and associated cough. In general, however, there is a gradual growth of papillomata, and acute respiratory distress is not common. Notwithstanding, in regions with poor access to health care and/or resource constraints, patients may present *in extremis*, since referral to specialist care is often delayed.

It is also not uncommon for patients to be misdiagnosed with asthma, recurrent croup or bronchitis, or other inflammatory causes of the larynx. In endemic regions, laryngeal tuberculosis (TB) is a consideration. Less commonly, patients can present with chronic cough, recurrent pneumonia, dyspnea, hemoptysis, dysphagia, failure to thrive, and apneic events. Clinicians who practice in health care systems with poor HPV vaccination coverage should always consider RRP in the differential diagnosis for patients not responding to medical therapy.

## Evaluation

Following history and examination, a flexible fiberoptic laryngoscopy (FFL) is performed to view the nasal cavity, pharynx, and larynx (Fig. 22.1). Presence and location of lesions are recorded. If the FFL does not reveal RRP, the underlying pathology is appropriately treated (Pearl 22.1). If lesions are concerning for RRP, then a direct laryngotracheobronchoscopy (DLTB/DLB) is performed, and tissue biopsy is necessary for histological confirmation. Viral subtyping can be requested.

**PEARL 22.1**

In patients with a history of endotracheal or bronchial disease, or symptoms suggestive of such, a tracheobronchoscopy is warranted.

Fiberoptic laryngoscopy findings to be documented include the following: (Video 22.1)

- Nature of the lesions – sessile, pedunculated, if obstructive, or ball-valving.
- Proximity of lesions to anterior/posterior commissures.
- True vocal cord mobility. If mobility is not observed or is equivocal, this is also documented.
- Presence of a glottic gap and patency of distal airway.

Imaging of the chest and trachea is recommended for symptoms suggestive of distal involvement. This includes respiratory

No disclosures/no conflict of interest

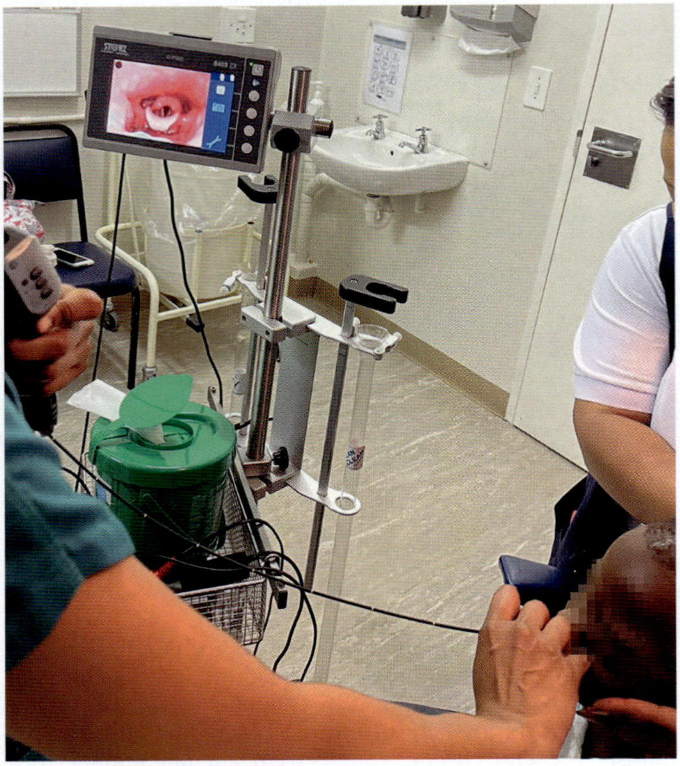

• **Fig. 22.1** Awake flexible fiberoptic laryngoscopy (FFL) in a clinical setting to view upper airways.

distress that is out of keeping with FFL findings, intraoperative or postoperative hypoxia that is unexpected, biphasic stridor, prolonged expiration, or wheezing (Fig. 22.2).

In a patient assessed to be unstable based on vitals, oxygen saturation, and clinical examination, it is necessary to decide on timing and safety of FFL evaluation–operating room as opposed to clinic or emergency room (Pearl 22.2).

**PEARL 22.2**

When possible, the operating room is the safest location for airway management in the setting of RRP. In an emergent situation where intubation is required outside of the operating room, there runs a risk of seeding disease distally and/or endotracheal tube obstruction by papillomatous tissue at the time of intubation. Always prepare for tube obstruction and reintubation, and for further management (typically in the operating room) immediately after intubation is performed. A tracheotomy tray should also be available.

This chapter focuses on the endoscopic clearance of obstructive papillomata that present at the various anatomical sites while preserving laryngeal structure and mucosa. Commonly used instrumentation is demonstrated along with technique for clearance. In selected patients, adjuvant intralesional therapy using bevacizumab is also included. Systemic bevacizumab therapy is an emerging treatment option but is beyond the scope of this chapter.

## Operative Approach

### Patient Selection and Informed Consent

All children with suspected papillomatosis need to have an airway assessment in the operating room under general anesthesia. Lesions are assessed macroscopically and tissue biopsied for histological confirmation (Fig. 22.3).

Tissue may be sent for HPV typing if offered by the institution. The extent of disease is confirmed and documented using the Derkay-Coltrera Staging Score.[1]

Patients and caregivers are shown images/videos of the condition, a description of what they may anticipate during surgery and recovery, including "red flags" for urgent return (Box 22.1).

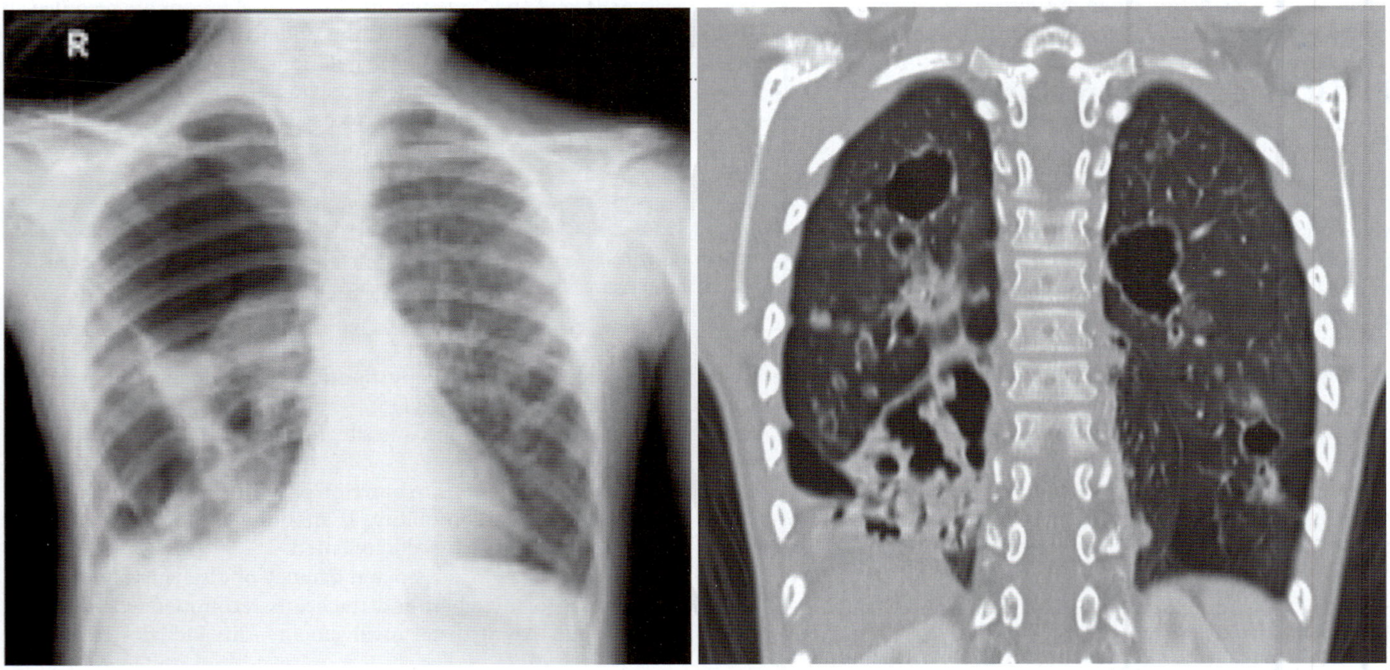


• **Fig. 22.2** Chest imaging depicting lung involvement.

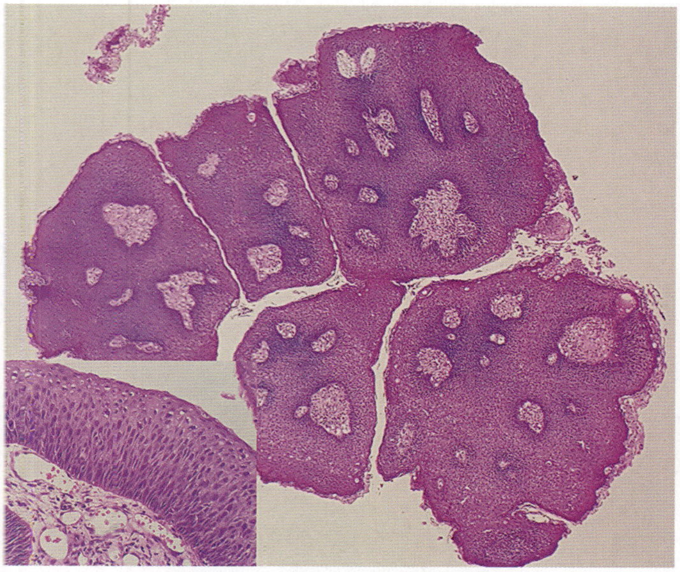

• **Fig. 22.3** Histology of respiratory papillomatosis *(image courtesy Dr. Shivani Singh)*.

**• BOX 22.1 "Red Flag" Symptoms for Urgent Return**

Dysphonia
Stridor[a]
Respiratory distress[a]
Feeding difficulties
Obstructive sleep apnea (OSA)
Nonresolving cough (>2 weeks)

[a]Baseline/on exertion/asleep (more importantly note any change/deterioration in symptoms)

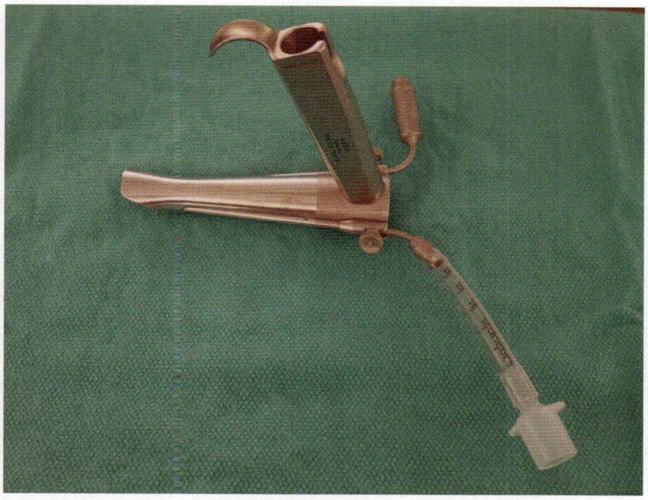

• **Fig. 22.4** Benjamin-Lindholm laryngoscope with side ports for oxygenation and light carrier.

## Equipment

1. Direct laryngoscopy is performed in suspension, with or without the use of a microscope. The author uses an age-appropriate Benjamin-Lindholm laryngoscope. The side port closest to the anesthetic machine is connected to a trimmed 5.0 uncuffed endotracheal tube (ETT) for passive oxygenation. The other side port is connected to a fiber optic bifid light carrier, accommodating laryngoscope and telescope (Fig. 22.4).
2. The standard set of microlaryngeal instruments are prepared (18 cm and 23 cm length), including cupped forceps, graspers, and Kleinsasser triangular jaw upward-curved forceps. A ball-ended suction is also recommended (Fig. 22.5).

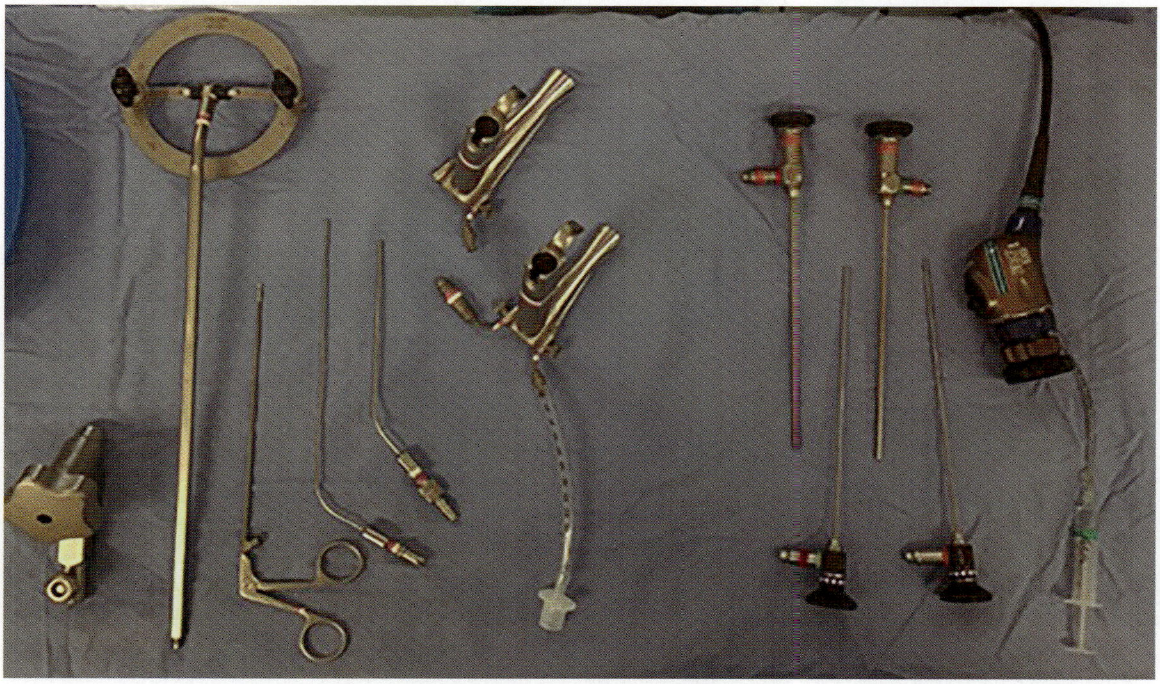

• **Fig. 22.5** Microlaryngeal instruments.

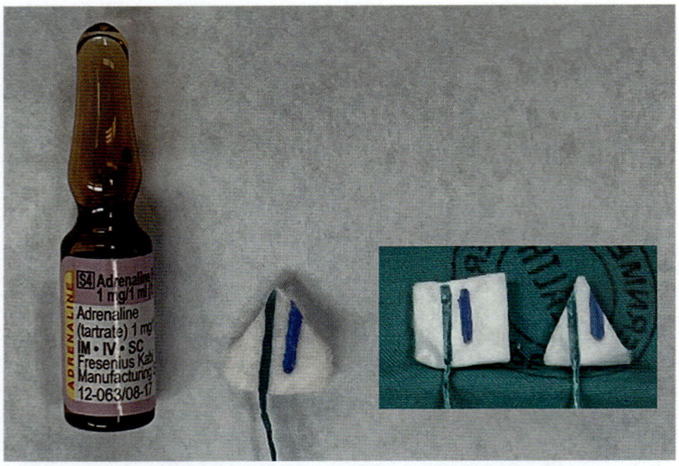


• **Fig. 22.6** Adrenaline-soaked neurosurgical patties cut into a triangular shape.

3. A gum guard and age-appropriate cuffed and uncuffed ETTs are made available. Smaller sizes are also necessary in anticipation of a narrower, obstructed airway, should a rescue intubation be necessary.
4. Neurosurgical patties/pledgets soaked in Adrenaline 1:1000 (undiluted) are prepared, 5 mm × 5 mm sized, some triangle-shaped for anterior commissure placement. (Fig. 22.6).
5. Topicalization with lidocaine is prepared using a luer-lock syringe attached to an atomizer. The maximum total dosage is calculated for the patient (7 mg/kg of 2% lidocaine). For greater volume, consider diluting with 0.9% normal saline to 1%. It is not advisable to dilute it beyond 1% because this would compromise effectiveness (Fig. 22.7).
6. Equipment for airway rescue by intubation is prepared in advance. (Fig. 22.8) Depending on the patient's level of respiratory distress, the main concern is losing the airway and having to successfully rescue it by intubation without dislodging any papillomata. Papilloma disruption with or without bleeding may risk further airway compromise, through obstruction distally or by ETT occlusion (blood and/or tissue).
7. In acute respiratory distress, a tracheotomy set with age-appropriate tracheotomy tubes on hand is recommended.

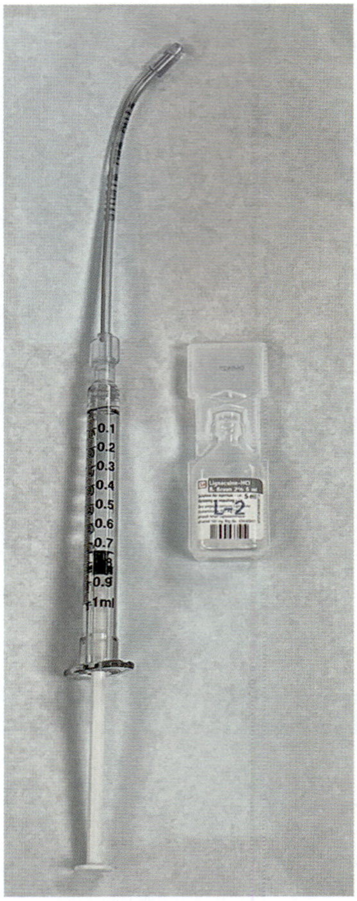


• **Fig. 22.7** Lidocaine prepared in a luer-lock syringe and atomizer for topicalization.

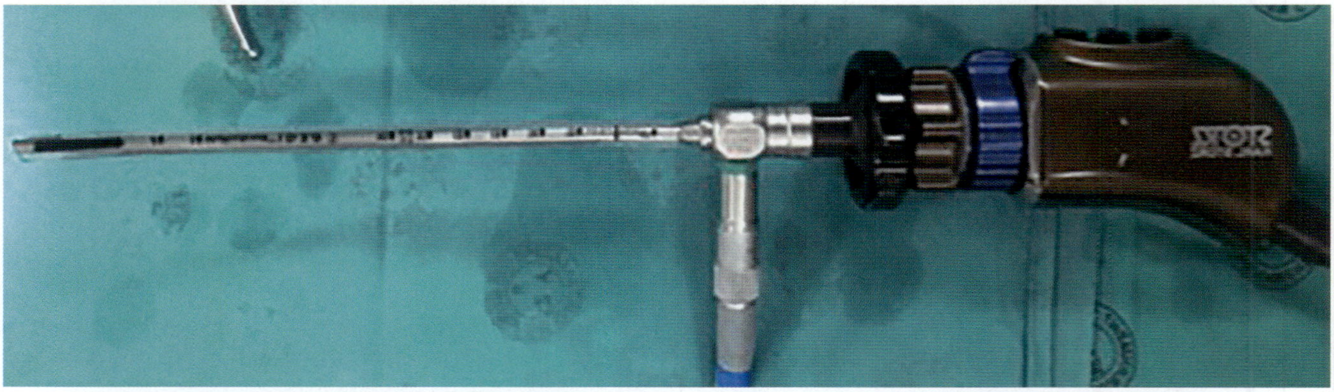

• **Fig. 22.8** Airway rescue intubation tool. An endotracheal tube is loaded onto a rigid telescope to create a "camera stylet."

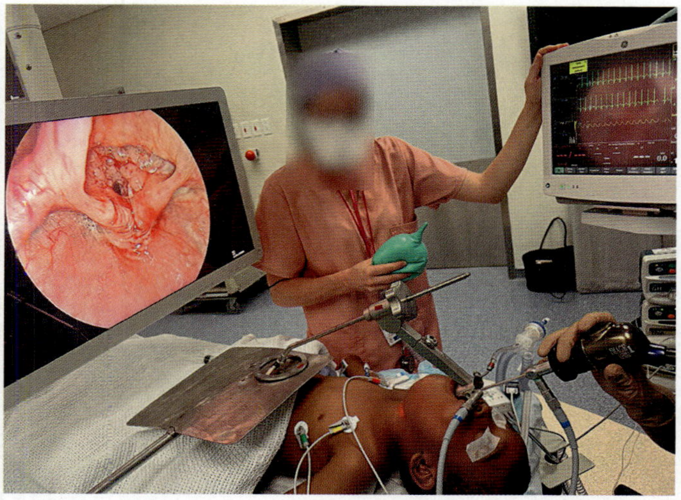

• **Fig. 22.9** Patient positioning in suspension with Benjamin-Lindholm laryngoscope onto tray.

## Patient Positioning

Patient is gently placed in suspension (Fig. 22.9).

## Steps of the Procedure (Including Tips and Tricks)

### Preparation

***Discussion with Anesthesia prior to commencement*** is recommended as in any shared airway procedure. Discussion should include information about the anatomical level(s) of obstruction, plan for restoring ventilation during surgery, and postoperative recovery (Intensive Care Unit [ICU] / high level of care may be indicated).

Depending on the patient's respiratory status and the experience of the surgeon and anesthesiologist, various options for ventilation are available, including spontaneous versus apneic approaches, jet ventilation, or with an indwelling laser-safe ETT in place for the duration of the operation. It is the author's preference to have the patient breathing spontaneously for the duration of surgery, or at least until the extent of disease is determined.

***A general anesthetic is commenced following the surgical checklist.*** This begins with a gas induction using sevoflurane, followed by establishing intravenous access and commencing total intravenous anesthesia (TIVA). In older patients, intravenous access can be established prior to induction of anesthesia, to increase safety. A propofol infusion titrated to the patient's weight is used. Simultaneous preoxygenation and spontaneous ventilation with bag-mask ventilation continue (Fig. 22.10A). Observe for chest rise, abdominal distension from over insufflating air, and cessation of breathing or apnea.

***For continued oxygenation,*** use the laryngoscope's side port to supplement oxygenation. Other methods include transnasal humidified rapid-insufflation ventilatory exchange (THRIVE) or a fashioned ETT placed along the alveolar ridge for passive oxygen administration.

***First look*** with an anesthetic laryngoscope (age-appropriate blade) to topicalize the larynx with lidocaine. This will allow for a quick view of the supraglottis and glottis to determine if intubation will be challenging (Fig. 22.10B). A gum guard is recommended to protect the teeth.

The Benjamin-Lindholm laryngoscope is then gently inserted, and the suspension arm is clicked in and fixed into place while resting on a Mayo table or suspension tray. Time of suspension is noted (Fig. 22.10C).

Topicalize the airway further, down to trachea, enough to trickle down to carina (Video 22.2). Apply adrenaline-soaked pledgets to the papillomata (Fig. 22.11A and 22.11B, Video 22.3). ***Second look*** is now possible, using a zero-degree, 4-mm telescope to view distally (Fig. 22.11C) (Video 22.3).

***Extent of disease*** is documented. Where to commence, and what instruments to use, is now decided. Clearance from proximal to distal can be pursued, or by targeting individual sites.

### Principles for Surgical Clearance

These are tabulated later (Box 22.2).

### Instruments for Debulking

Depending on the availability of equipment at the institution, various surgical options are used. Advantages and disadvantages of each are briefly tabulated (Table 22.1). All instruments present a unique surgical learning curve. Without proper training or supervision and without knowledge of the mechanical settings, serious and potentially irreversible airway injury, or worse, may occur. Always keep the tip of the wand/blade/fiber in the airway, visible at all times, and especially when activated. When necessary, a 30-degree angled telescope can help provide additional visualization of the lesions and instruments tip.

1. **Cold steel instruments**

   Utilization of already available microlaryngeal instruments makes for the most cost-effective option. Debulking and pausing to suction is a two-step process and can be time consuming in an already high-risk procedure.

   Kleinsasser triangular jaw and upturned forceps are preferred to remove the bulky portion of the papilloma close to the stalk while avoiding injury to adjacent normal mucosa (Fig. 22.12, Video 22.4) Tactile feedback is excellent with these forceps, as softer papillomata easily detach from the epithelium when compared to underlying tissue. Right, left, and upturned forceps are recommended. Cupped forceps, by design, are for tissue biopsies. The cut end bites down with closing of the cups. One must be careful, as this instrument can bite into deeper uninvolved tissue.

   Aim to achieve hemostasis with each laryngeal unit using pledgets, thereby reducing blood loss and repeated distal suctioning (Fig. 22.11A and 22.11B).

2. **Laryngeal Microdebrider**

   This powered instrument consists of a handpiece, disposable laryngeal blade, foot pedal, and a console (Video 22.5). Technology uses suction and saline irrigation to draw tissue into the distal opening or aperture, housing

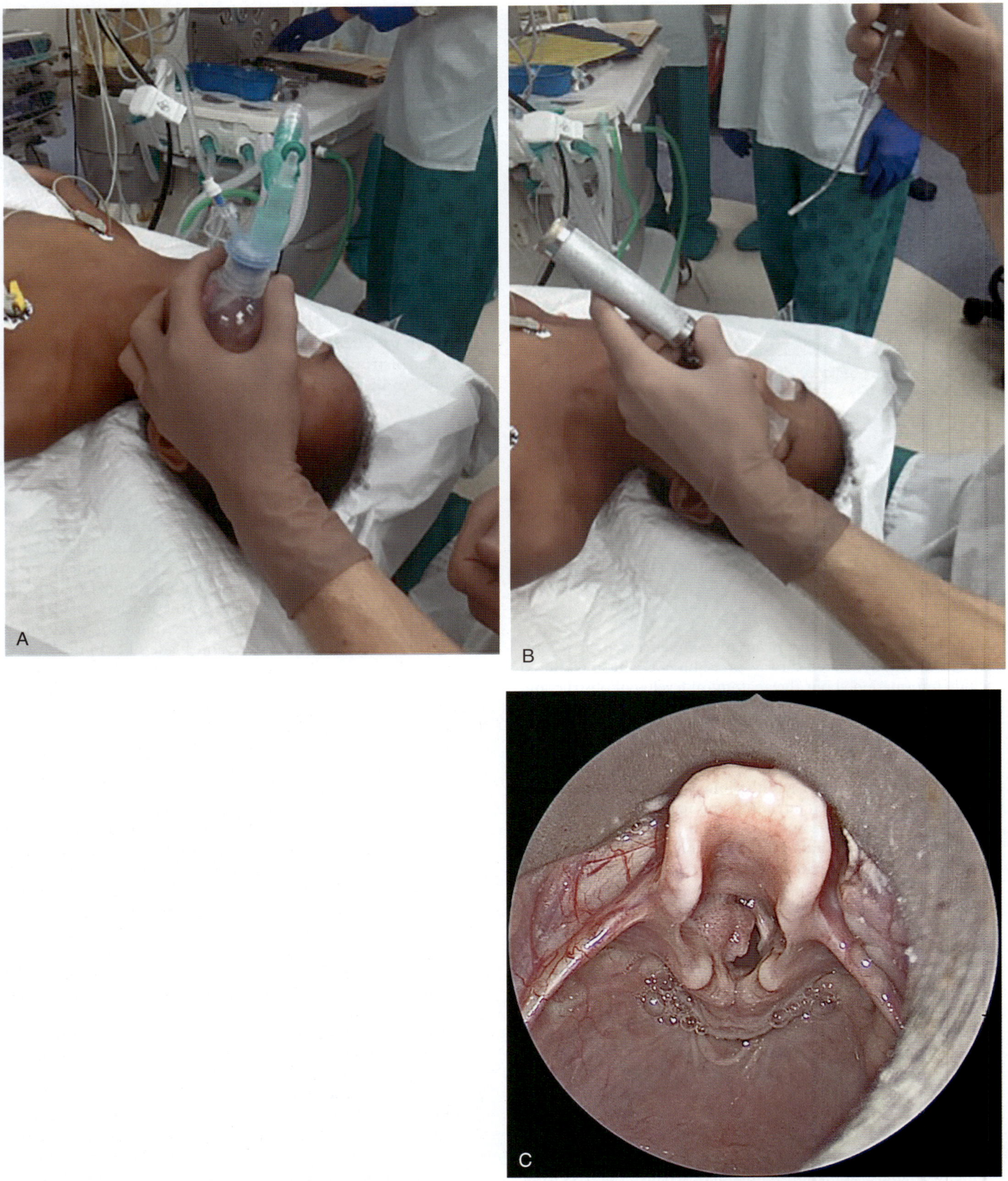

• **Fig. 22.10** General Anesthesia. (A) Bag mask ventilation. (B) Topicalization of local anesthetic with atomizer onto vallecula. (C) Glottic view in laryngeal suspension.

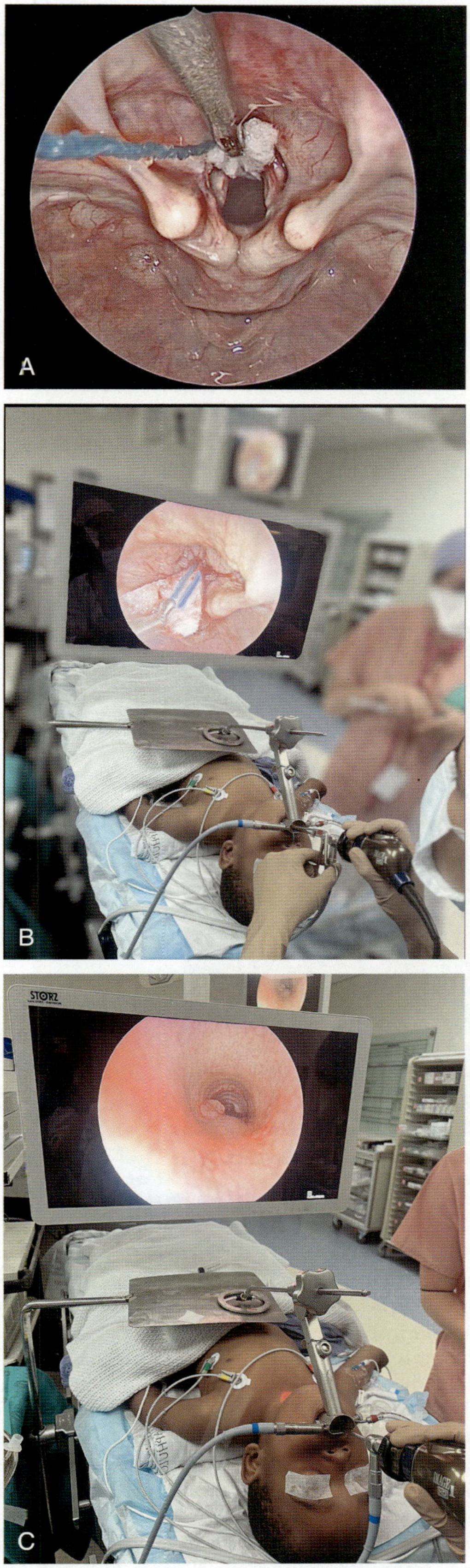


• **Fig. 22.11** Application of pledgets. (A) Placement of pledget. (B) Application. (C) Second look – discrete papilloma in trachea.

**• BOX 22.2 Principles of Clearance**

1. First, remove papilloma bulk obstructing/intruding lumen, without mucosal breach. For example, an anterior or lateral papilloma ball-valving into the lumen (Videos 22.10 and 22.11).
2. In glottic disease with papillomata extruding from the medial margin of both true cords, choose one side to debulk. Debulk the opposite side at the following surgery.
3. Maximally preserve normal adjacent mucosa
   a. Avoid mucosal injury by exclusively handling the papillomata
   b. Be careful with vital structures—anterior/posterior commissure, vocal process, laryngeal surface of epiglottis, and subglottis, if involved.
   c. Remain superficial when biting papillomata.
4. Papilloma-involved tissue and surfaces
   a. Use controlled instruments to debulk around delicate structures
   b. Avoid
      i. leaving opposing raw edges/surfaces for synechia to develop
      ii. Deep bites, prolonged penetration of vocal process, stripping mucosal lining. This can lead to hemorrhage and unintentional tissue loss and subsequent scarring. Bleeding occurs with retained papillomata or injury to adjacent mucosa
      iii. Exposed cartilage
      iv. Using laser to bulky tissue
      v. Aggressive removal of papillomata on trachealis or near carina. Ensure instruments are parallel to airway, especially, when entering through tracheostoma. Patient may cough, and unintentional tissue loss can occur.
5. It is not necessary to remove every lesion at every surgery—discrete, mural, sessile, nonobstructive lesions can remain if not causing secondary infection/granuloma.
6. Biopsy any lesion that appears suspicious, or if dual pathology is suspected.

the rotating blade that amputates any suctioned tissue (Video 22.6). Tissue and blood are swiftly suctioned away. The blade has a 15-degree angled tip that rotates with finger-wheel control, allowing additional precise tip placement. Blades used on the larynx are typically 2.9 mm in width, with an 18- or 23-cm working length (Video 22.5).

The microdebrider works gently and quickly to shave papilloma bulk close to vital structures while minimizing mucosal damage. The console is set to 60 to 500 revolutions per minute (RPM) on forward oscillation. On entry, always insert blade with a closed aperture, to avoid indiscriminate suctioning of tissue. The author recommends the double-curved skimmer blade, ideal for meticulous excision of papillomata in fragile areas, that reportedly provides shorter procedure times and quicker patient recovery (Pearl 22.3).

**PEARL 22.3**

Under circumstances wherein the papilloma is abutting or involving a vital structure such as the lamina propria, the blade can be rotated to the open position immediately above the papilloma to be debrided. The papilloma is then elevated with the suction, and a single tap of the foot pedal will excise only what is in the suction port. This can be repeated until the majority of the lesion is debulked.

**TABLE 22.1 Advantages and Disadvantages of Each Modality**

| Technique | Technology | Advantages | Disadvantages |
|---|---|---|---|
| Cold steel | Oldest | Available, affordable, safe, less pain | Time consuming, blood in field |
| Microdebrider | Mechanical/powered tool | Time efficient; less pain, quicker recovery, better immediate, and early postoperative voice outcome<br>2.9 mm width and rotatable tip | Costly consumables<br>Not reusable |
| Coblation | Newer | Time efficient, less pain | More expensive<br>Large tip end and width –3.8 mm<br>Standard length |
| CO2/YAG laser | Older<br>Thermal | Time efficient, standard management for years | Expensive, painful, significant heat dissipation into surrounding tissues, edema, scar formation, vapor plume, carbonized tissue<br>Laser precautions |
| Trublue laser | Thermal<br>Newer | Time efficient, less pain, portable, reusable, cheaper consumables | Still more expensive than other tools, laser precautions |

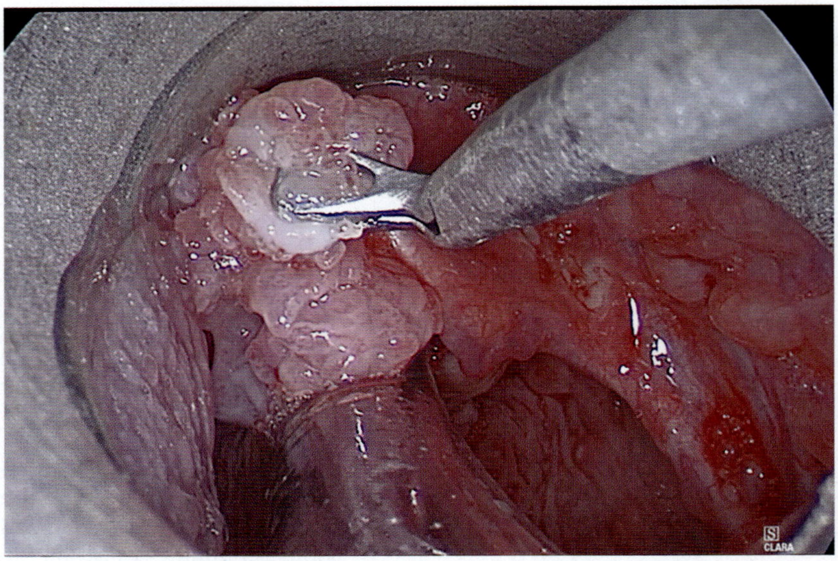

• **Fig. 22.12** Debulking cold steel. Kleinsasser forceps used to debulk papillomata.

3. **Coblation**

Plasma-mediated radiofrequency ablation (coblation) creates and applies an energy field through an isotonic sodium chloride medium. By coblation, the medium is dissociated into free sodium ions that are ultimately responsible for tissue dissociation and breakdown. Coblation is applied to the tissue with a disposable wand connected to a controller using pedal function – ABLATE (debulking) and COAG (hemostasis). Preferred papilloma settings are 5 (ABLATE) and 3 (COAG). Furthermore, the shaft of the wand can be modified for a better angle, and there are different tip constructs and geometries. Excess saline entering the distal airway is suctioned with an additional suction instrument.

Coblation is therefore able to reduce mass, making bulky exophytic papillomata the ideal lesion to benefit from its use (Fig. 22.13A and 22.13B). Low heat generated from the instrument, and the lack of a spark or an ignition medium, reduces risk of airway fires when compared to laser. Tissue penetration limited to the lamina propria adds further safety advantage.

Use suction from the wand tip to gently pull the papilloma away from underlying tissue (Videos 22.7 and 22.8). The

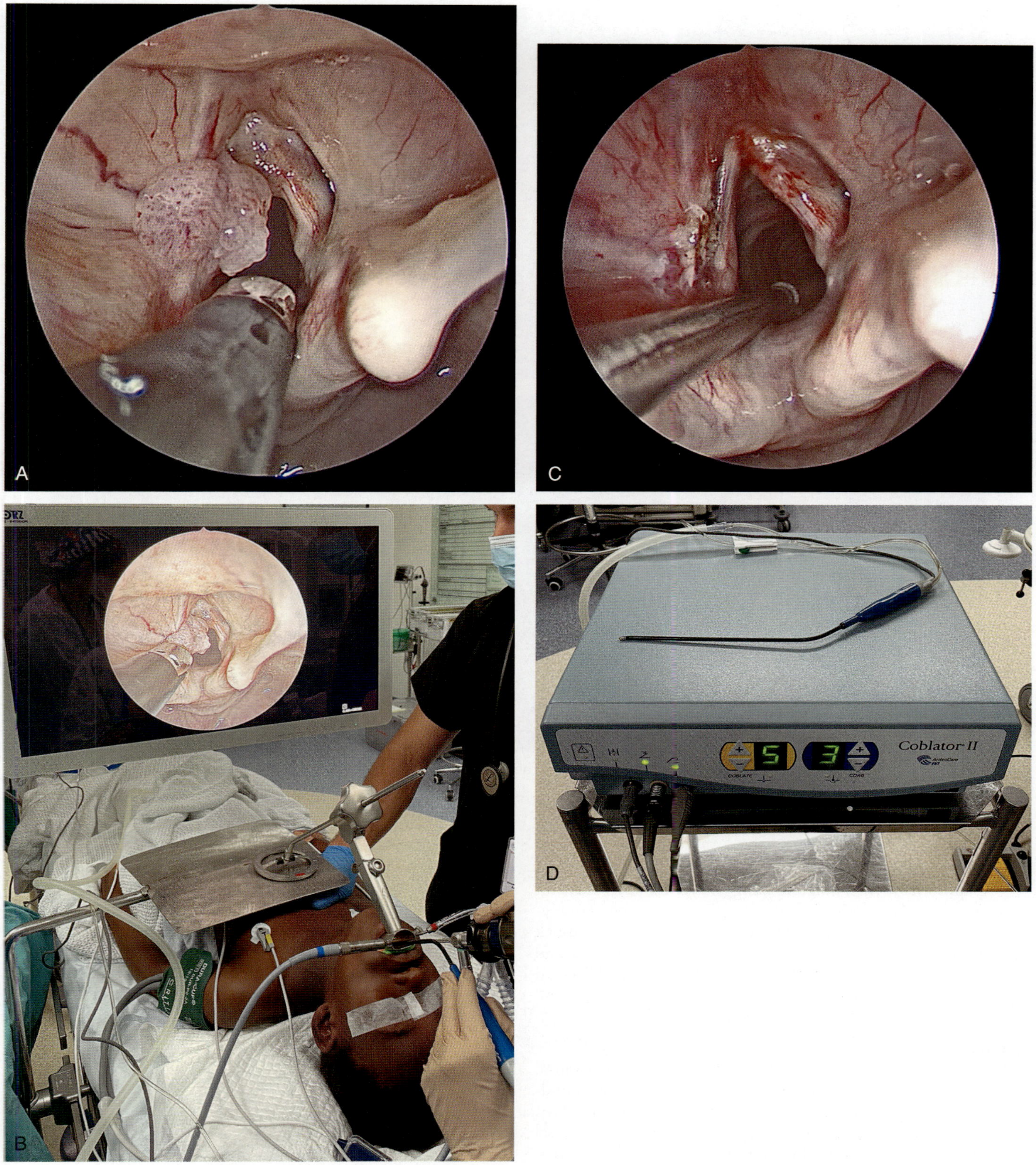


• **Fig. 22.13** Coblation. (A) First remove obstructive lesion in airway. (B) Image of coblation. (C) Final view after clearance. (D) Machine and wand connection.

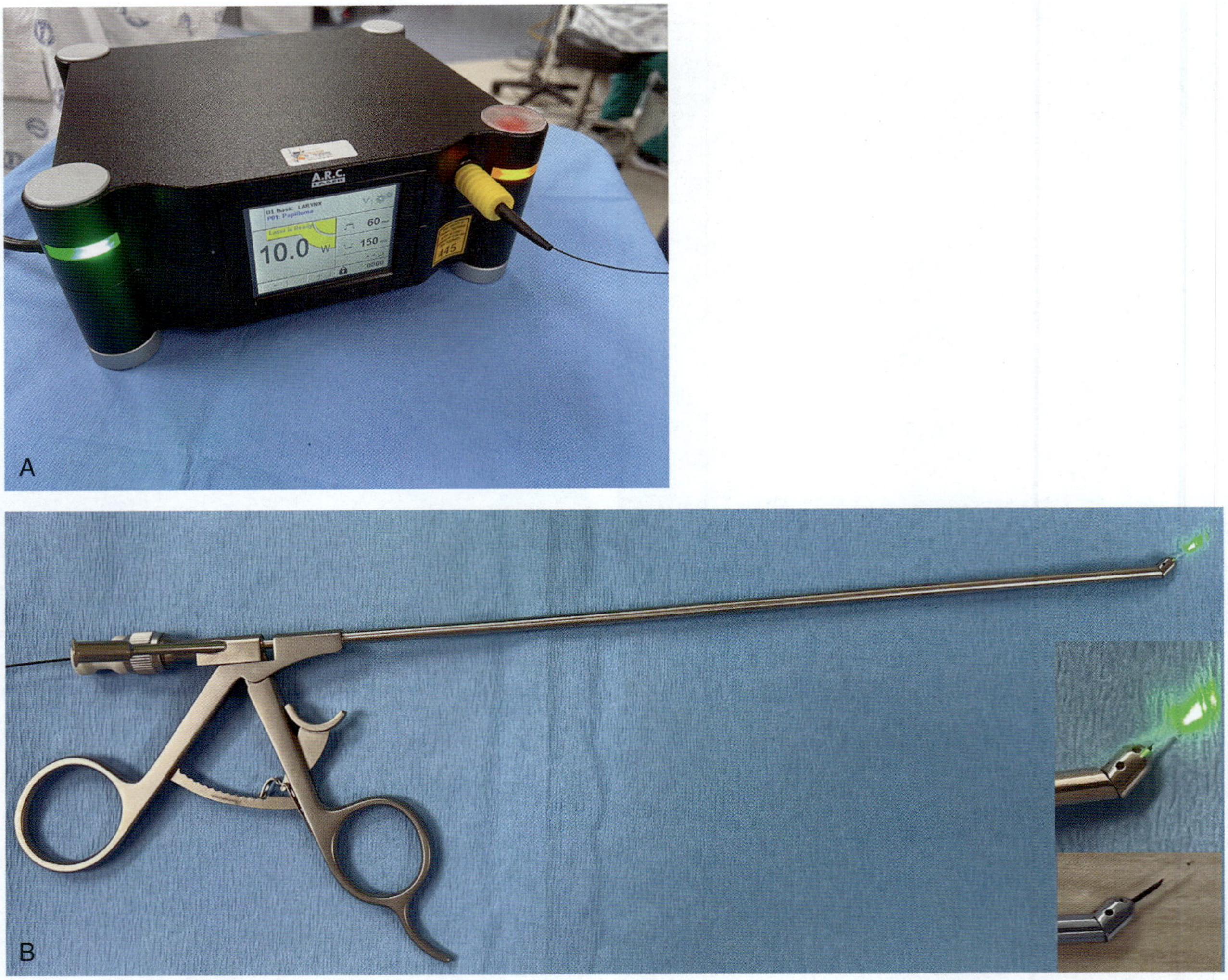


• **Fig. 22.14** Blue Light Laser 445 nm. (A) Console and settings. (B) Karl Storz forceps with rotating tip for upward fiber direction.

papilloma is then ablated using the yellow ABLATE foot pedal while exerting minimal to no trauma on underlying tissue (Fig. 22.13C). Short bursts of ablations in quick pulses, on and off, in 0.5-second intervals, are safe and effective. The author recommends the Procise LW wand (Fig. 22.13D). The wand's outer diameter is 3.8 mm and may pose a challenge in very small patients.

4. **Laser**

   Carbon dioxide ($CO_2$) laser, previously the mainstay of surgical clearance, carries the risk of heat dissipation into surrounding tissues and resultant consequences of thermal injury. Recurrent use also caused significant scar and laryngeal organ damage, prompting other debulking modalities that ablated and minimized bleeding, as mentioned earlier. The introduction of fiber-delivered laser systems like KTP and Nd:YAG lasers are as effective as $CO_2$ laser in papilloma ablation, with bendable tip, ideal for maneuverability.

   More recently, blue-light laser with a wavelength of 445 nm light technology providing photo-angiolytic and cutting properties was introduced (Fig. 22.14A). This flexible optical fiber inserts into a laryngeal forceps that precisely directs the tip to target infraglottic or very anterior lesions (Fig. 22.14B). Some centers may have laser-specific handpieces that similarly allow precise control of the fiber. Settings are adjustable, depending on context-baseline settings: range 4 to 10 W, 30 to 60 ms on, 120 to 150 ms off, using 300 microfiber (Fig. 22.14A).

   Laser precautions are required to avoid airway fires; fraction of inspired oxygen ($FiO_2$) must be <30% prior to the commencement of laser use in all cases.

### *Tracheotomized Patients*

A general anesthetic with gas induction is commenced via the tracheotomy. Upsize the tube for the duration of surgery, to optimize

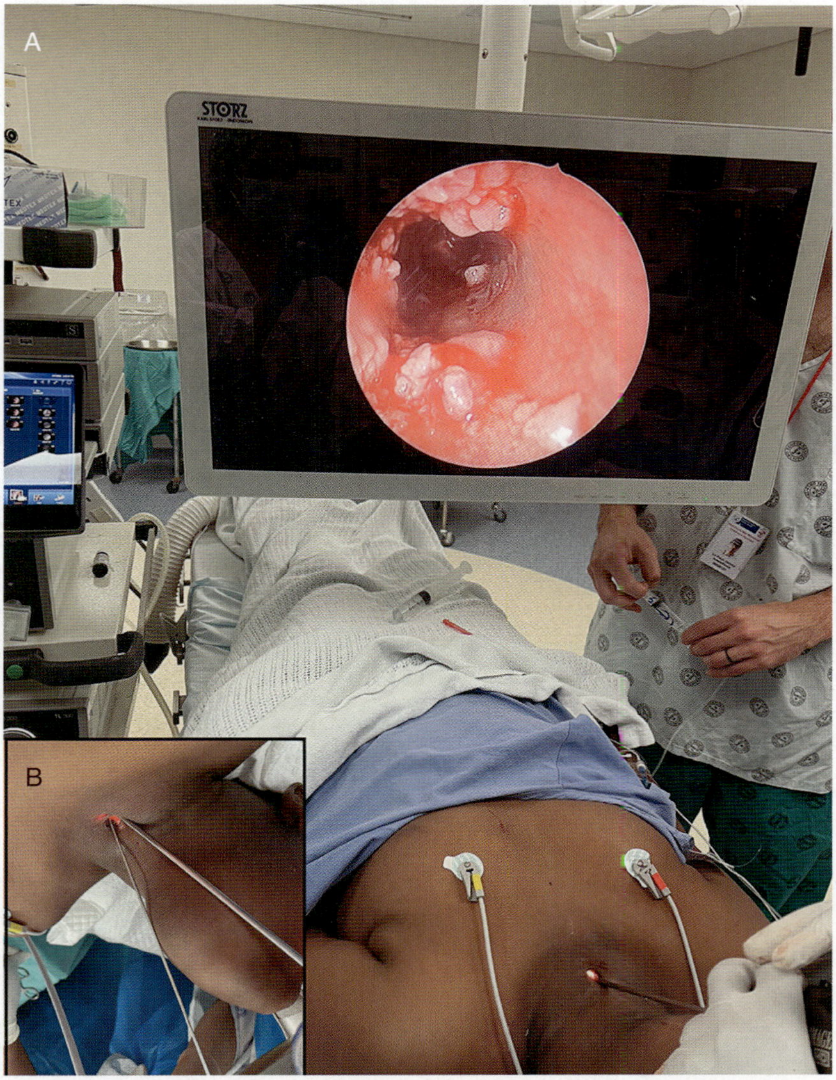


• **Fig. 22.15** Tracheotomized patient. (A) In suspension with Parsons laryngoscope. (B) View through stoma distally.

ventilation with a big leak. Once anesthetized, the patient is gently put into suspension (Fig. 22.15A and 22.15B).

Proximal clearance aims to improve voice quality by establishing retrograde flow. Mucosal preservation is key. Leave nonobstructive residual disease behind to prevent scarring. Removing papillomata around or distal to stoma requires preoxygenation, serial removal, and reinsertion of tracheotomy tube.

The author prefers cold steel over powered tools in the trachea (Video 22.9). Care must be taken not to damage trachealis. If possible, insert an ETT from the oral cavity to just above the stoma, permitting oxygenation (Fig. 22.16, Video 22.9).

### *Adjuvant Therapy With Bevacizumab (Avastin)*

A minority of cases require intralesional therapy. Indications are for serviceable voice, to vulnerable areas prone to scar formation, to prevent web formation and irreversible scarring. Single-site injection can be sublesional or intralesional and is performed after debulking. Using an orotracheal injector (Fig. 22.17) with a 1-mL slip-tip syringe of 0.5 mL (12.5 mg) Bevacizumab is loaded and injected (Fig. 22.18). This can be repeated every 4 to 6 weeks to monitor response to therapy before spacing the injections further apart.

## Tracheotomy

Tracheotomy is seen as a last resort. However, in patients with rapidly recurring disease, it may be lifesaving. There are reports of seeding with tracheotomy insertion, but this is not proven. In some patients with aggressive disease, it may facilitate longer intervals between debulking procedures.

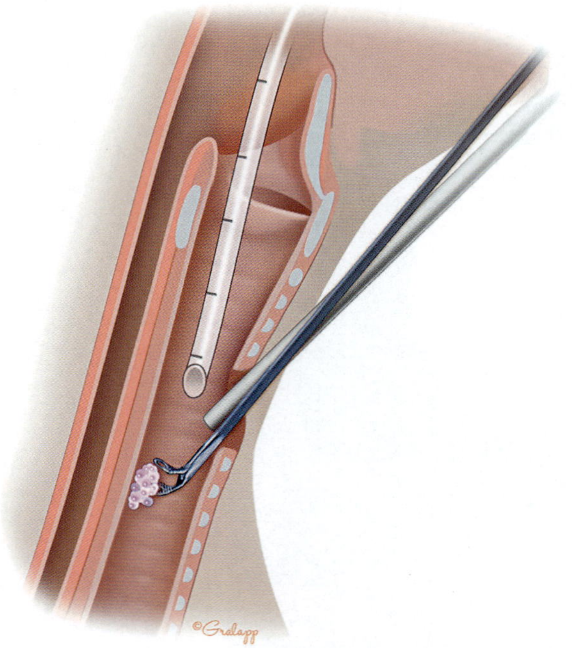


• **Fig. 22.16** Telescope with forceps through stoma to retrieve obstructive papillomata. Oxygenation permitted proximally with endotracheal tube above stoma. (© 2024 Chris Gralapp.)

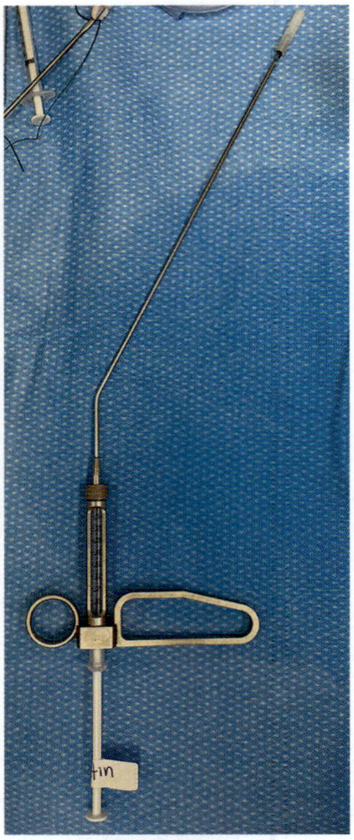

• **Fig. 22.17** Orotracheal injector for Bevacizumab intralesional therapy. *(Image courtesy Dr. Karthik Balakrishnan).*

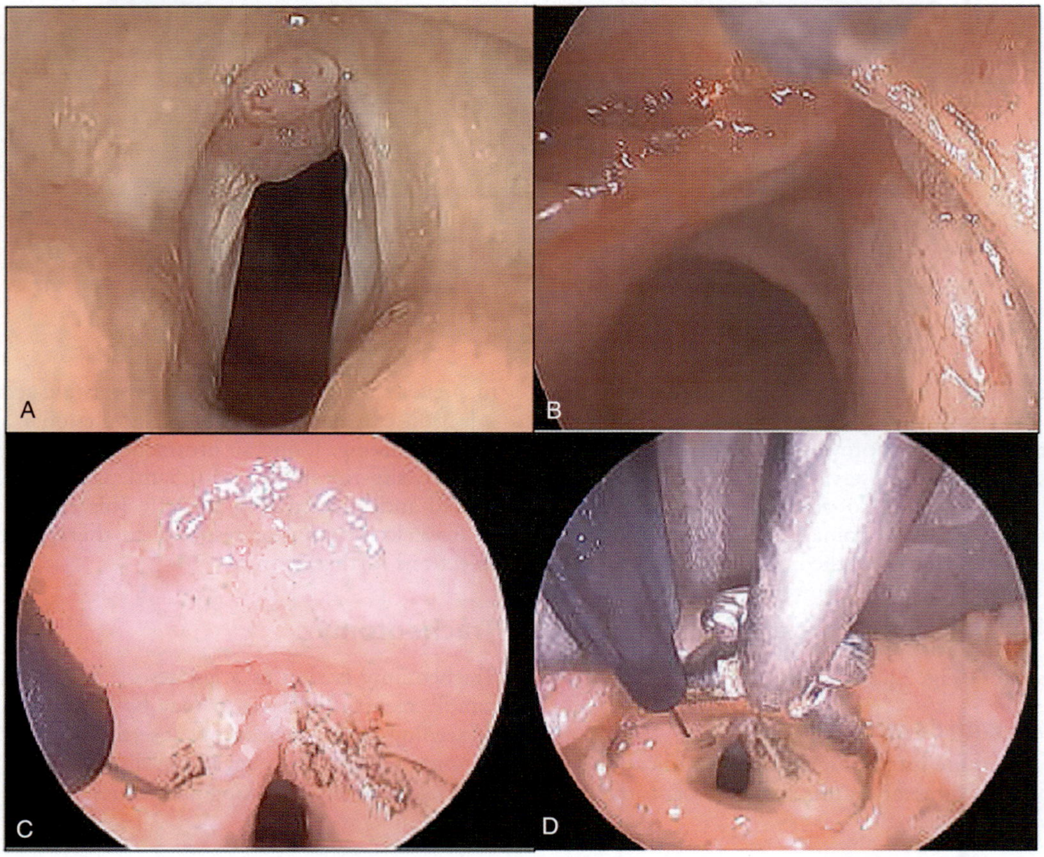


• **Fig. 22.18** Injecting of Bevacizumab. *(Image courtesy Dr. Karthik Balakrishnan).*

## Reference

1. Derkay CS, Malis DJ, Zalzal G, Wiatrak BJ, Kashima HK, Coltrera MD. A staging system for assessing severity of disease and response to therapy in recurrent respiratory papillomatosis. *Laryngoscope.* 1998;108:935–937. http://www.ncbi.nlm.nih.gov/pubmed/9628513.

# Index



*Note:* Page numbers followed by "*f*" indicate figures, "*t*" indicate tables, and "*b*" indicate boxes.

## F



## G



## H



## I



## K



## L



## M



## N



## P